Also by Richard Chun:

Tae Kwon Do—The Korean Martial Art

Moo Duk Kwan Taekwondo—The Korean Art of Self-Defense

Advanced Moo Duk Kwan Taekwondo

Tae Kwon Do Spirit and Practice—Beyond Self-Defense

Advancing in
TAE KWON DO

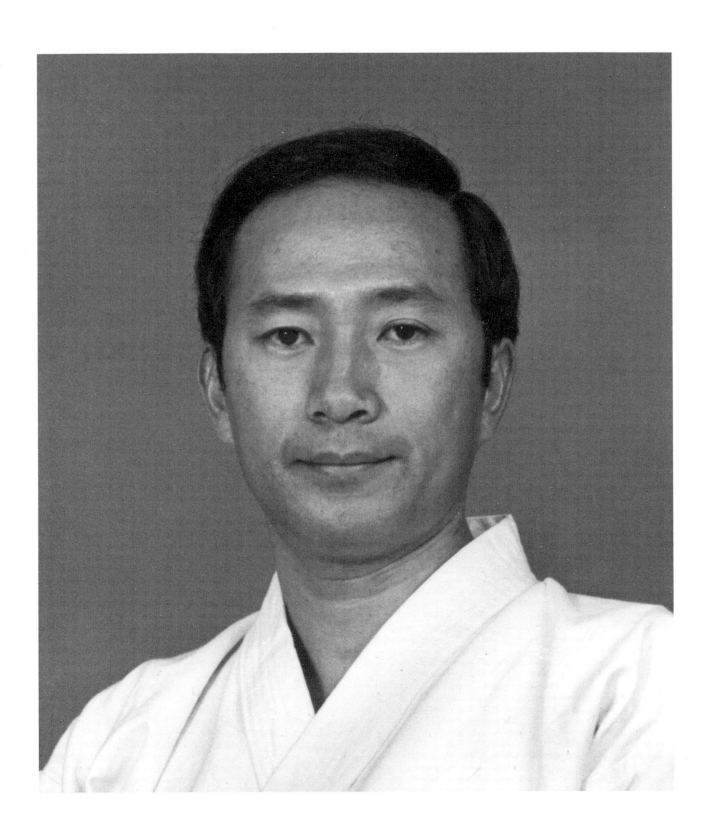

Advancing in TAE KWON DO

RICHARD CHUN

YMAA Publication Center
Boston, Mass. USA

YMAA Publication Center, Inc.
Main Office
4354 Washington Street
Boston, Massachusetts, 02131
1-800-669-8892 • www.ymaa.com • ymaa@aol.com

Cover Design: Richard Rossiter

ISBN-10: 1-59439-072-x
ISBN-13: 978-1-59439-072-2

Second edition, originally published by Harper-Collins.

10 9 8 7 6 5 4 3 2 1

Publisher's Cataloging in Publication

Chun, Richard.

Advancing in tae kwon do / Richard Chun. -- 2nd ed. -- Boston,
Mass. : YMAA Publication Center, 2006.

p. ; cm.

ISBN-13: 978-1-59439-072-2
ISBN-10: 1-59439-972-X
1st ed. published: New York : Harper & Row, c1982.
"Includes nine black belt forms required by the World
Taekwondo Federation for rank promotion."--Cover.
Includes index.

1. Tae kwon do. 2. Karate. 3. Martial arts. I. Title.

GV1114.9 .C48 2006   2006934017
796.815/3--dc22   0610

Editor's Note:
Spellings of certain words in this second edition have been changed to match the modern usage of
the World Taekwondo Federation. However, the spelling of 'Tae Kwon Do' has been retained in
the title (only) of this book for both editions.

Disclaimer:
The author and publisher of this material are NOT RESPONSIBLE in any manner whatsoever for any
injury which may occur through reading or following the instructions in this manual. The activities,
physical or otherwise, described in this material may be too strenuous or dangerous for some people, and
the reader(s) should consult a physician before engaging in them.

Printed in Canada.

Contents

Author's Note for the Second Edition

Since this book was first published in 1983, much in the world of Taekwondo has changed just as much has remained the same. As we shall see, both are positive aspects relating to this ancient and evolving art. Within the past two decades Taekwondo has won status as a fully-recognized Olympic sport. This is due in no small part to the tireless efforts of the World Taekwondo Federation—initially through the leadership of Dr. Un Yong Kim, and presently under the direction of Dr. Chung Won Choue. We have witnessed significant changes in the way the competitive sport is administered with WTF officials announcing—even at this writing—new and exciting programs that will carry us into the future. Updated safety measures have been instituted to protect the athlete from injury while retaining the ability to compete effectively. The role of the referee has been simplified, and judging made more accurate through the refinement of electronic scoring. Moreover, athletic performance has benefited from advances in physiology, nutrition, and exercise. Recognized as the most popular martial art in the world today, many American universities now sponsor Taekwondo teams at the collegiate level. Simply put, it is apparent that Taekwondo is keeping pace with the future.

But, does this mean that the ways of the past are to be discarded in favor of modernity? On the contrary! It is said that five thousand years ago a venerable Taoist sage created the *I Ching,* or *Book of Changes.* The key to this ancient classic revolves around the Um/Yang (Yin/Yang in Chinese), a celebrated symbol representing balance between two opposing forces yielding to constant change. As martial artists, we appreciate the necessity of change and, furthermore, embrace it due to its timeless nature. However, there are components of Taekwondo that should and will remain unchanged in the interest of tradition.

Forms or *Poomsae,* for example, represent the essence of any traditional martial art and once established should be altered only within the scope of one's personal performance, but never in technique. Furthermore, Taekwondo is supported by an ancient philosophy embedded in Asian culture that cannot be ignored if the art is to be practiced diligently. From these philosophical paradigms are drawn the ethical guidelines that act as a moral compass for those seeking a deeper meaning from their training. These teachings reach back to antiquity and are reflected later in this book through the execution of Poomsae and the philosophical elements that underscore them. Time cannot amend these doctrines just as it cannot annul the existence of *Ki,* the universal life force that courses through the human body. Any advanced explanation of Taekwondo needs to take into consideration the manipulation of this vital life force and its use by the martial artist to intensify technique. Meditation, too, a practice that has been studied since time immemorial, needs to remain an intrinsic element of the practitioner's routine in order to calm the mind and maximize potential.

All of these components relating to Taekwondo both as a world sport and a traditional martial art are discussed within the pages of this book. While some new data has been added in an effort to expand on my earlier thoughts, nothing of substance has been eliminated since the value of the original text has been proven through its use as a reference manual in schools around the world. I feel it is essential, however, to mention those who have assisted me in preparing this work for reissue. First and foremost, I would like to thank my senior student Master Doug Cook, an author in his own right, for his editorial contributions and for his dedication to making this work a success. Furthermore, I would like to express my sincere appreciation to Patricia Lurye, Virginia Ratsep, Christine Indorato, Elizabeth Quasius, John Jordan III, and Raoul Ratsep, for their efforts in transcribing the original edition of this book into a digital format. I also wish to convey my gratitude to my students for their diligence and to the many members of the United States Taekwondo Association whose mission it is to promote the ancient and evolving art of Taekwondo. Moreover, I would like to thank David Ripianzi and Tim Comrie of YMAA Publication Center for making this second edition possible. Finally, I would like to recognize and praise Dr. Un Yong Kim, Dr. Chung Won Choue, past-president and current president of the World Taekwondo Federation respectively, and Woon Kyu Uhm, president of Kukkiwon, for their vision in shepherding Taekwondo into the future.

—Richard Chun

Preface

Taekwondo, the art of punching and kicking, is not merely a fighting skill; it is a way of life and a way of thinking. In order to truly master the essence of the art of Taekwondo, one must learn to master oneself, to be totally committed to the mental as well as the physical discipline demanded.

As you diligently practice the physical techniques, you must internalize the philosophical principles of Taekwondo. If you do not do this, you are studying the art superficially, and you will not derive the full benefit from it. By combining the two equally important aspects of Taekwondo, you will gain confidence and a feeling of well-being in a non-aggressive, non-violent manner.

The study of Taekwondo can improve you as a person. It will teach you to control your own *Id*—your aggression, your temper, and your insecurity. It can make you extremely sensitive to your environment, so that you cannot be taken unaware, and it will help you to truly know yourself, so that you will be in full command of your own strengths and weaknesses and able to perceive the strengths and weaknesses of your opponent or opponents as well as those inherent in any situation.

Everything in nature is interdependent, including ourselves. We must try to learn to live in harmony with the Universe and not try to manipulate it for our own gains. At the same time we must cultivate and preserve life along with our individuality.

We must endeavor to avoid a confrontation before it becomes a physical threat. If attacked, we should not use excessive force to defend ourselves. Moderation is an important principle that we must develop, and this can only be done by knowing our strengths, our weaknesses, and ourselves. Only then can we know our opponent, his strengths, and his vulnerabilities. Our worst weakness is fear. Once we serenely accept the fact that in defending our life we may be killed, we eliminate panic, and we no longer have anything to fear.

The Um and Yang principle teaches us that we can allow an attacker to overextend himself and thereby provide a means for his self-defeat. Where there is action, there is reaction; this is the constant balance found in nature.

We must strive for harmony by developing strong character to withstand adversity and to conform to the social order in which we live. We must respect family members and the authority of society. This should be carried into the Taekwondo class, which is like family. Respect, humility, and trust must be shown to the teacher, who is the father figure and to the students and place of practice. We should harmonize with society yet not allow the impersonal forces to limit our individuality. We should not attempt to dominate, nor should we allow fear or other forces to dominate us.

Meditation can help us to eliminate distractions, so that we can know ourselves by penetrating our self-created illusions. This self-knowledge will help us to understand and overcome our opponents.

Patience is absolutely necessary to the study of Taekwondo. Through patience and discipline we can develop better concentration while practicing our physical techniques. The mind must be calm and the will determined, in order to increase our moral courage. A troubled or distracted mental attitude will blur our perception, and this can spell

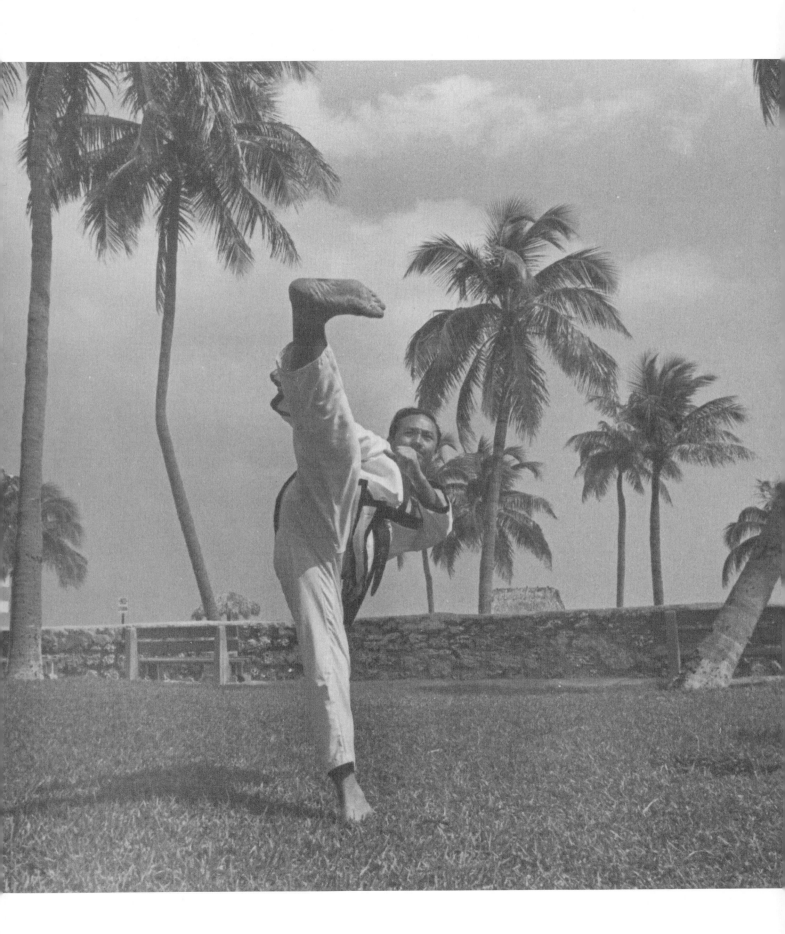

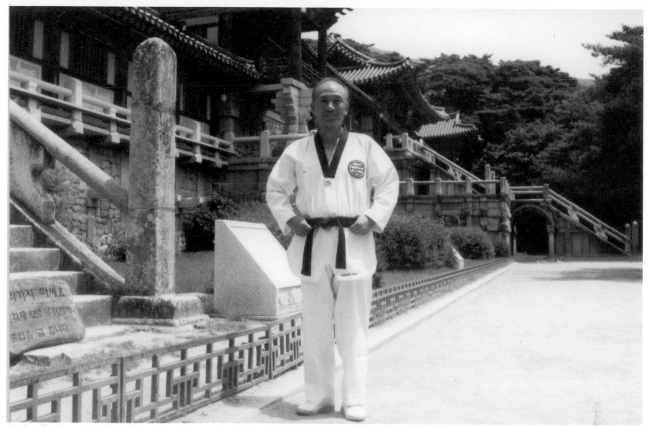

Richard Chun at Bulkook Temple, Kyung Joo, Korea. Young aristocrats called *Hwarang dan* trained Taekwondo 2000 years ago.

defeat. Once we have perfected our physical techniques and combined them with the proper mental attitude, we will react properly to an attacker without having time to stop and think. The parts of the body will flow as they are totally attuned to our mind, our instincts, our senses, and our perceptions.

This is one of the meanings of total awareness in Taekwondo. It flows naturally and automatically out of the concept of oneness with the Universe and the shedding of ego and worldly thoughts.

This is the Way of Taekwondo.

There is great emphasis on forms in this advanced book. There are several reasons for this. Forms are the basics of Taekwondo. Diligently practiced, they provide you with strong defensive and offensive positions as a foundation for advanced combinations.

As you learn your advanced forms, you are learning advanced hand techniques and kicking techniques that occur in combinations and can be used in free fighting. All of the advanced techniques and combinations are explained in Chapter 10.

Due to the confines of space, I have not delved into the most basic kicking, punching, falling, and self-defense techniques of Taekwondo. These are exhaustively covered in my first book, *Tae Kwon Do: The Korean Martial Art* (Harper & Row, 1976). I strongly suggest that you refer to that volume for detailed explanations and illustrations of basic and advanced kicking, punching, blocking, and self-defense techniques.

I wish to express my deepest appreciation to the following people for their efforts in the preparation of this book.

I wish to thank Dr. Un Yong Kim, past-President of the World Taekwondo Federation, for making this book possible. His example, devotion to the art, untiring efforts to make Taekwondo an international sport have been an inspiration.

I wish to thank Richard Jackson for his help in editing this book, Herb Fogelson and Marco Vega for the photography, Sheba Emerson for her artistic drawings, and my students who have helped make this book what it is.

CHAPTER 1

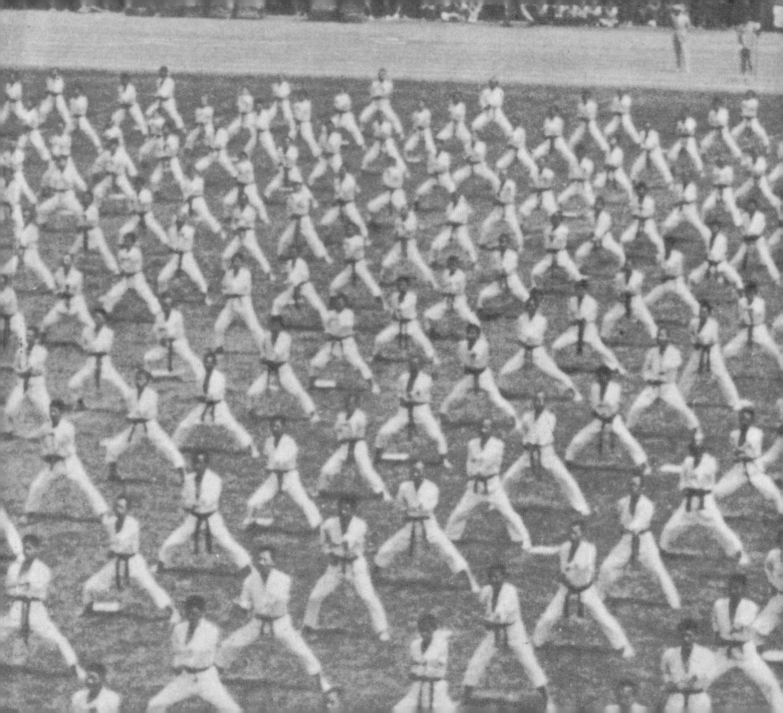

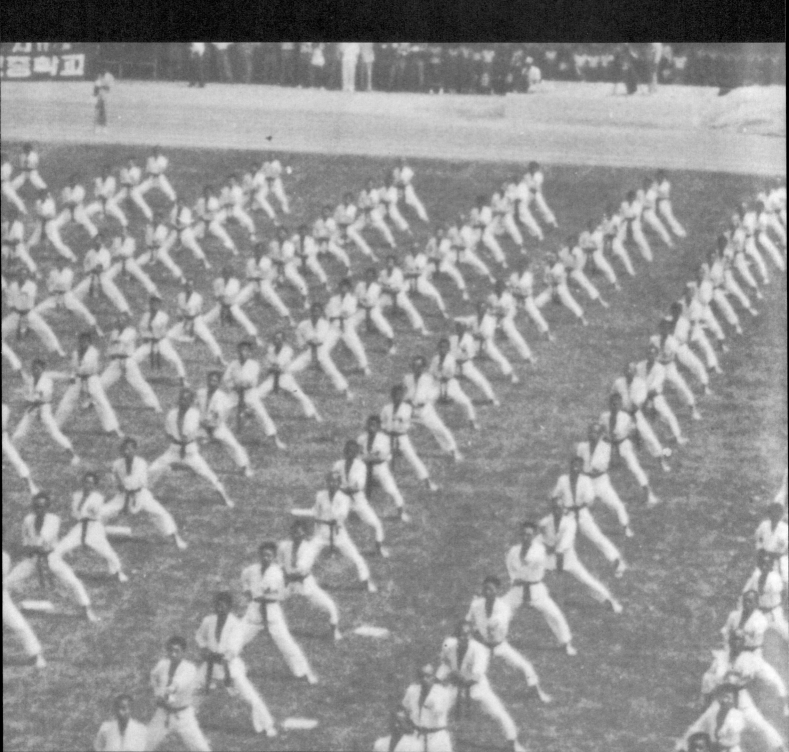

WITH THE EXPLOSIVE GROWTH in popularity of the Asian martial arts all over the world, Westerners have been exposed to a wide range of martial arts systems and styles.

There are weapons systems and weaponless systems, sport and non-sport systems, hard and soft styles. Even a person with only a passing acquaintance with the concept of martial arts has come across names like karate, kung fu, jujitsu, judo, aikido, hapkido, tai chi chuan, kendo, and Taekwondo. Yet only one person in perhaps five hundred is equipped to explain the philosophical and physical differences between these very different arts.

One logical distinction is the difference between "hard" and "soft" styles.

The "hard" styles rely on techniques that direct maximum instantaneous power to a target in attacking and defending. Karate is one of these. Muscles are tensed and focused at the instant of impact. Movements are powerfully executed, and the kick or punch is intended to drive through the target.

"Soft" styles shun this approach. They rely on relaxation, evasion, pliability, and yielding to avoid a direct attack, while using *Ki* energy to throw the attacker off-balance, using his own momentum against him. Tai chi chuan is a good example of this kind of "soft" style.

Taekwondo, "the art of kicking and punching," incorporates the abrupt linear movements of karate and the flowing, circular patterns of kung fu with its own incomparable kicking techniques to form an integrated system unique to Korea.

Taekwondo is an exact system of symmetrical body exercises designed for unarmed self-defense and counterattack. This definition, however, is only superficial, for Taekwondo, is more importantly a state of mind. Thus, the control of one's own mind, self-restraint, kindness, and humility must accompany physical grace. Taekwondo develops the speed and power to kill instantly with bare hands and feet. But it is the art of the discipline to develop such control, coordination, and balance that the punching and kicking movements can be stopped just centimeters short of their mark on an opponent's body.

The "Do" in Taekwondo means "the Way," or "a way-of-being-in-the-world." This Way is not chosen arbitrarily, but in accordance with one's own temperament, as qualified by the notion of what is Good—creative rather than destructive—and in harmony with the immutable laws of the Universe. The Way does not impose; it nurtures.

As you study this book, you will learn more about the history, the philosophy, the principles, and the science that makes Taekwondo unique in the world. It is an ancient and venerable art, born of necessity, tempered in adversity, and perfected through dedication, discipline, love, and understanding.

It is a lifelong study.

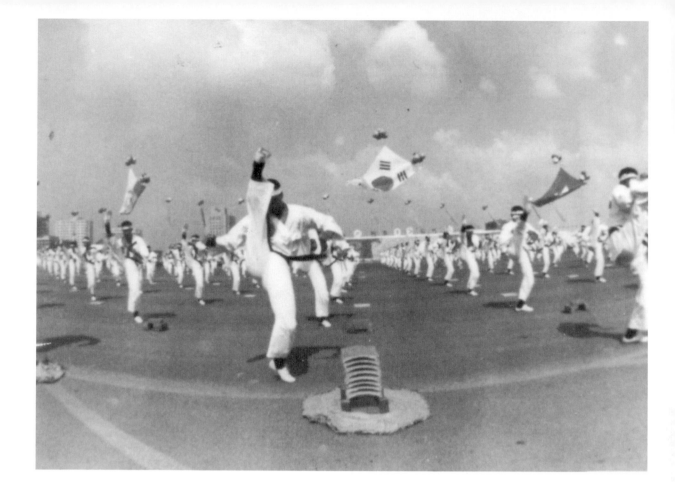

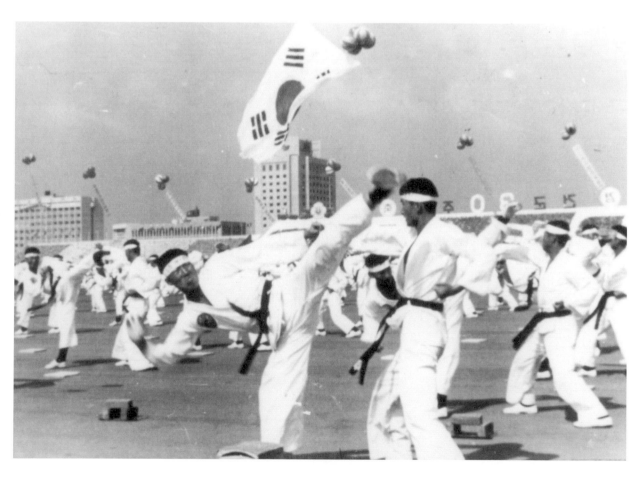

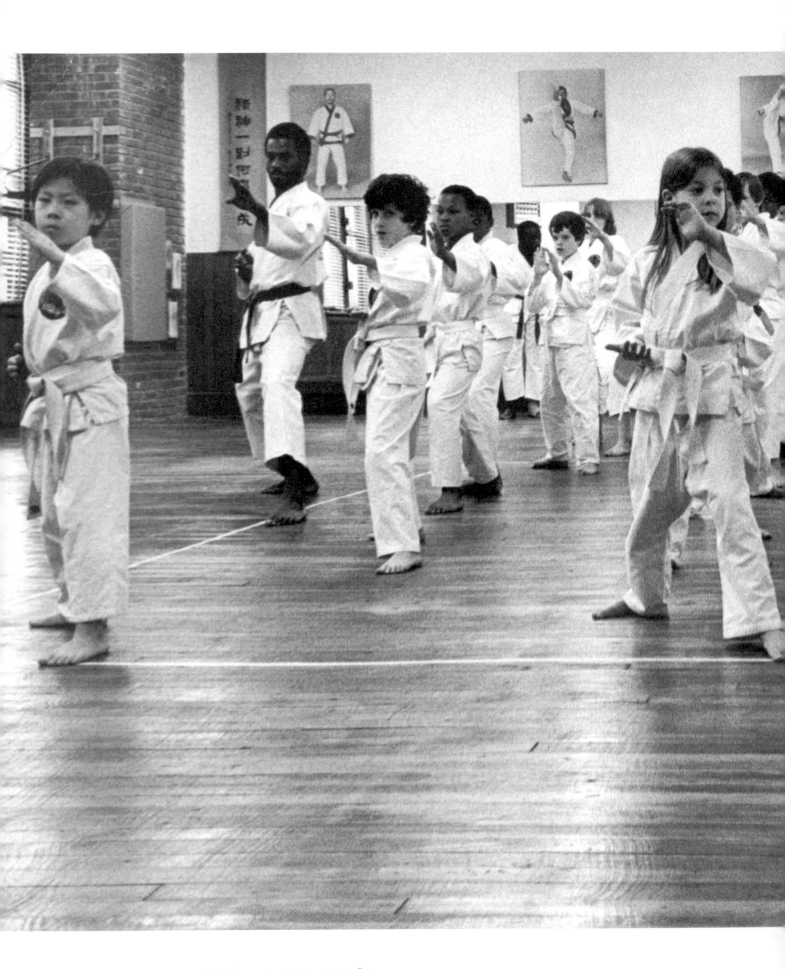

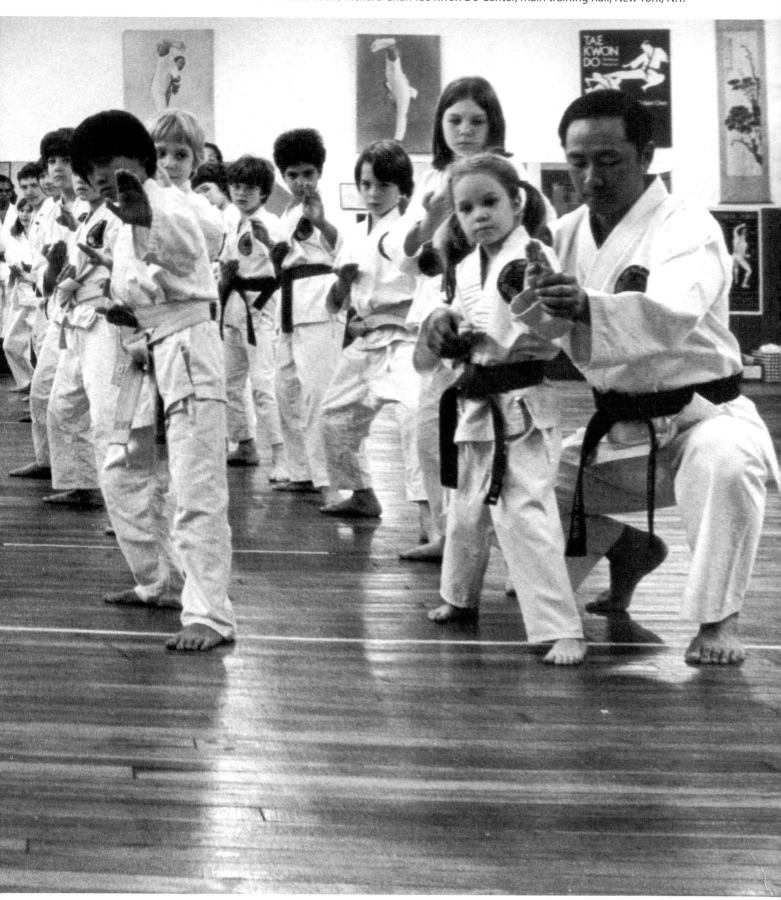

History

Taekwondo was originally the national martial art of Korea; it is now an *international* art and sport.

Tae means "to strike with the feet," *Kwon* means "destroying with the hand or the fist," and *Do* means "Way" or "method," so *Taekwondo* etymologically means "the art of kicking and punching."

At this writing, Taekwondo has over 100 million students in more than 115 countries around the world. Taekwondo is believed to be one of the oldest Oriental arts of unarmed self-defense. It was widely practiced during Korea's Three Han era, 300 years before Christ.

In 1935, a team of Japanese archeologists unearthed a royal tomb of the Korean Koguryo dynasty and found a mural believed to have been painted between 3 A.D. and 427 A.D. The mural clearly depicts men practicing primitive forms of Taekwondo, then called *Soo Bak*, "punching and butting."

The art was refined and perfected during Silla dynasty, which began in Southeastern Korea in 57 B.C., and was incorporated into the discipline of *Hwarang Do*, "the way of the flower of youth." In this way, Taekwondo became part of the ethical, mental, and physical philosophy of the young men who were trained to become the ruling backbone of Korea.

During its long and embattled history, Korea's spirit of Hwarang Do grew and evolved, borrowing from the great religions of its world. From Confucianism it drew filial piety, empathy with one's fellow man, and loyalty to the state. From Taoism it drew the concept of action through non-action. And from Buddhism it gained the philosophy

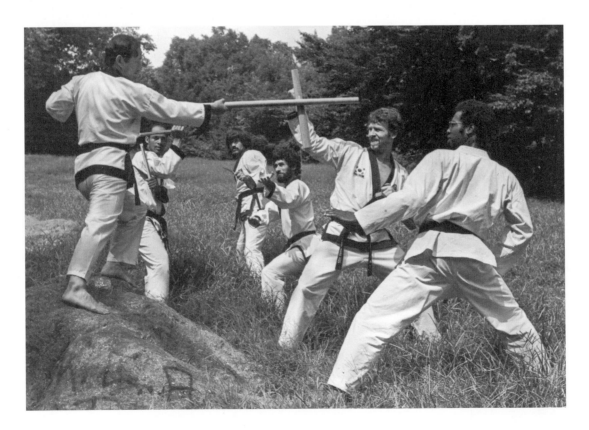

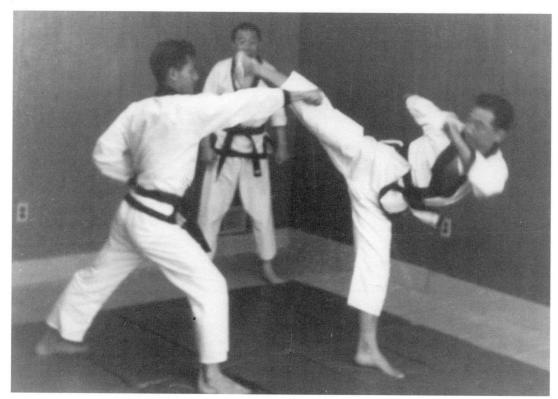
Right to left: Grandmaster of Richard Chun, Ki Whang Kim in training.

of rejecting evil and acting for good, and respecting the sanctity of life. But the history of Taekwondo goes back much further than the first century A.D. and Hwarang Do.

There is archeological evidence of an ancient proto-Korean people which dates back over thirty thousand years. However, the beginnings of true Korean culture are believed to have developed in 2332 B.C. with the establishment of the Ancient Korean State. This takes us back over four thousand years. Since that time, the Korean people have to fight to protect or regain their independence from the Chinese, the Scytho-Siberians of Central Asia, the Mongol Hordes, and the marauders—later the armies—of Japan. This created in the Korean people a fierce warrior spirit, intense national loyalty, and an indomitable will to survive—characteristics which are the source of the martial art of Taekwondo.

In the sixth century A.D., the Chinese Sui dynasty fielded armies of over a million men to invade and occupy Korea. These Chinese armies were so severely defeated that the Sui dynasty fell in 617 A.D., to be replaced by the T'ang dynasty.

During the Koryo dynasty, founded in 918 A.D., and the Yi dynasty that followed it, Taekwondo, then known as Subak, was not only practiced as a skill to improve health and as a sport activity but was also encouraged as a martial art of considerably high virtue.

Subak is believed to have gained its greatest popularity during the reign of King Uijomg, between 1147 and 1170 A.D. This period roughly corresponds to the Chinese Sung and Ming dynasties, during which Chinese kung fu became widely popular. Taekwondo, however, is purely Korean in origin, having achieved independent development throughout the long history of Korea.

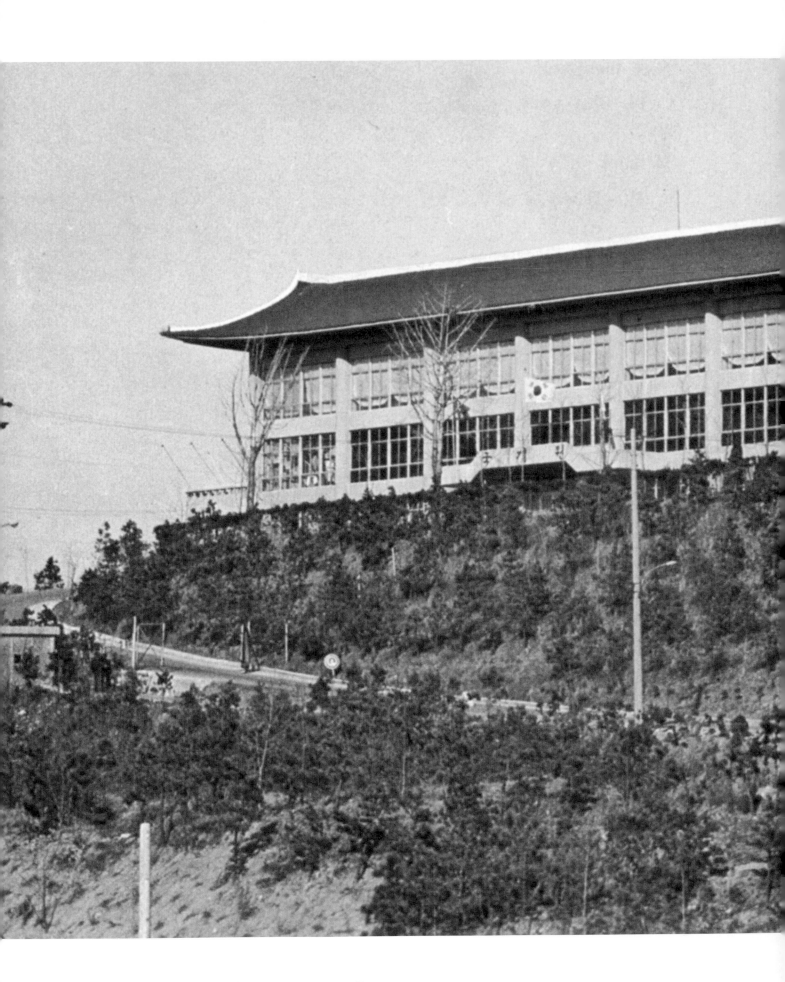

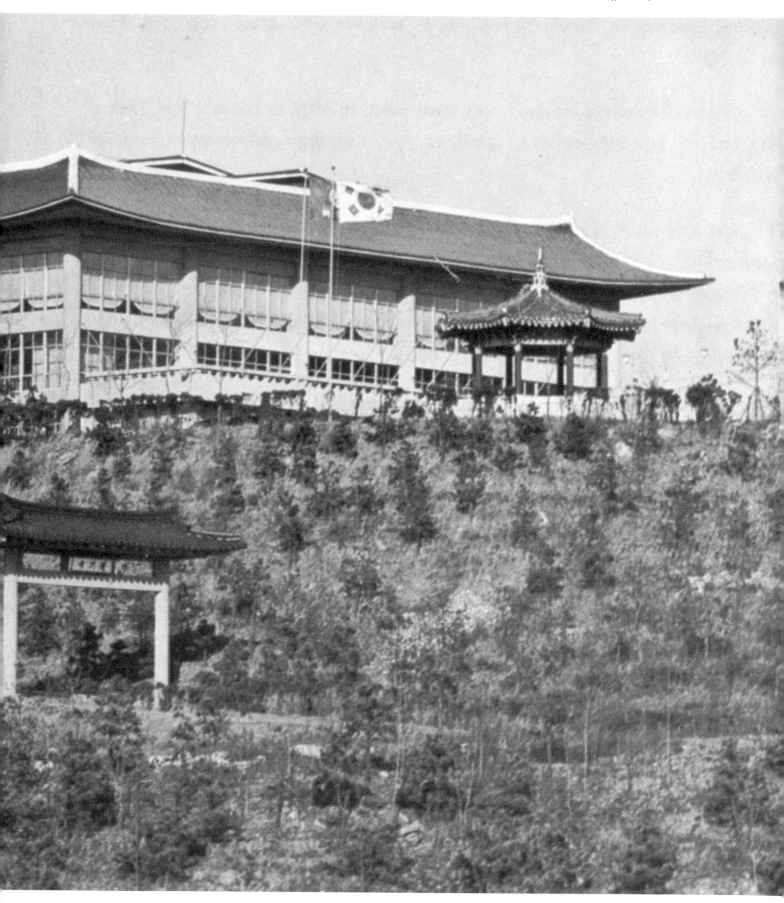

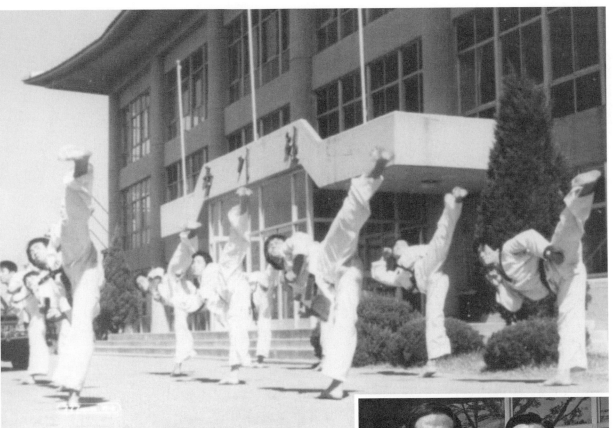

The Koreans are a very inventive people. This can be seen in their art of self-defense, their invention of the first ironclad fighting vessels in 1592, and in another invention of which most Westerners are not aware. Koreans were printing books with moveable metal type in 1443 A.D., a full ten years before Johann Gutenberg. Movable type had been used in China since 1045—four hundred years before Gutenberg—but that type had been made of clay.

In the more recent history of Korea, the importance of Taekwondo began to decline because of the negligence of the royal courts, which were disturbed by the strife between feuding political factions. It was cut back to its roots and stayed alive as a recreational activity for ordinary people.

At the turn of the twentieth century, Taekwondo was outlawed by the ruling Japanese occupiers of Korea. It then went underground, where people practiced it secretly and once again kept it alive.

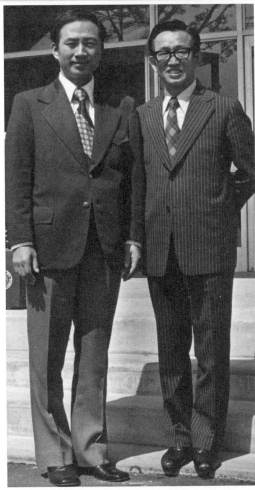

Richard Chun with Grandmaster Woon Kyu Uhm, President of Chung Do Kwan at Kukkiwon.

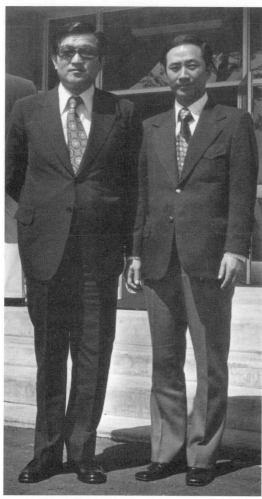 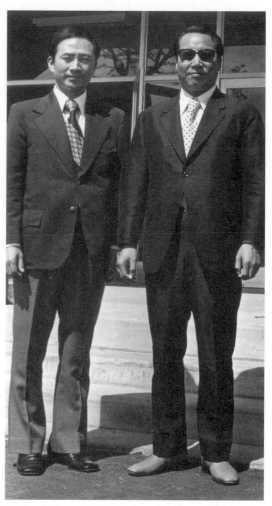

Richard Chun with Grandmaster Chong Woo Lee, President of Ji Do Kwan at Kukkiwon.

Richard Chun with Grandmaster Chong Soo Hong, President of Moo Duk Kwan at Kukkiwon.

In 1945, when Korea was liberated from the Japanese, a number of Koreans who were interested in Taekwondo took steps to revitalize this ancient and traditional martial art. About ten schools were founded by masters with different particular philosophies and different emphases on techniques to express their differences in style.

Between the period of Japanese occupation and the Korean War, from the turn of the century to 1950, the name of for the Korean martial art changed several times. It was first known as *Kong Soo* ("empty hand"), and the *Tae Soo* ("Tang hand"), then *Hwarang Do* ("warrior hand"), and then *Tae Kyun* ("kicking and punching").

In the early 1950's and 1960's, there were several associations formed for the development of Korea's unique and indigenous martial art—a Korea Tang Soo Do Association, a Korea Soo Bakh Do Association, a Korea Tae Soo Do Association, and a Korea Tae Kwon Do Association.

On February 23, 1963, the Tae Kwon Do Association joined the Korean Athletic Association and began to participate in national tournaments. Since then Taekwondo has flourished and spread in popularity, becoming the national sport of Korea. It is now included as part of the school curriculum from first grade through college and is required for military service.

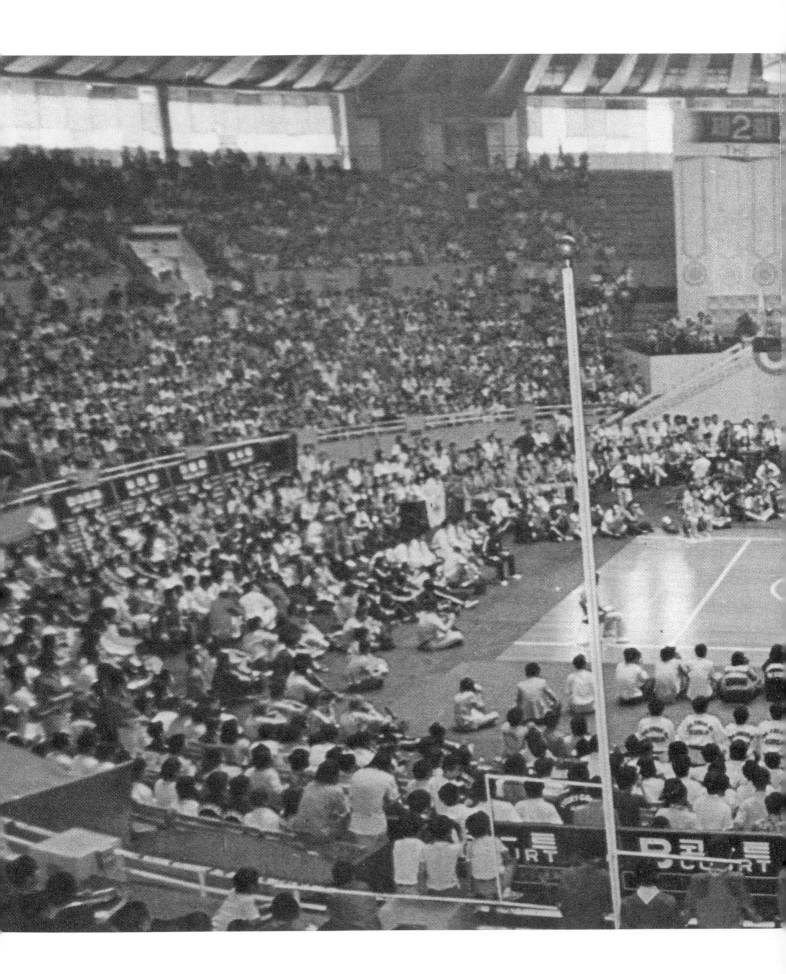

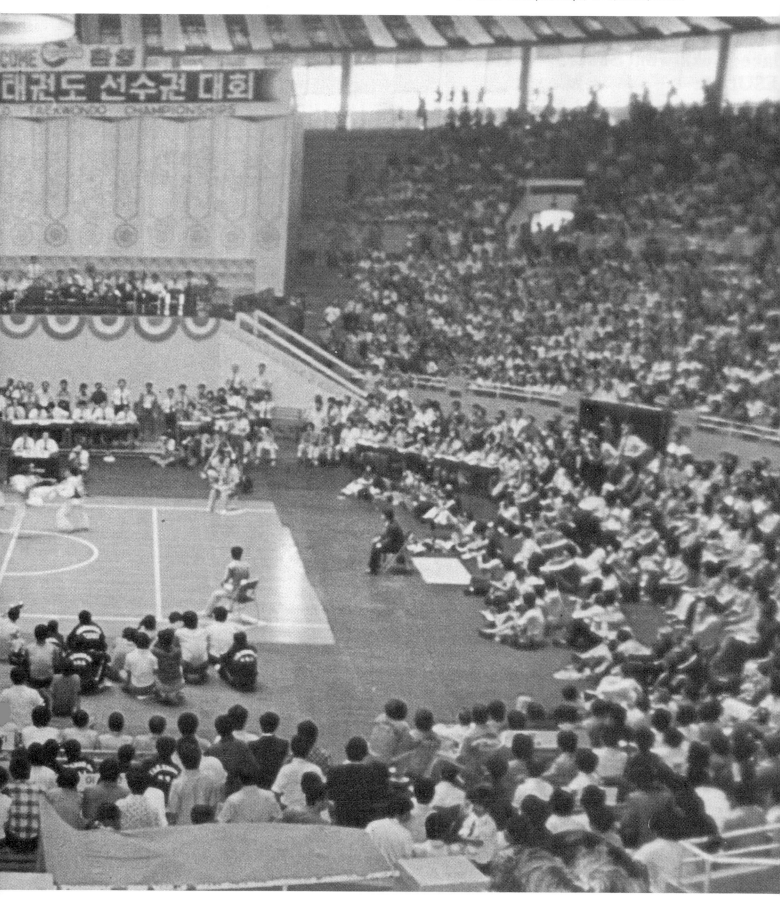

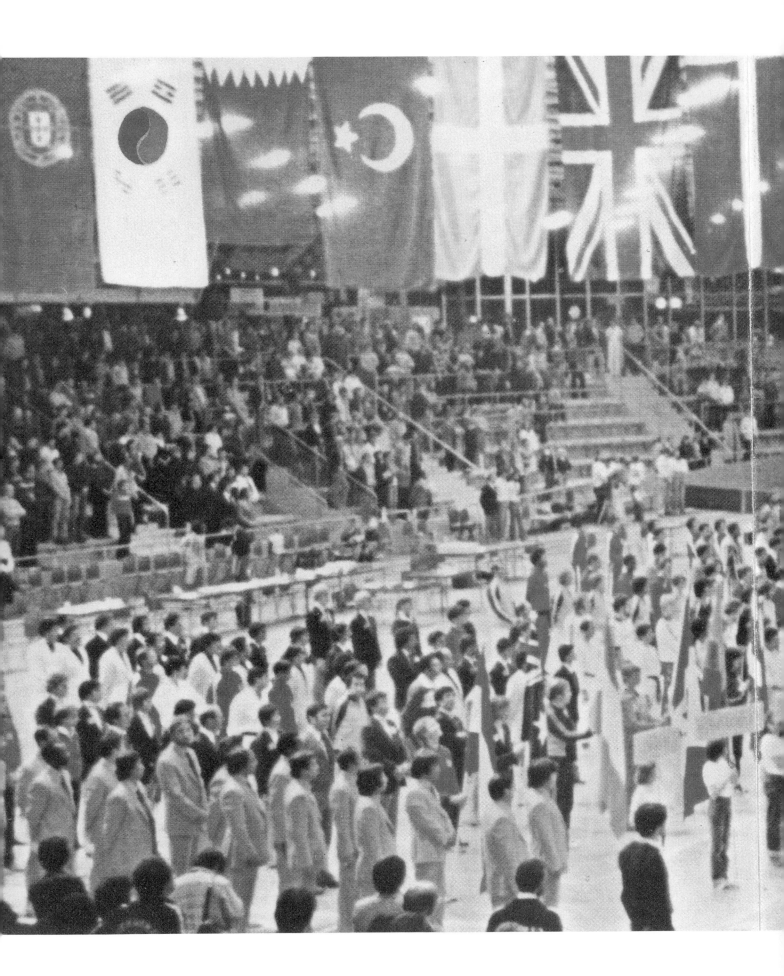

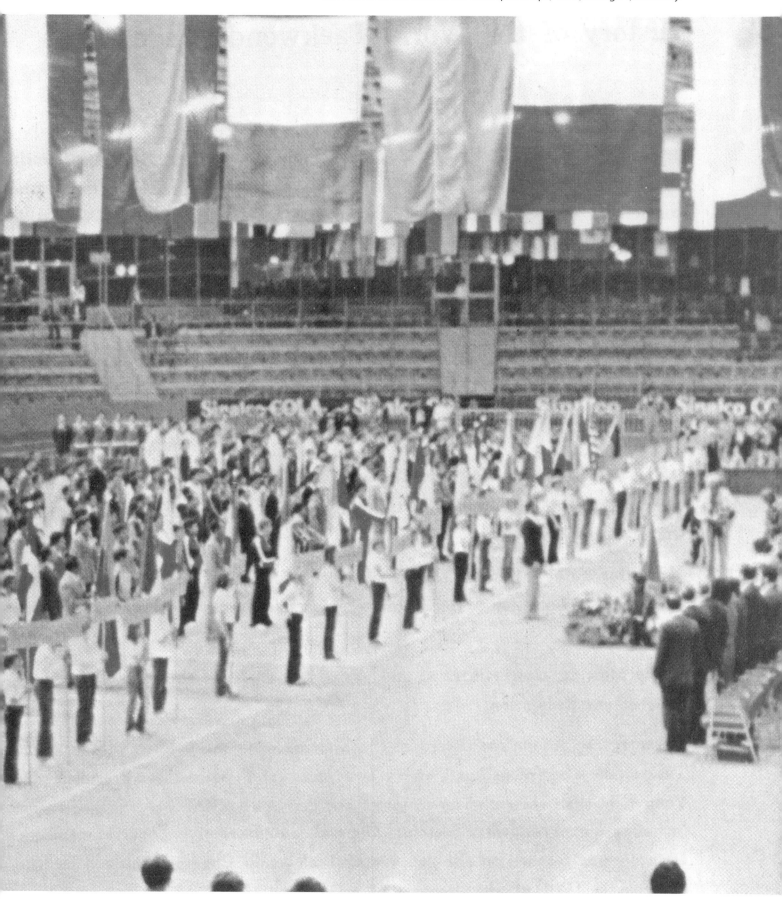

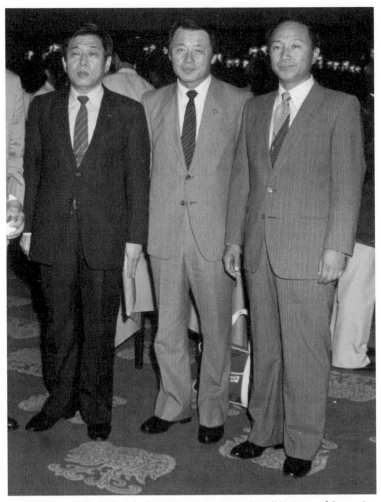

Right to left: Richard Chun, Dr. Young Woo Lee (Minister of Sports),
Dr. Un Yong Kim (Vice President of IOC) at the championships.

In 1965, the Tae Kwon Do Association was recognized by the other associations and the Korean government, and was adopted as the organization to bring different groups and schools together into one.

Young Chai Kim was elected president.

In 1970, the Board of Directors at the Tae Kwon Do Association elected Dr. Un Yong Kim their next president.

In 1972, Kukkiwon (the World Taekwondo Center) was built in Seoul to train advanced students from all over the world. Dr. Un Yong Kim was elected president of Kukkiwon. Kukkiwon serves as a research center for the advancement of Taekwondo as a scientific sport, provides a testing center for black belt promotions, and is used to hold national and international Taekwondo championships.

In May 1973, the First World Taekwondo Championships were held at Kukkiwon, Seoul, Korea. Thirty countries participated. In team competition, Korea won first place, the United States won second place, and Mexico and the Republic of China tied for third place. The world championships are held biannually.

Following the 1973 tournament, all of the officials representing their countries at the championships formed the World Taekwondo Federation and elected Dr. Un Yong Kim president.

Since the formation of the World Taekwondo Federation and the successful first World Taekwondo Championships, there have been many international championships held annually all over the world, such as the European TKD Championships, the African TKD championships, the Middle East TKD Championships, the South American TKD Championships, the Pan American TKD Championships, the Asian TKD Championships, and many invitational international championships.

1973	1st Taekwondo World Championships	Seoul, Korea
1975	2nd Taekwondo World Championships	Seoul, Korea
1977	3rd Taekwondo World Championships	Chicago, USA
1979	4th Taekwondo World Championships	Stuttgart, Germany
1982	5th Taekwondo World Championships	Guyaguil, Ecuador
1983	6th Taekwondo World Championships	Copenhagen, Denmark
1985	7th Taekwondo World Championships	Seoul, Korea
1987	8th Taekwondo World Championships (1st Women's)	Barcelona, Spain
1989	9th Taekwondo World Championships (2nd Women's)	Seoul, Korea
1991	10th Taekwondo World Championships (3rd Women's)	Athens, Greece
1993	11th Taekwondo World Championships (4th Women's)	New York, USA
1995	12th Taekwondo World Championships (5th Women's)	Manila, Philippines
1997	13th Taekwondo World Championships (6th Women's)	Hong Kong, China
1999	14th Taekwondo World Championships (7th Women's)	Edmonton, Canada
2001	15th Taekwondo World Championships (8th Women's)	Jeju City, Korea
2003	16th Taekwondo World Championships (9th Women's)	Garmisch Partenkirchen, Germany
2005	17th Taekwondo World Championships (10th Women's)	Madrid, Spain
2007	18th Taekwondo World Championships (11th Women's)	Beijing, China

Taekwondo has increased in popularity and has contributed to the spirit of competition and sportsmanship internationally. Much of this has been due to the untiring effort of Dr. Um Yong Kim, whose contribution enabled Taekwondo to be recognized and to grow as a world sport in a very short period of time.

In October, 1979, Dr. Um Yong Kim was elected president of the non-Olympic International Sports Federation of the General Assembly of the International Sports Federation (GAISF). The GAISF is comprised of twenty-six Olympic Federations, and twenty-seven non-Olympic Federations.

Dr. Kim was also elected president of the Executive Committee and Council of World Games I, which was held in Santa Clara, California, in August 1981. The pre-World Game Taekwondo Championships were held in June 1978 in Seoul. Forty countries competed. Korea took first place, the Republic of China took second, Germany took third, Mexico took fourth, and the Ivory Coast fifth.

In July 1980, at the Eighty-Third International Olympic Committee Session meeting in Moscow, the World Taekwondo Federation was granted IOC recognition and became a member of the Olympic Games.

In October 1980, Taekwondo, which had been accepted as a member of the Conseil

International Sportive Militaire (CISM), held its first international championship tournament in Seoul. Korea won first place.

In October, 1980, Dr. Un Yong Kim was elected to the six-member Executive Council of the GAISF at the Fourteenth General Assembly meeting in Monaco. In the five short years since Taekwondo became a member of the GAISF, it was adopted as an Olympic sport, and the World Taekwondo Federation was recognized by the International Olympic Committee to supervise all Taekwondo activities.

In May 1981, the IOC approved the inclusion of Taekwondo in the 1988 Olympic Games to be held in Korea. Since the country chosen to sponsor the event is traditional-

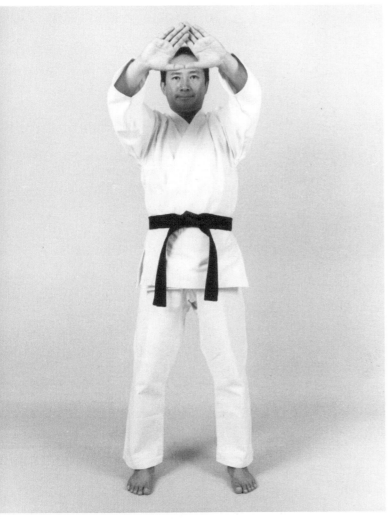

ly entitled to choose a demonstration sport, the Korean leadership, including Dr. Kim, who had become Vice President of the Seoul Olympic Organizing Committee and a member of the International Olympic Committee by 1986, naturally chose to display Taekwondo with great success. Row upon row of seasoned Taekwondo practitioners performed basic techniques and breaking skills on the field of the newly-built Olympic Stadium that was filled to capacity. This honor united the hearts and minds of the Korean people and catapulted their national martial art to world prominence.

Dr. Un Yong Kim, who in 1992 became vice president of the International Olympic Committee, continued promoting Taekwondo on an international level through his affiliation with various sports organizations. Named an Executive Board Member of the IOC in 1997, it is largely due to Dr. Kim's untiring efforts that Taekwondo debuted at the 2000 Sydney Olympics as a full-medal Olympic sport and then again in the 2004 Athens games.

In 2004, after more than three decades of service, Dr. Un Yong Kim stepped down from his post as the de facto leader of sport Taekwondo. Succeeded by Dr. Chungwon Choue as president of the World Taekwondo Federation, a man who had served as vice president of the organization for many years, and Woon Kyu Uhm as president of the Kukkiwon, the future participation of taekwondo as an Olympic event was suddenly thrown into doubt. However, as of this writing, through the leadership ability, wisdom, and diplomatic skills exhibited by Dr. Chungwon Choue in harmonizing differing factions of the sports community, sport taekwondo, along with judo, will once again share the honor of being the only two Asian martial arts with competitors vying to place at the 2008 Olympic Games in Beijing, China and then again in 2012 at the summer games to be played in London, England.

Philosophy of Taekwondo

Taekwondo is the unique product of the time and the place of its development. It evolved in an environment that was constantly changing. The art was developed and polished throughout the long history of Korea and is therefore like no other martial art in the world.

Its environment and its development were spiritual as well as physical. It was not shaped merely by physical competition. Every master, whether or not he is remembered today, brought his own skills and perspective to what has become Taekwondo. This process has brought about a spiritual evolution of the art.

Historically, those who held power in Korea lost it through physical, political, or spiritual weakness. They lost out to others, perhaps more hardy, who continued the gradual but inevitable evolution.

The evolution of Taekwondo continues, changing to meet modern conditions and demands. Yet it builds upon its ancient and venerable foundation.

Modern Taekwondo is a means of individual freedom and expression. Properly practiced, it purifies the spirit as it trains the muscles and the mind. It enables one to focus unrestricted and to concentrate on the natural movements of the body and on the regulation of one's own breathing patterns. It builds character and leads to a love for mankind and a desire for peace.

To the initiated, Taekwondo may appear to be an aggressive art. This is an easily understood misconception, since it is a martial art. Its techniques are designed to maim or even kill an opponent, if necessary. Blows with the hands, feet, elbows—even the head—can break bones, boards, roof tiles, and stones. Clearly, this is no peaceful art!

Yet it *is* a peaceful art, a paradox expressing the Um and Yang theory of eternal duality which exists within nature. Taekwondo teaches its practitioners to live in harmony with nature, in oneness with the Earth and the Universe. It helps one develop an acutely sensitive awareness of the aspects and forces of nature. In Korea, students of Taekwondo will go out into nature, near a waterfall, or a calm lake, and purge their bodies and souls, to emerge with a clean, clear heart. In this way, they aspire to become like water, which, because it possesses tremendous inherent forces—life-generating as well as terribly destructive—is all the more beautiful and reassuring when you see it as a gentle stream, flowing around rough rocks in its path.

The simplicity of this philosophy is profound and subtle. It develops the warrior's sense of mercy and benevolence, and teaches courtesy, politeness, modesty, and calmness, without vulgar pride or arrogance. It builds a nobility of character, self-restraint, and courage, as well as a posture of alertness and vigilance.

It is possible to achieve skill and technique without building character, but when you meet an opponent who possesses a direct, hard, and pure spirit with real moral fiber that gives him supreme confidence; your technique will be useless.

A story is told of a master swordsmith whose technique in making blades was excellent but whose character was weak. This weakness came out in combat, when the blades he made would cause their wielders to get into bloody fights in which both they and their opponents would get killed or badly hurt.

One warrior, on receiving one of these swords, decided to test it before he used it. He placed the blade in a swiftly flowing stream in which autumn leaves were floating. Every time the blade touched a leaf, the leaf was cleanly sliced in two.

Then, another warrior tried the same test with a different blade that been made by

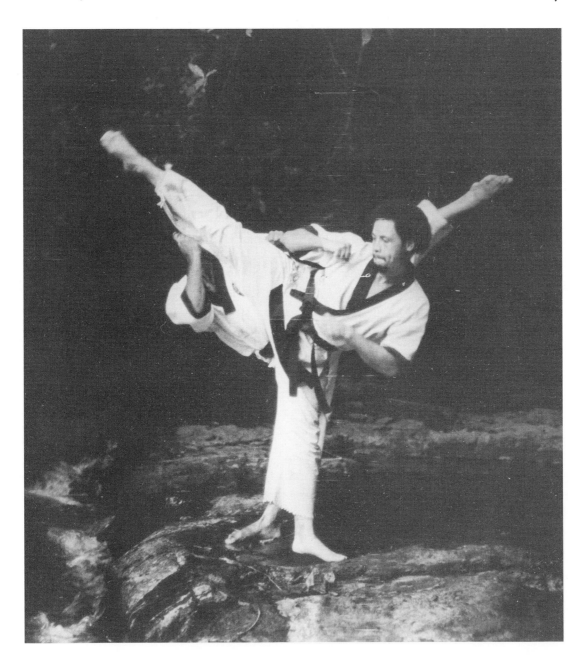

the greatest of swordsmiths, a man of great spiritual power. The fearful leaves avoided the blade.

In human relations, Taekwondo demands sacrifice, self-restraint, kindness, humility, patience, forgiveness, and love of one's fellow human beings. Like the great religions, Taekwondo teaches you not to cause pain and suffering but to actively prevent them. It is up to you to learn to control a hot temper, for instance, and to develop a reserve that leaves you indifferent to the abuse of others, even though you know you can destroy them if you choose to.

For practitioners of Taekwondo, victory through dishonor is despised. One must fight honorably or be dishonored. The ultimate good lies not in winning a hundred battles, but in overcoming a man or an army without a conflict.

Taekwondo has been described as a state of mind. It goes far beyond physical speed, strength, and grace. It is a way of life. In its simplest sense, Taekwondo is doing anything perfectly, without ego, and in harmony with the Universe. The goals sought are three:

1. to achieve a concentration of power
2. to realize one's own true nature (this is the real meaning of enlightenment)
3. to achieve the realization of the truth of enlightenment in everyday life

The goals are achieved through meditation, or positive training of the mind. Enlightenment does not come easily. Even the ancient Zen masters spent a many as twenty years groping toward it. (Although there is a tradition that the great Zen master Shakkyo achieved it in but a single hour!)

One of Taekwondo's most important principles is its reverence for all forms of life. The power we learn is awesome, and it carries with it an awesome responsibility, which cannot be takes lightly. Remember, if you harm someone; you will have to answer for it—and live with what you have done.

Taekwondo's rule is to use the *minimum force necessary* to subdue an assailant, defeating him with minimum harm to his body. A human being is not a punching board.

You can train yourself into calm detachment and fearlessness in the face of stress, avoiding the obstacles of anxiety, indecision, ambition, and unchecked passion, and replacing them with serenity and self-control. You must concentrate your power. This will give you an incalculable psychological advantage over your opponent.

In Korea, there was a hot-tempered champion swordsman who no one had ever beaten, but he knew that he was not a good person and that this would one day catch up with him. So he submitted to being bound, hand and foot, to a tree for three months. Exposed to the elements, he began to train his mind and work at building a mild character. In this way, he came closer to being a perfect person.

Students of Taekwondo in Korea are not taught any techniques for the first two

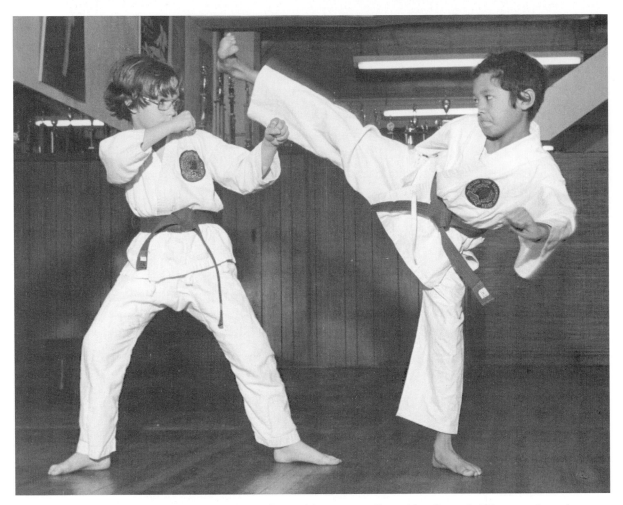

weeks. They are made to clean the cold training floor barefooted. This teaches them to respect the school as their home, and it teaches them patience, humility, and sacrifice.

As you learn the true philosophy of Taekwondo, you will find that it helps you, as a black belt, to teach it to others more easily. You will find that the study of Taekwondo is a continuing process in which the master is forever a student. This is a humbling realization, but it is true that only through humility can you hope to achieve understanding.

When you act as a teacher, you will experience pleasure instead of jealousy when you see a student advancing more rapidly that you did when you were at his or her stage. You will gain satisfaction at having imparted the skill and knowledge which you have learned for a purpose greater than yourself. Humility as a teacher will beget patience and bring you closer to truth, loyalty, dignity, compassion, genuine virtue, and true courage.

The chapters that follow will train you in your career as a black belt. You will find that you have to unlearn much of what you thought you had learned and to relearn it in a totally new way.

There is a reason for this. Until you reached your current level of mental and physical ability, you could not have begun to master the tiny nuances in each and every one of the movements of the art. You were simply not prepared to do so. Your attainment of this level brings you to a new beginning at a higher plateau. This is the meaning of First Dan.

The difficulty of going from one Dan to the next higher Dan increases geometrical-

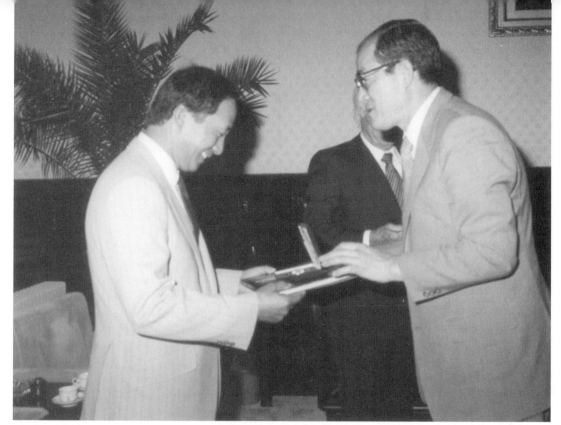

Master Richard Chun (left) receiving a special medal for promoting the art of Taekwondo as a world and Olympic sport from the mayor of Seoul Special City, Seoul, Korea, May 1982.

At the award ceremony (right to left): Dr. Un Yong Kim (president of the World Taekwondo Federation and I.O.C. member), Honorable Sung Bae Kim (mayor of Seoul), Honorable German Rieckehoff (chairman of the Caribbean Olympic Commitee), Master Richard Chun.

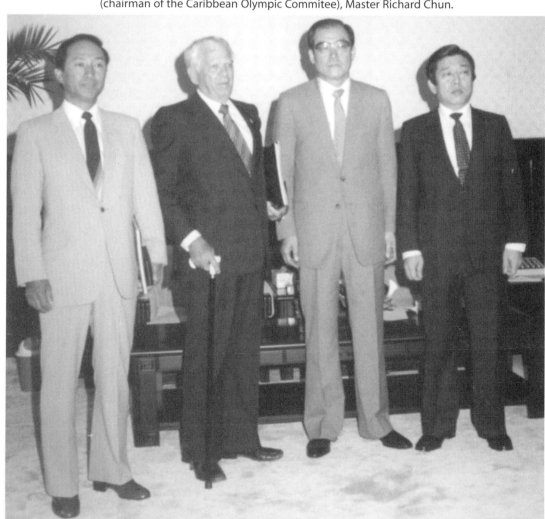

ly. Unlearning and relearning are much more difficult than learning in the first place, but they offer the only path to the goal.

You will have to redouble your concentration and your disciplined practice until you are totally absorbed in the act and you become part of the unified spirit, which overcomes disorder. Just as a beam of sunlight can be focused by a laser into an irresistible beam, so your strengths can be sharpened and concentrated, and focused onto your opponent's weaknesses, so that the desired end is achieved.

The path on which you have embarked is an arduous one that will make great demands on your body and your spirit, but you can be encouraged by the realization that others have gone this way before you and that they can help you on the journey.

If the task seems difficult, remember—once you have started it, it is not so hard. Most people are born with natural ability and strength, and life is not easy for any of us. However, if you keep applying yourself with diligence and determination, you will find yourself getting closer and closer to your goal. All worthwhile things are as difficult as they are rare.

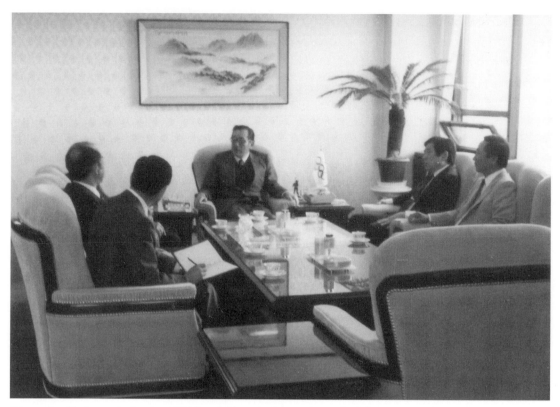

Discussing Taekwondo for the 1988 Seoul Olympic Games. From the left: Master Richard Chun, Dr. Un Yong Kim (president of the World Taekwondo Federation), Honorable Yong Shik Kim (president of the Organizing Commitee for the 1988 Seoul Olympic Games), Seoul, Korea, May 1982.

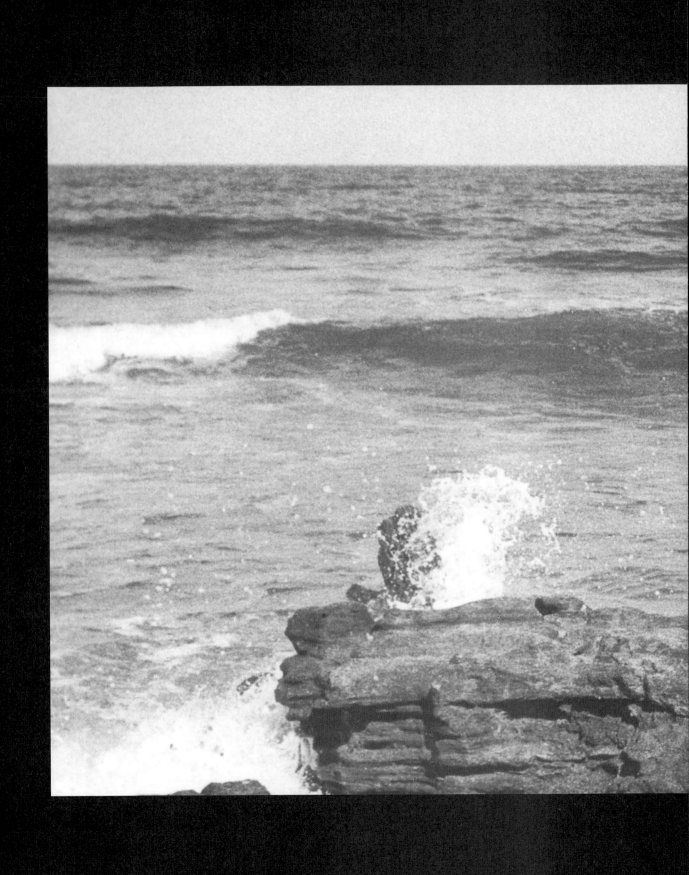

CHAPTER 2

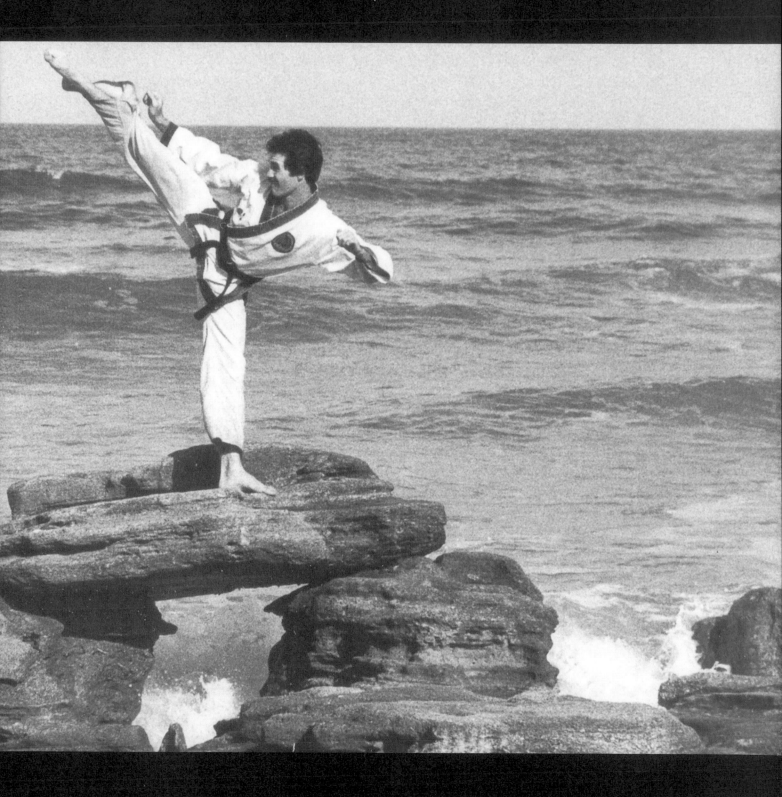

Principles of Taekwondo

TAEKWONDO is based on two governing principles—the first is the *principle of Um and Yang*, the second is the principle of *Ki*, or vital energy.

In looking at the Um and Yang symbol, we see that the circle represents the Unity of the forces in the Universe. This Unity is made up of two opposite but complementary forces which we find in every object and every process. These are the forces of the Um and Yang. They are the forces of light and darkness, of left and right, of ebb and flow, positive and negative, male and female, matter and anti-matter, warp and woof, good and evil. We see them in the change of seasons, in the movements of the tides, and in the existence of a harmonic Universe.

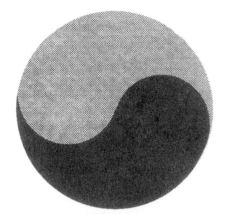

The Korean Um/Yang.

The polarities of Um and Yang are in constant interaction and flux. The Um is a passive, receptive force, and the Yang is an active, assertive force. Both are necessary in the Universe and in our lives.

The boundary between these forces creates the harmony and balance from which everything is created. A balance between Um and Yang is necessary for the proper functioning of any living thing, and all things consist of both Um and Yang as related to one another. Um and Yang are symbolic of eternal change and the natural rhythms of life: the symbol for them is not static, but kinetic and flowing. It depicts a serene cycle of constant flux.

The sine-curve boundary between Um and Yang is a high-energy vibration—the *Ki* or "vital life force." Ki is the cosmic ocean in which everything exists. It is kept in balance by the Um and Yang, working in rhythm. It is at its best when it flows freely, neither too active nor too passive, but in perfect harmonic balance.

The Ki provides your basic bioenergy. When you accept and understand your Ki, the universal flow and balance of nature works through you. You can accept the natural rhythm of any situation and move naturally and strike naturally.

It is important to understand that Ki, being energy, cannot be created or destroyed. It exists. It can be changed, transmuted, or transformed, however—once you understand how to tap it.

Taekwondo recognizes that there is no separation of body and mind. There is, instead, a balance between the physical, the emotional, and the intellectual. Once you are truly aware, you can see a situation for what it is and see how it can be transformed to achieve your goal.

The concept of Um and Yang leads, in Taekwondo, to hard and soft techniques. We learn from nature. The soft summer breeze is pleasant and friendly; the tornado can drive a sliver of straw six inches into solid oak. So in Taekwondo, we learn the dual attributes of the wind—its force and speed, and also its elusiveness and its invisibility.

Taekwondo began to teach you its principles long before you were ready to understand or accept them. It did so through techniques which were practiced relentlessly. You found yourself building inner strength, stamina, and commitment. Thus your formal techniques were a form of meditation and had a cleansing effect on your spirit. They also build concentration.

Concentration of power requires that you focus your personal Ki energy and become totally absorbed in your activity. You must be aware of everything—distracted by nothing. You learn to perceive without self-conscious thinking. This mental concentration increases physical power tenfold and directs it with maximum efficiency. When timing and focus are precise, there is no waste of power or effort. You can act spontaneously, rather than react.

Concentration leads to spontaneous knowledge of every action—wisdom independent of thought. This has a practical use. One can train to make quick decisions, to perceive those things which cannot be seen. Perception is strong, sight is weak.

Observers of Taekwondo are sometimes led to believe that the master moves through reflex. This is a misperception. The master moves with the *speed* of reflex and *appears* to be unthinking. This reflects the supreme importance that Taekwondo gives to intuition rather than to the verbalizing intellect. This is the principle of "no thought." It shows its perfection. The master controls the event, and this is one of the fruits of true mastery Taekwondo.

So the student learns not only technique but "heart." If the heart is strong and technique is faulty, the blow will miss the mark. But if technique is strong and the heart is weak, the student will lack the crucial fluidity, flexibility, and creativity to adapt to the situation as water adapts to its container. Thus, drill becomes increasingly important. You must strive to make your techniques as natural as breathing, so that if you are caught unaware, you will respond in the proper way. If you have to "remember" a technique, it will come too late to do you any good.

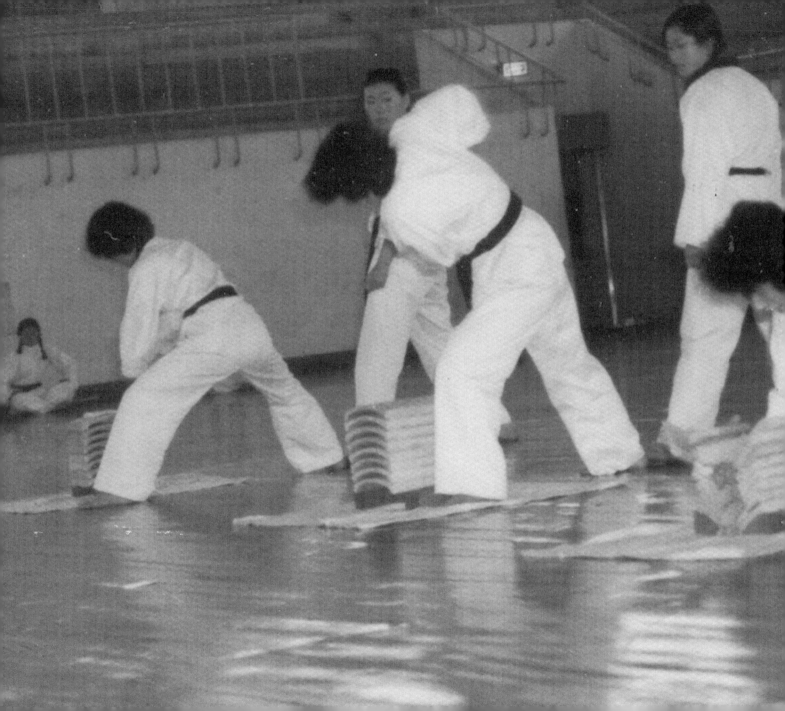

CHAPTER 3

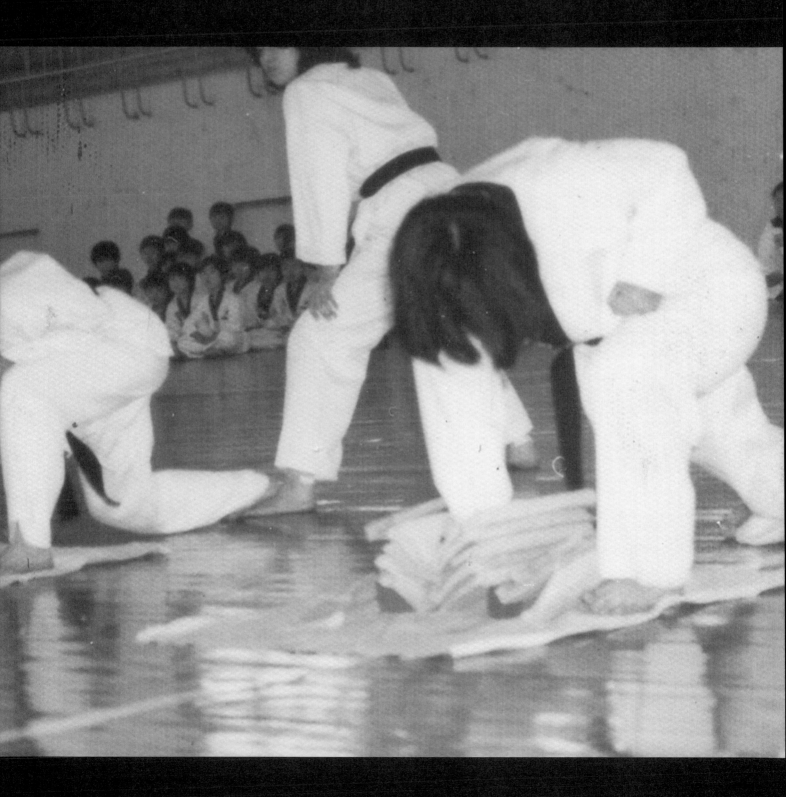

The Science of Physics

TAEKWONDO is both science and art. For over twenty centuries, it has made instinctive use of the principles of classical mechanical physics, which were intuitively understood but not codified until Isaac Newton did so less than three hundred years ago.

Newton's Three Laws of Motion state:

1. A body at rest tends to remain at rest, and a body in motion tends to remain in motion—unless some outside force acts. (This is the Law of Inertia.)
2. Force equals mass times acceleration. ($F=ma$. A mass exerts no force when it is moving at a constant velocity. The velocity must be increasing—accelerating—to create force. Acceleration is defined as the increase of velocity with time.)
3. Every action has an equal and opposite reaction.

Newton's First Law of Motion explains why it doesn't hurt when you drive your knuckles through a pine board. The key is inertia. Inertia is the phenomenon which makes it harder to get a car rolling by pushing it than it is to keep it rolling. Inertia also explains why the car is difficult to stop once it gets rolling.

We have all had the experience of doing push-ups on our knuckles. It hurts. It hurts because the layer of fluid and flesh (which is mostly water) between the skin and bones of the knuckle deforms, or gives way, under the slow, steady pressure of our weight. Then, it's bone against nerve, which equals pain.

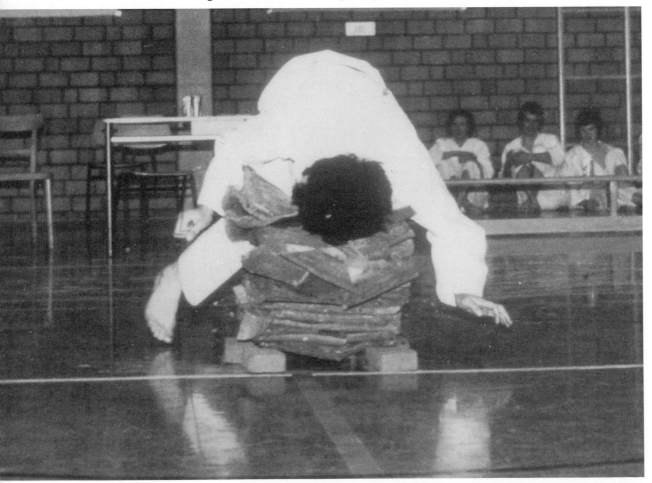

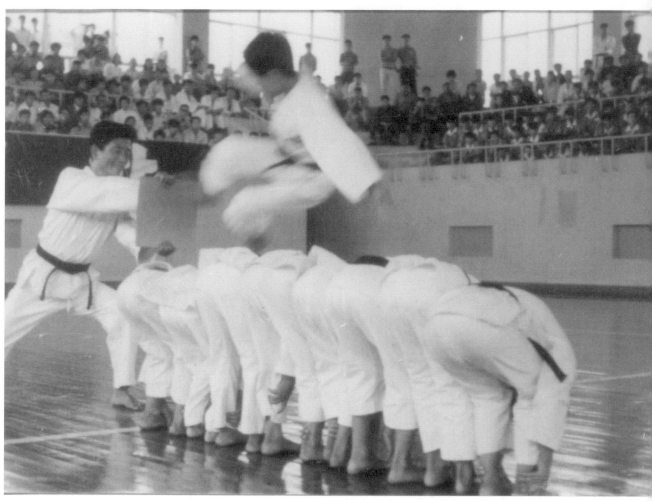

Now, take the case where you break the board with those very same knuckles. Because of the velocity of the blow, the layer of fluid simply *doesn't have time* to deform, and for that instant, it behaves like a tough, rigid body. The board is more brittle, and since it doesn't have time to deform either, it breaks. The damage to the board occurs in the first $\frac{1}{64}$ inch of contact.

There are numerous other examples of fluids acting like rigid bodies on impact. When an airplane crashes at sea, the plane doesn't simply sink. Rather, it smashes at the surface, as if it had hit a brick wall.

Another example is the woodchuck your car hits at 60 mph. The hapless woodchuck dies from *internal* injuries. Most of the time, his skin isn't even broken. But look at your car—four hundred dollars worth of damage to your bumper and your fender, all because the soft woodchuck didn't have time to deform.

Thus, soft is hard, because of inertia. And a known weak material can break a strong object.

In Taekwondo, we use Newton's First Law in many ways. When an attacker is in motion, we use his inertia against him. (Remember, a body in motion tends to remain in motion.) We allow his inertia to get him off balance. Sometimes, we help a little by tripping him or throwing him. Or, as he comes headlong at us, we kick—providing the outside force mentioned in the First Law.

In the same way, we use our own static inertia to give us maximum stability. This is the function of our basic stances: Horseback Stance, Front Stance, and Back Stance.

We use Newton's Second Law in as many ways as the First Law, primarily in our hundreds of striking techniques. The law says force equals mass times *acceleration*. Every punch, kick, or strike we learn is effective, not because it is moving along at a nice, uniform velocity, but because it is accelerating. The velocity itself is increasing at a measurable rate.

When the Forward Middle Punch, for instance, is used to break a board, the striking first begins at the hip. It is at rest, the body relaxed. When the Forward Striking Punch is thrown, the fist picks up velocity very rapidly. When the fist has traveled about 85 percent of the distance to the full extension of the arm, it has achieved maximum

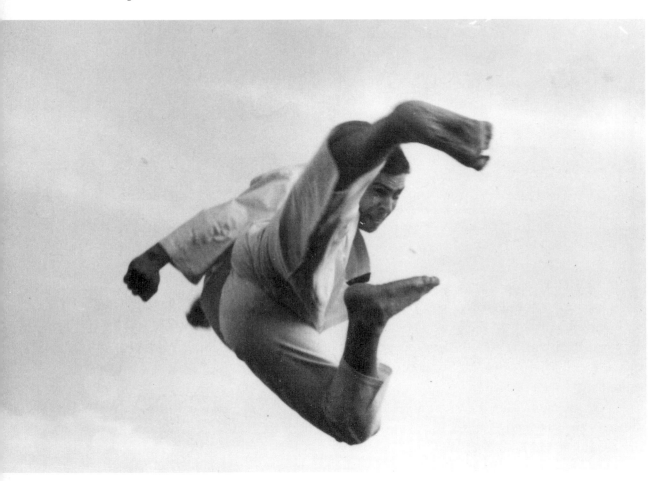

velocity. This velocity has been measured for a black belt student at Taekwondo by a stroboscopic camera with a strobe flashing at 120 flashes per second. The maximum speed of the punch was measured at velocities up to 9.8 meters per second! Once the fist hit the board, it decelerated at a rate of 3500 meters per second. This translates into impact energy on the order of 100 joules. A board will break at 6.4 joules of energy. A concrete patio block measuring 40 centimeters by 90 centimeters by 4 centimeters and weighing 6.5 kilograms requires only 8.9 joules to break it.

The energy created by other kinds of blows is even more impressive. The peak velocity of a downward Knife-Hand Strike was measured at 14 meters per second. The Roundhouse Kick reached 11 meters per second, and both the Front Thrust Kick and the Side Kick reached maximum speeds of 14.4 meters per second.

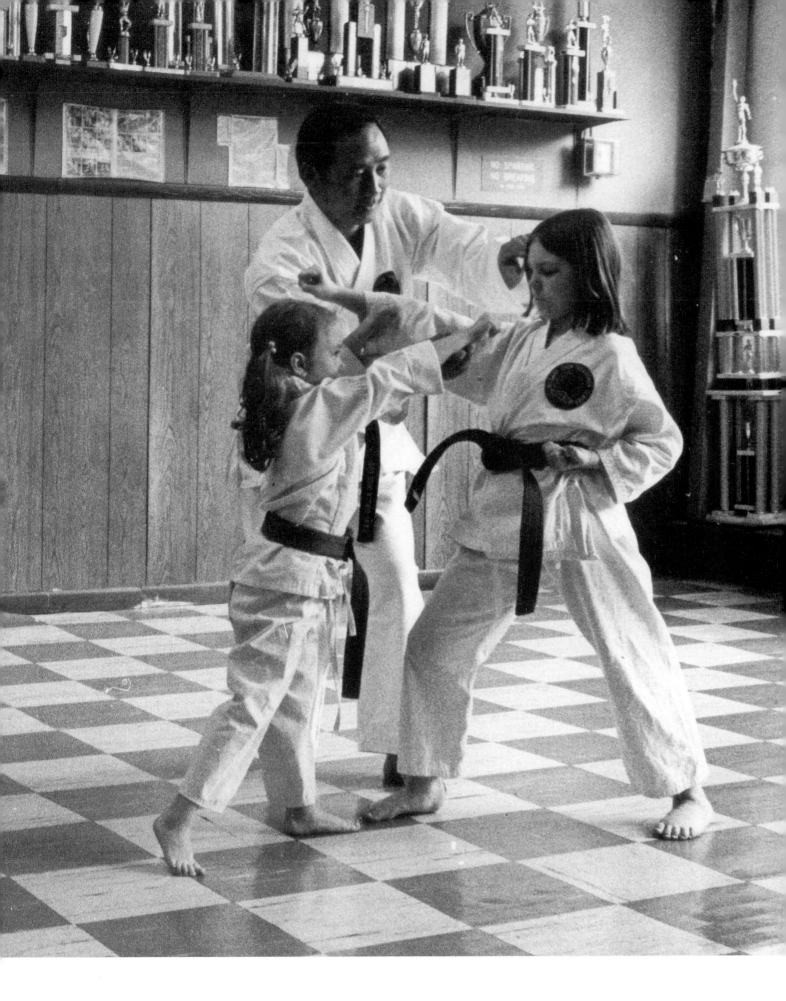

At 14 meters per second, the Knife-Hand Strike exerts an impulse force of 675 pounds on the unfortunate board.

Newton's Third Law finds expression in the pull/push techniques of our punches and kicks. Using the Forward Middle Punch as an example, we pull the non-striking fist simultaneously with the strike. This creates a "coupling" effect, which doubles the force of the punch while neutralizing our own inertial forces and compensating for the equal and opposite reaction, which would steal power from the blow.

All of this is very instructive, but many people who routinely use these techniques and break boards, roof tiles, bricks, and even stones are not even dimly aware of the classical physics involved. Yet it is important, in our modern world, to recognize that our ancient art is founded upon scientific principles, which although relatively newly discovered, have nonetheless been operating since before our planet was formed.

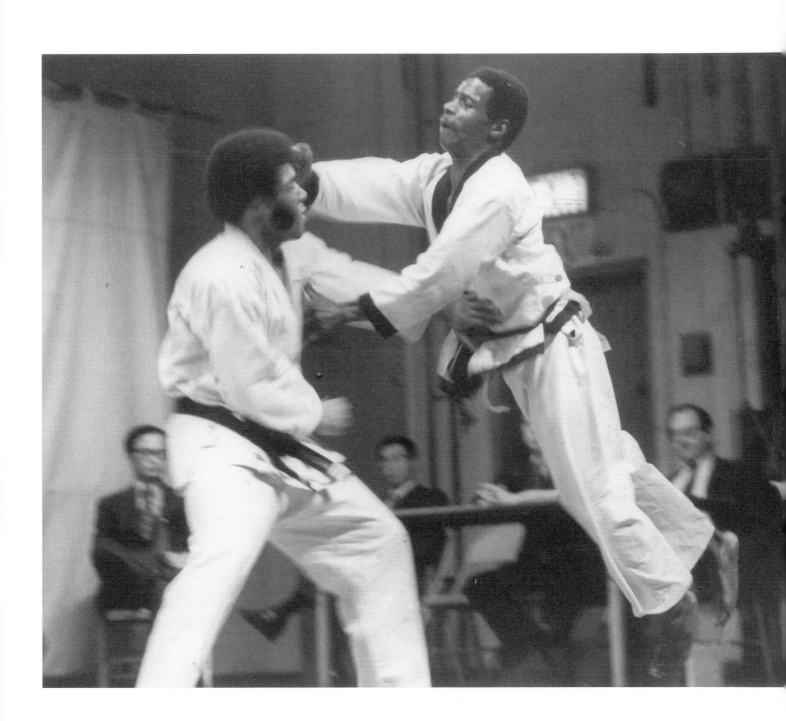

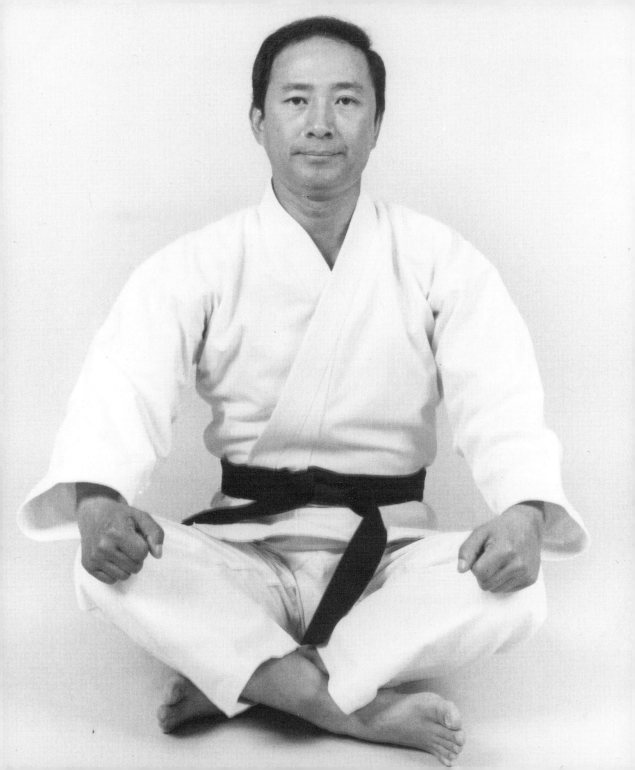

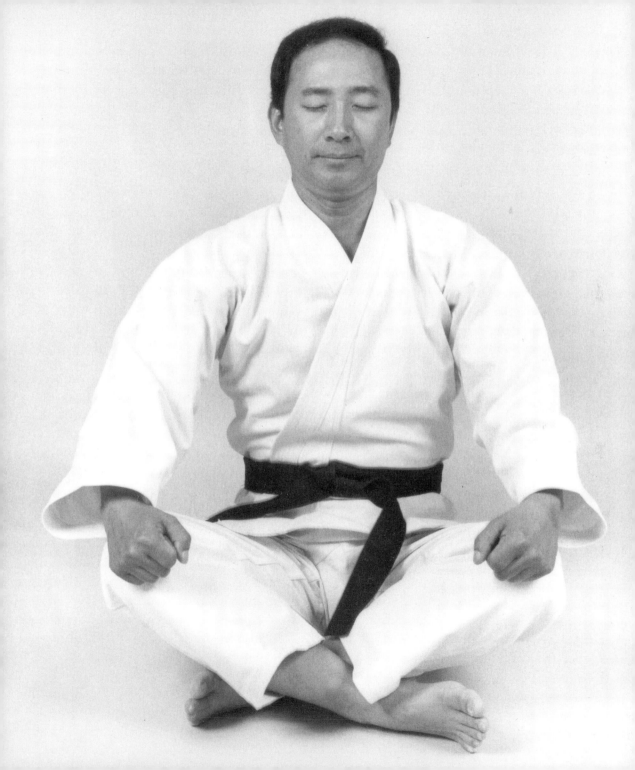

IT HAS BEEN pointed out earlier in this book that Taekwondo is spiritual and comprises mental as well as physical training. It is essential that the serious student of Taekwondo recognizes this fact.

As we have seen, Taekwondo originated far back in the history of mankind. It was originally developed and used against strong, power-hungry men who consistently intimidated weaker ones. As men learned to use Taekwondo to defend themselves against physical attack, they found that their new skill eliminated fear of attack and intimidation. Only then were they able to occupy their minds with the higher goals of spiritual enlightenment and individual self-expression.

But mental training in Taekwondo has an even more immediate value to the application of the martial art.

In our normal lives, our minds are constantly being overrun by what has been called "stream-of-consciousness" thoughts. Random thoughts constantly intrude on our purposeful thinking. Focused concentration is replaced by polyphasic thinking, and our mental efficiency is reduced immeasurably. Thus, we never get to realize our true powers.

In a self-defense situation, this state of affairs can be fatal. When your life is threatened, you cannot afford the luxury of random thoughts wandering willy-nilly through your mind. Your full attention must be focused on one moment—the only moment that matters. If your mind is not focused, you lose the effectiveness of concentrated inner strength and power, and your ability to devote your full *Ki* to the task at hand.

What you need is total concentration—total attention to the job to be done. Meditation strips your mind of extraneous thoughts and helps you to focus on a single thought and action. Your "empty mind," once achieved, permits you to enjoy spontaneity of action and full creativity.

Unfortunately, this mindlessness does not come easily. It requires constant practice, sometimes for years. The average individual cannot think of anything for even five seconds. Ten seconds of "serene mindlessness" seems like an eternity. Yet with sincere and diligent effort, meditation that lasts for fifteen minutes at a stretch can become second nature.

Such meditation opens up a universe of consciousness and a state of "being with the world." Its results are confidence, understanding, tranquility, serenity, self-knowledge, and the knowledge of others. There is a famous saying:

> *If you know your opponent and know yourself,*
> *then in a hundred battles you will always win.*
> *If you do not know him, but know yourself,*
> *you will win half the time, and lose half the time.*
> *If you know neither him nor yourself,*
> *you will always lose.*

This is why philosophy and meditation are vital to the student of martial arts. You must learn to understand yourself as well as your aggressor, and meditation is the means to this understanding.

The physical side of meditation helps achieve the spiritual result. The very *position* you assume when preparing to meditate strengthens your body by developing muscle tone. It helps your abdominal muscles grow strong, regulates and controls your breathing, and stretches your leg muscles. In the process, you learn to relax completely, banishing body tension, and you concentrate on your vital center, your Ki.

You begin by sitting with your back ramrod straight. Your legs are either crossed in front of you or tucked under your body, so that you rest on your shins and insteps. Your eyelids are half-closed, and you are lazily looking at the tip of your nose. Your mental "eyes" are turned inward. Your mind and your total consciousness are focused on your psychic center: a spot one inch directly below your navel. You breathe from your diaphragm. Your belly will expand as you inhale and contract as you exhale.

At first, you will have extreme difficulty keeping your untrained mind from wandering for even five seconds. Do not be discouraged. Practice for fifteen minutes at a time, day after day. Fight distractions as you would an opponent.

Focused meditation will also train you to respond rapidly in the face of a threat that has escalated beyond verbal mediation when the mind and the body must *react* rather than *anticipate.* This important distinction lies at the core of traditional defensive strategy. Making the false assumption that an attacker will execute a reverse punch when, in truth, his intention is to kick, may result in severe injury to the defender. To appreciate the value of meditation as it applies to this component of self-defense, one needs look no further than the stillness of a serene pool of water reflecting the image of a full moon. Because the surface is unbroken by ripples, the image is pure and undistorted. The mind of the martial artist can be taught to act in a similar fashion. Through the sincere and diligent practice of meditation, the Taekwondo practitioner will develop an uncanny ability to react to an unprovoked attack rather than anticipate a potential false move. How is this possible?

The mind, like an unbroken stallion, has a proclivity for galloping away when left to its own designs. Thoughts of daily activities, bills, work or school, all have the ability to intrude on a tranquil mind. Great effort is required to focus on nothing. Yet, nothing, no mind, or *mushim*, is what the martial artist seeks. Mushim is the mental state where one is unhindered by preconception. As difficult as this stage of consciousness may be to achieve, we do have an ally in our quest. Just as the Asian warriors of the past, who walked a razor's edge between life and death in the service of their king, meditated before battle, we too, as modern-day warriors can vanquish the dangers of anticipation by cultivating a clear and tranquil mind. However, there are many types of meditation. Which is appropriate to achieve the result we as martial artists desire? One approach, as a preface to self-defense training, consists of sitting cross-legged in the half-lotus posture on a folded blanket to promote comfort. The hands are positioned in a gesture known as a *mudra.* Again, there are a variety of mudras, each symbolizing and meant to amplify a spiritual concept. The *cosmic mudra*, where the back of the left hand is placed in the palm of the left hand (reverse for women), thumbs touching, is a simple yet effective mudra to begin with. Make a perfect oval rather then permitting the thumbs to create a "peak" or the palms to collapse into a "valley." Let the hands gently rest in the lap, close the eyes and sit erect with the nose in line with the navel. Aside from allowing for a smooth exchange of breath, this posture will encourage a free flow of *ki*, or internal energy, to circulate throughout the body. Using the breath as a focal point, slowly inhale through the nose and exhale through the mouth assigning a single count to each cycle. Count to ten only and then return to one. Invariably, as you meditate, stray thoughts will attempt to invade the mind. Briefly acknowledge these feelings and permit them to pass through your consciousness as would a gentle breeze, all the while returning to your breathing. Eventually, with patience and time, you may be able to abandon your counting altogether and simply focus on the breath. This basic method of meditation should serve to calm the mind prior to training and partially eliminate the distraction of anticipating rather than reacting.

Moreover, as mentioned previously, enhancing the flow of Ki throughout the body is yet another objective of meditation. Why is this seemingly abstract action important to the martial artist? The manipulation of Ki, the universal life force, can be used for both benign and punitive purposes. For instance, in order to promote health, the practitioner of *kiatsu*, or Ki therapy, applies massage to the various *acupoints* that cover the body in an effort to stimulate a flow of ki; when an abundant supply of Ki is present, a sense of well being pervades; when it is deficient, illness reigns. Likewise, the practice of *acupuncture* subscribes to the same principle by inserting needles at key points throughout the body to remove blockages in the series of pathways or *meridians* that traverse the human anatomy. The martial artist, on the other hand, channels Ki to a specific part of the body with the hope of projecting it through the striking surface whether it is fist or foot. This projection of Ki has the potential of amplifying the effectiveness of a technique many fold. Ki channeling can also be used to fortify the body at specific points thus preventing injury to the defender.

This effort requires determination and persistent work. It will be uncomfortable at first, even boring. It will frustrate you and make you angry with yourself. This, too, will be a distraction. But you must persevere. If you make a sincere and concerted effort, you will find that your periods of being able to control your own mind will grow measurably in duration day by day.

And then, one day, you will experience that brilliant flash of self-awareness that will come to you as an incandescent illumination as you meditate. Your awareness will be both within and outside of yourself. That is the goal.

Do not fight the process. Go with it. Become one with it. Relax into it, and allow it to take hold of that place where your primitive instincts live.

Advanced Taekwondo cannot be learned by means of intellect alone. It must be accepted, almost on an emotional, transcendent level. Sometimes a stubborn intellect can actually be a handicap in this. Through disciplined concentration, your entire consciousness can absorb the lesson.

Then you will discover your own humanity and awaken beyond your "self" into an external existence in harmony with your own true spirit and the Universe of which it is a part.

You will unleash your Ki, your vital spirit, and focus totally and exclusively at one target in one suspended instant. And someday that ability could save your life.

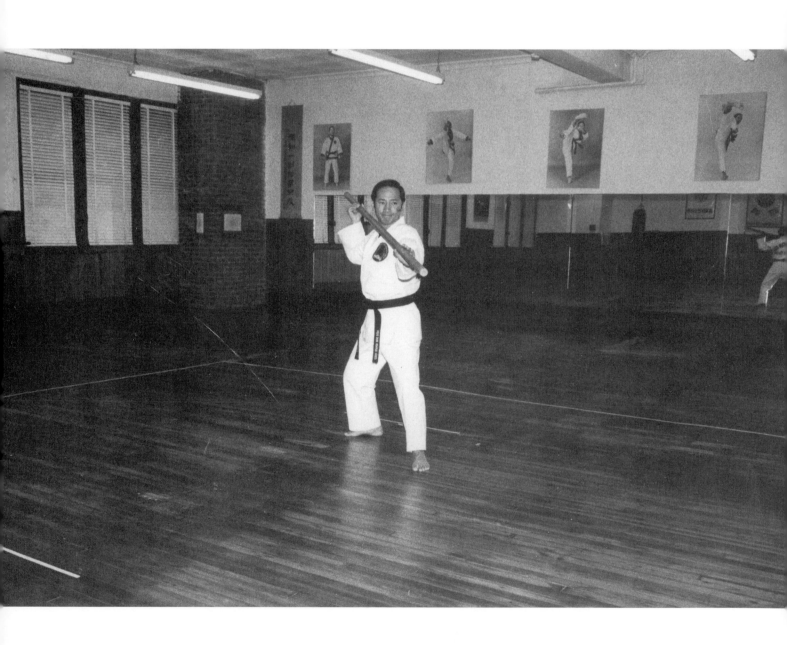

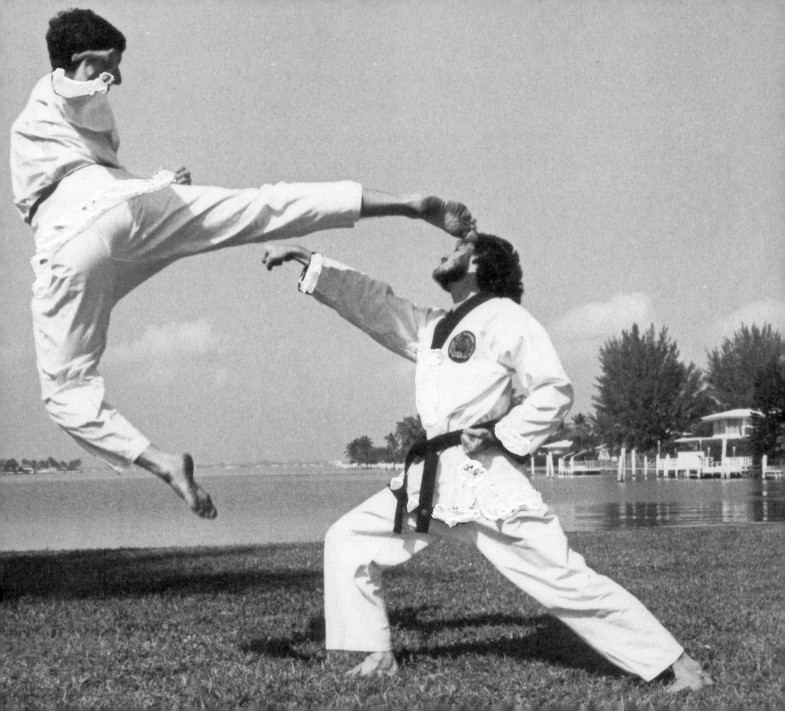

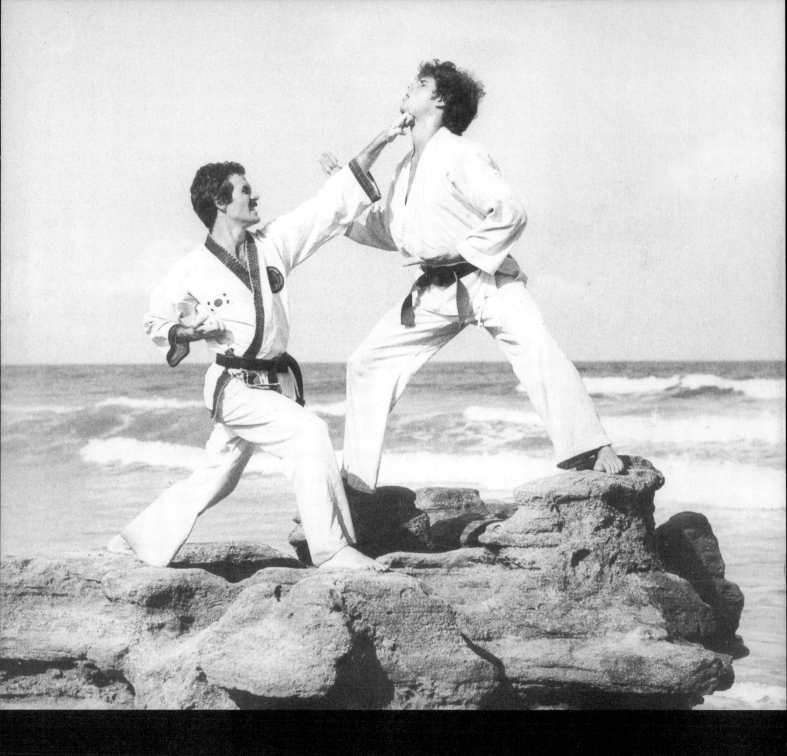

Training for Various
Hand and Foot Techniques

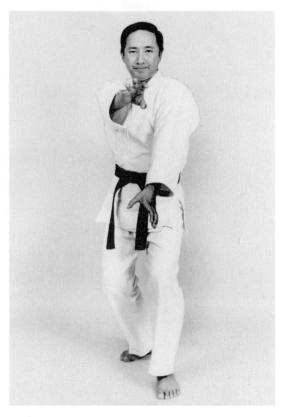

YOUR HANDS AND FEET are the ultimate human weapons. They have the advantage that they are always with you, unlike weapons that you cannot carry or would not wish to carry.

As you have progressed in your study of the art of Taekwondo, you have learned to use your hands and feet in ways that you would not have thought possible.

Now it is time for you to develop coordination, speed, and power, so that you can succeed in delivering effective blocks and attacks against several opponents, if necessary. Timing is critical to this.

As a beginning and intermediate student, you learned to deliver kicks and punches with power and precision. Now, as an advanced practitioner, you must train to be able to perform six different techniques with lightning speed, precision, and accuracy against one or multiple opponents.

You will learn to develop and apply multiple faking techniques to confuse and befuddle your opponents, and to develop effective combinations to adapt to your own condition and to the situation in which you may find yourself.

You will have to be comfortable enough with each technique that you will be able to improvise on the spur of the moment, even under the stress of attack. To accomplish this, you will have to practice each combination hundreds and hundreds of times, so that they will become as familiar to you in use as the Forward Punch.

Many advanced hand techniques and combinations are discussed in the forms section of this book. These can be applied in combat. Because of the limitations of space, I am presenting here several combinations of foot and hand techniques and a series of advanced leg-stretching exercises. These should provide you with a springboard for endless combinations and variations.

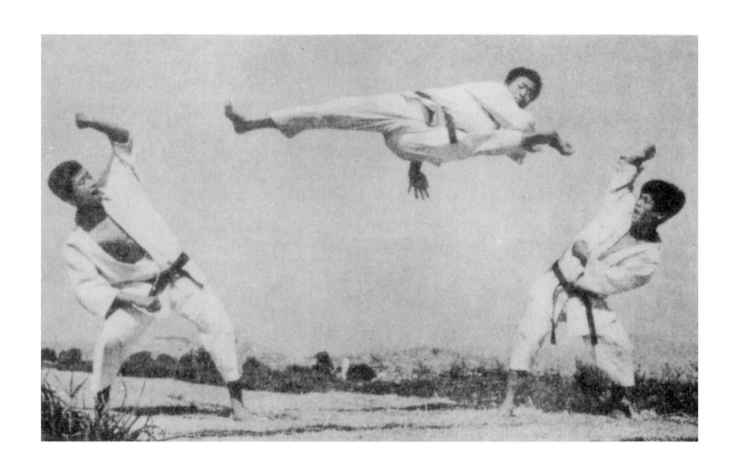

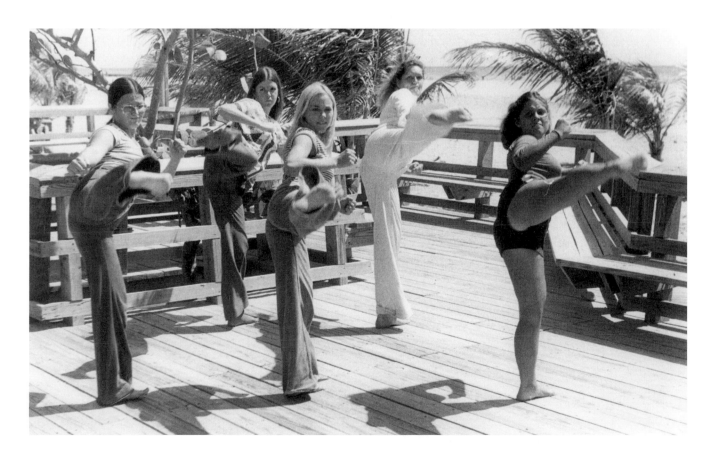

47 / Training for Various Hand and Foot Techniques

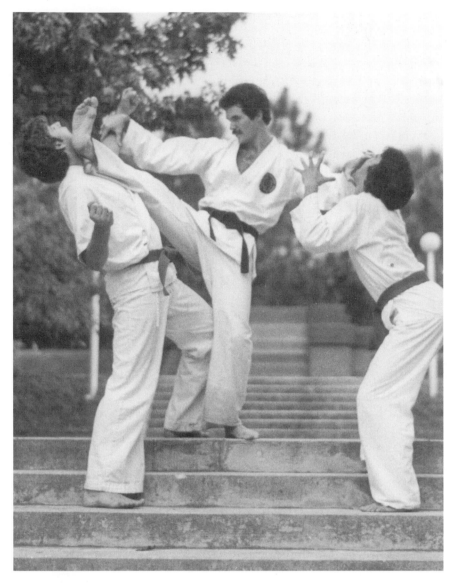

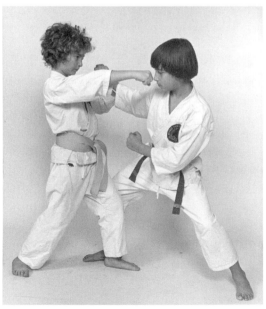

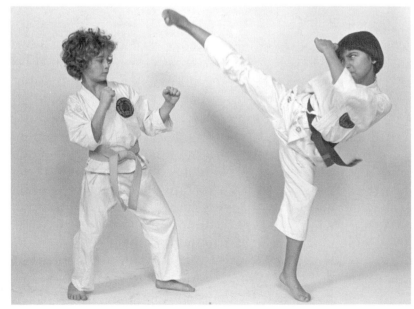

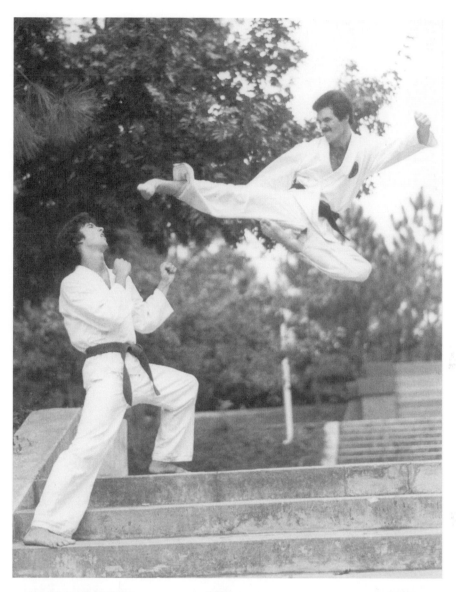

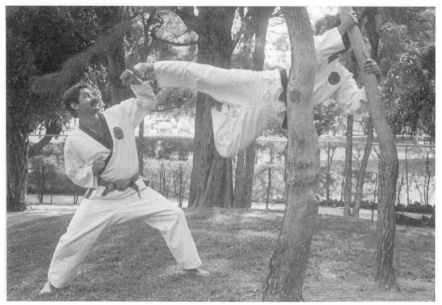

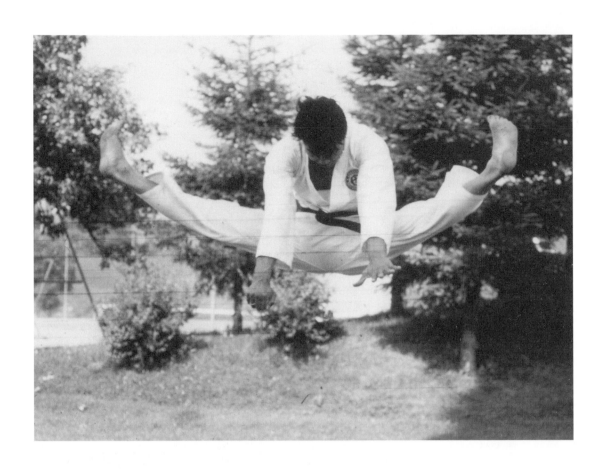

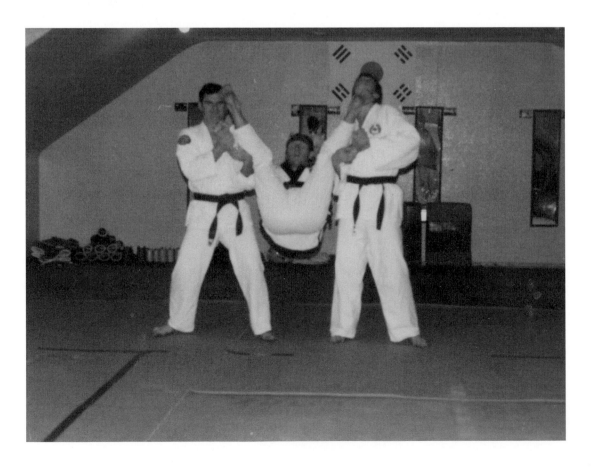

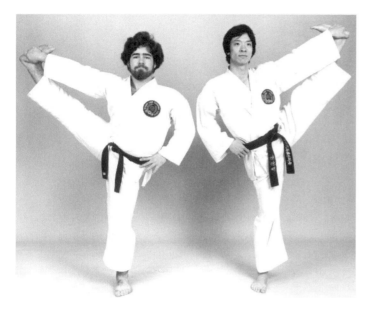

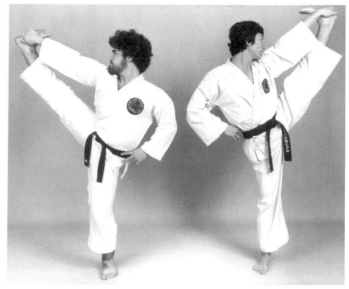

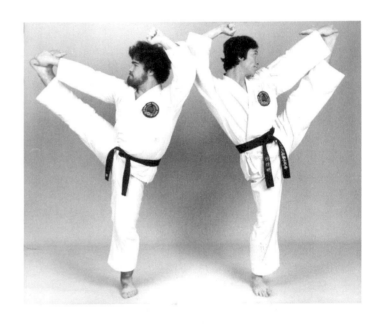

ADVANCED LEG-STRETCHING EXERCISES

1. Side Leg Stretch

Five different standing methods.

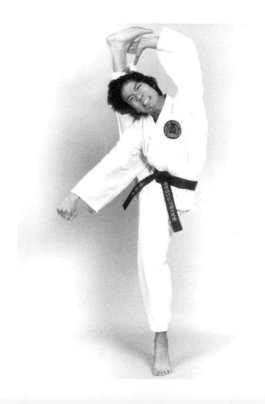

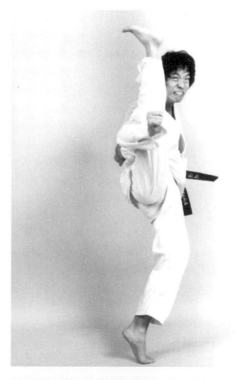

2. Leg Stretching
Two different floor methods.

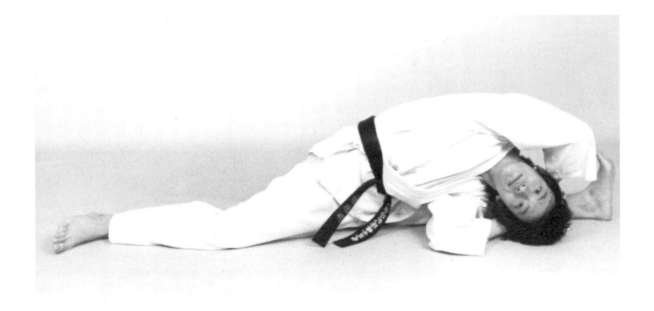

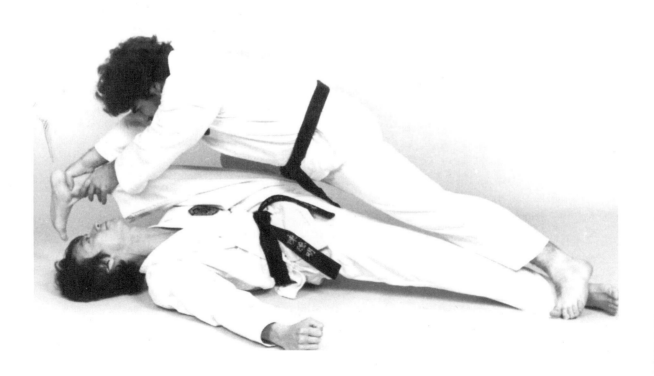

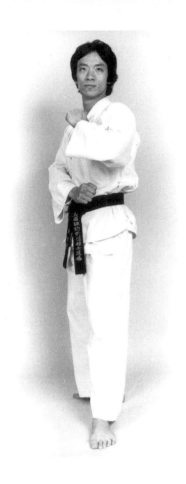

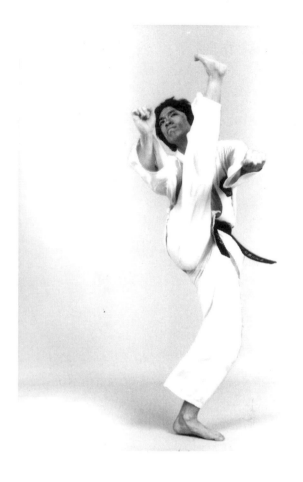

3. Stretch Exercise for Wheel-Kick

Practice.

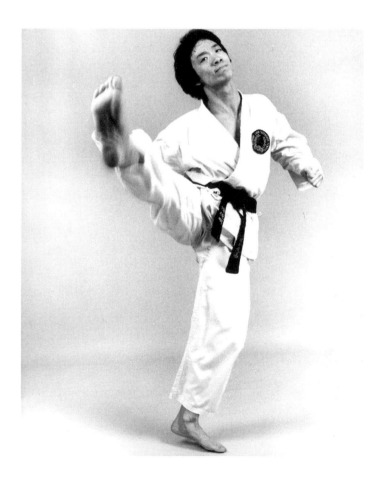

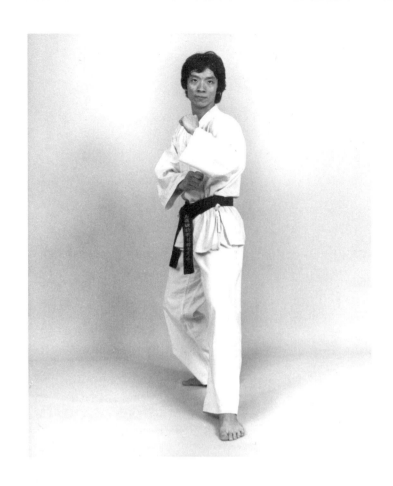

4. Stretch Exercise for Axe-Kick
Practice.

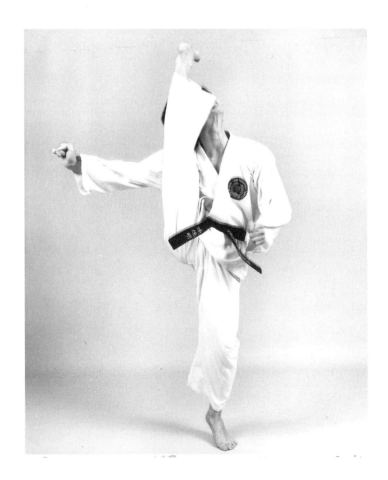

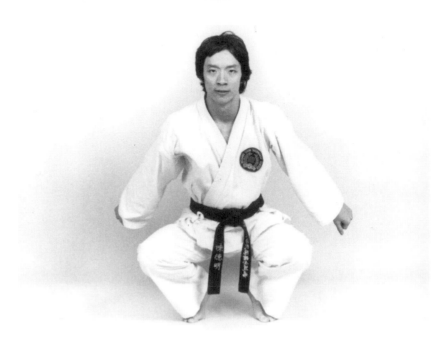

5. Two Jumping Side Stretches

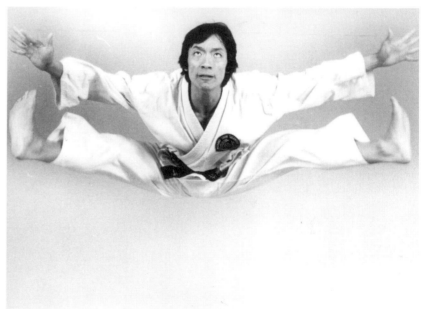

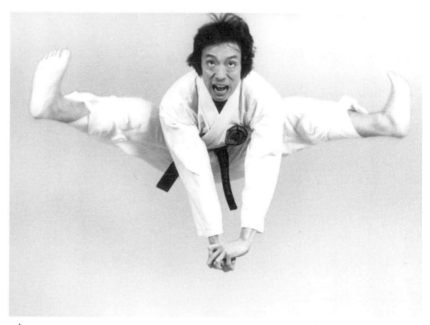

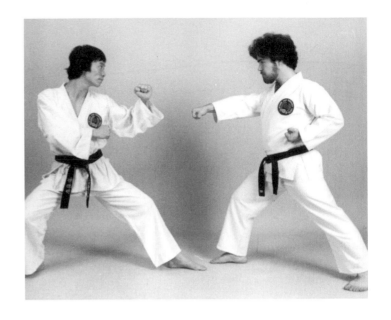

ADVANCED KICKING TECHNIQUES

1. Turning Wheel Kick

Turning your body to the right, pivot on the ball of the left foot, raise your right foot, and execute a Turning Wheel Kick, striking the opponent's face with the outside of your heel. Continue swinging with the knee locked.

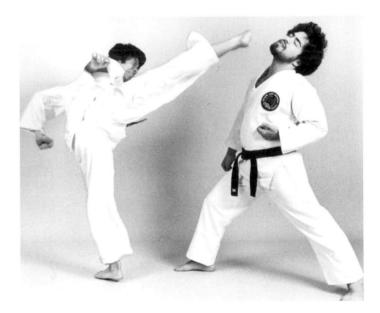

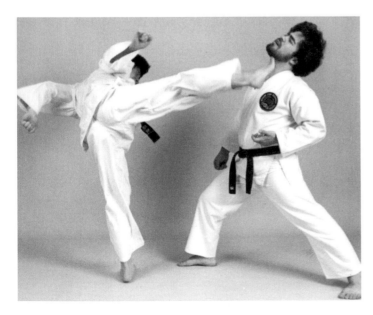

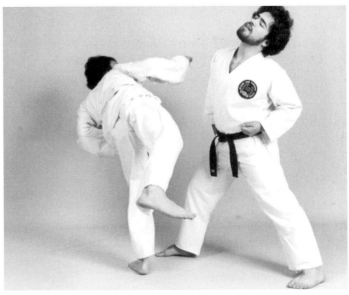

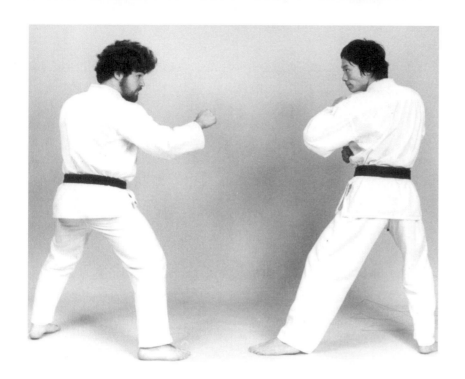

2. Standing Jumping High Front Kick

Jump as high as possible with both feet leaving the ground at the same time. Execute a High Front Kick with your back foot.

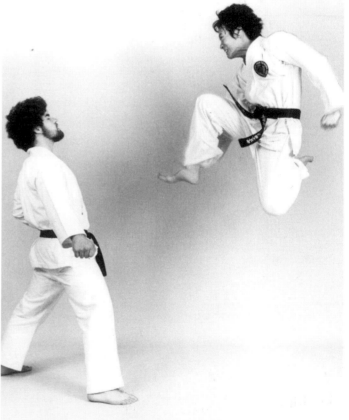

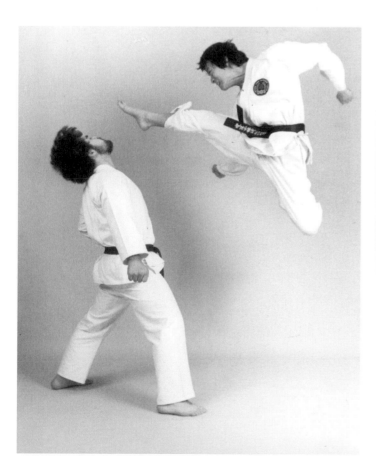

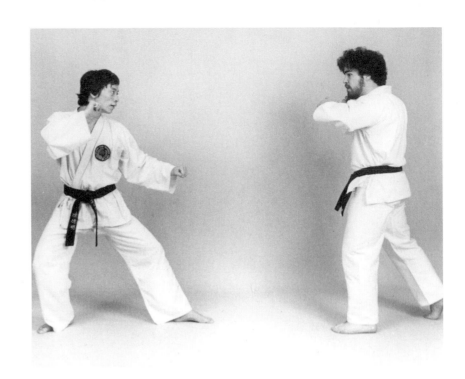

3. Standing Jumping High Instep Round Kick

Jump as high as possible with both feet leaving the
ground at the same time. Execute a Round Kick
with the instep of the back foot.

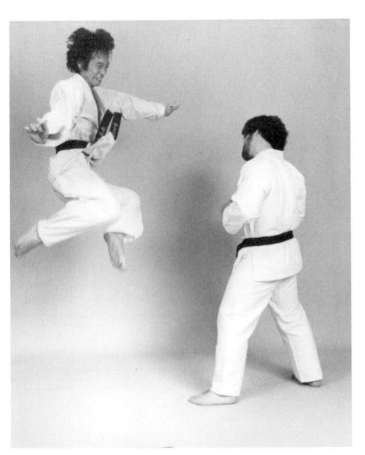

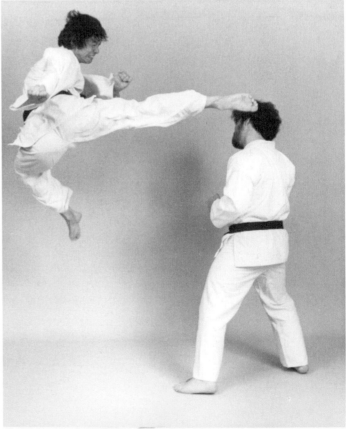

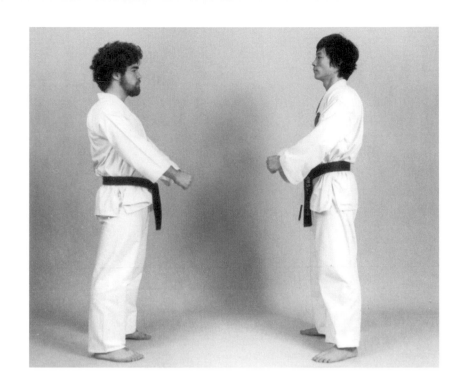

4. Standing Jumping High Round Kick

Jump as high as possible with both feet leaving the ground at the same time. Execute a High Round Kick with either foot.

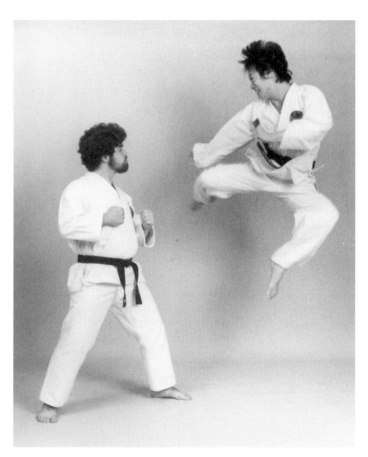

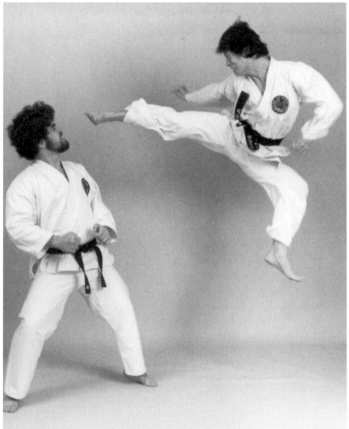

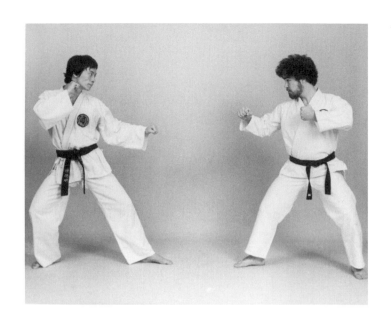

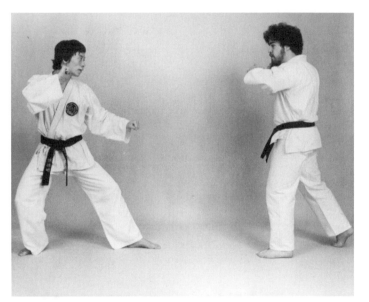

5. Jumping Double Side Kick

Step forward with your back foot, and jump as high as possible. Execute a Side Kick with both feet.

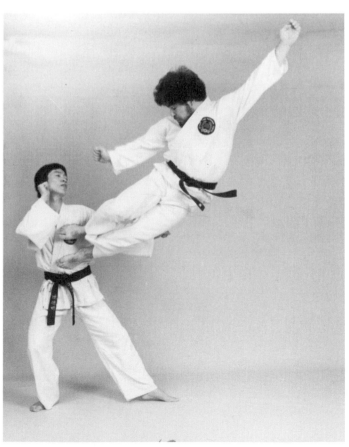

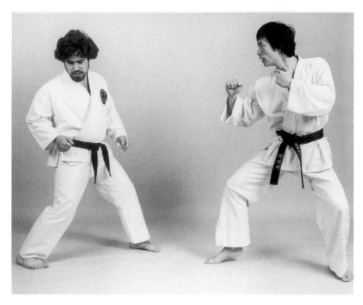 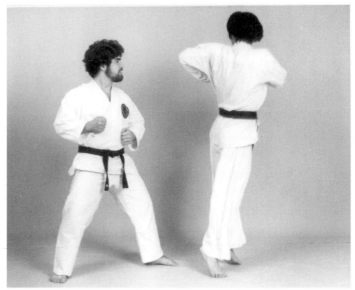

6. Jumping Turning Wheel Kick

Twist and pivot, and jump as high as possible, raising your left leg. Execute a Jumping Wheel Kick, striking the opponent's face with the outside of your heel. Continue swinging with your knee locked. Follow up with a Reverse Punch to the solar plexus.

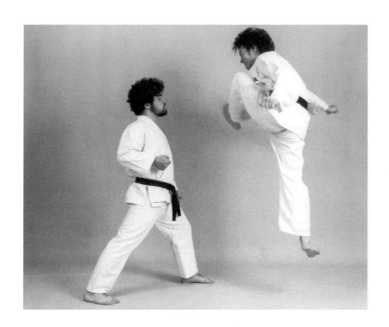

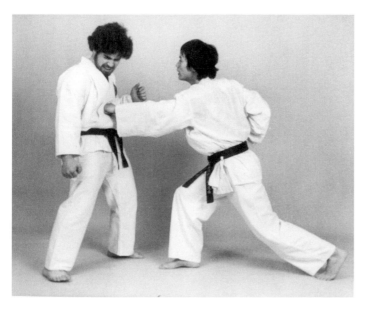 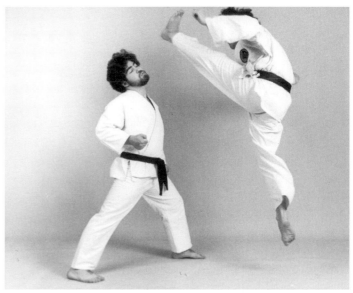

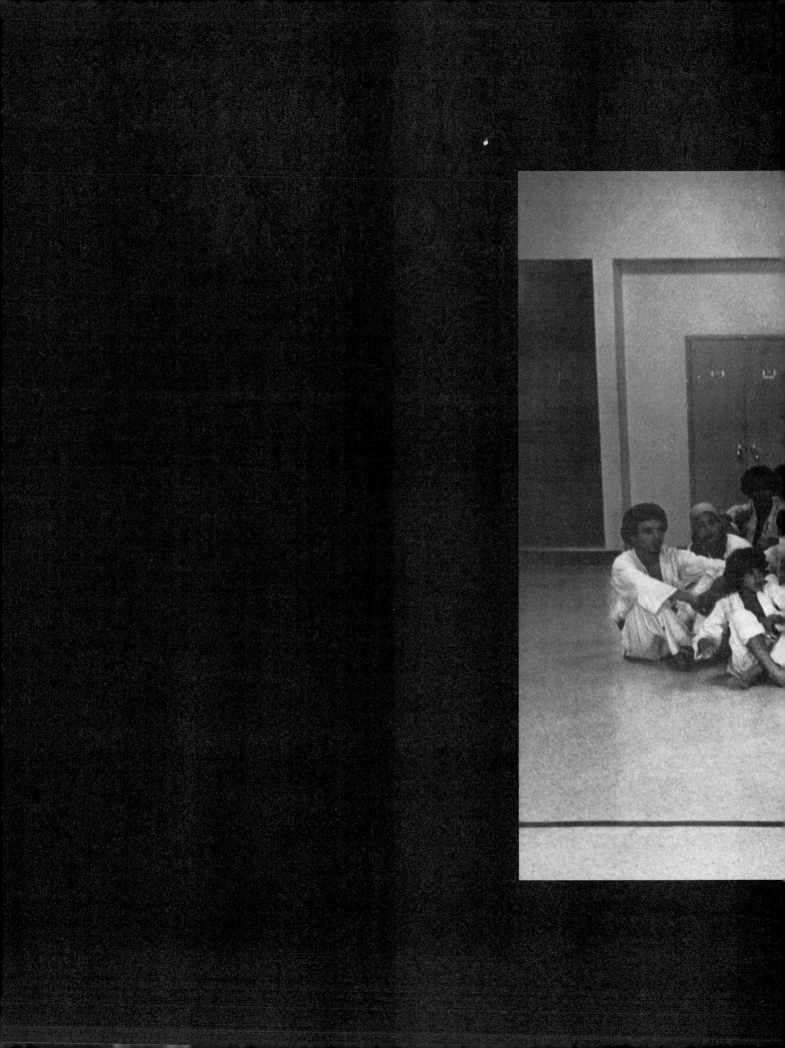

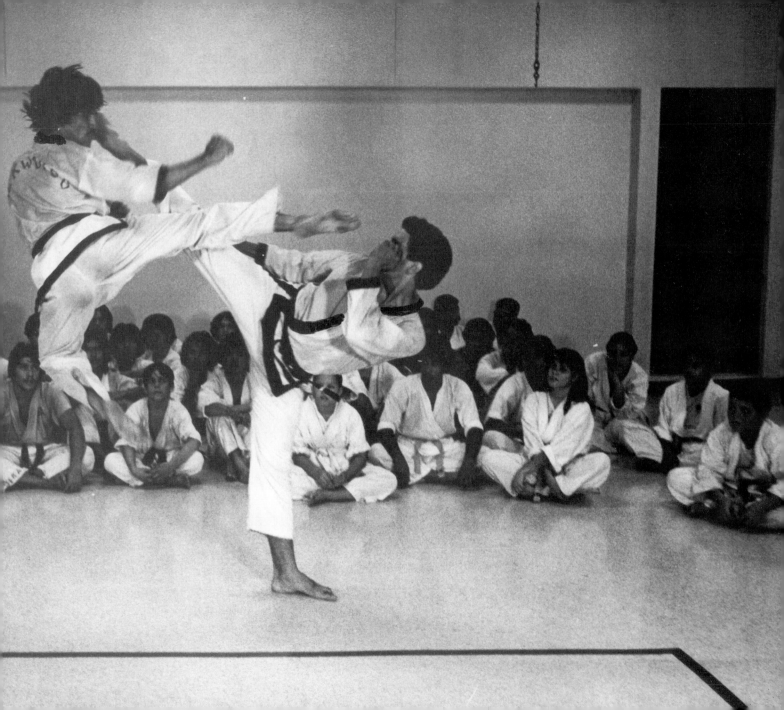

SPARRING IS SIMULATED COMBAT. Each participant starts with the same basic materials—the body and a basic knowledge of techniques and combinations. The outcome depends on his or her strategy in the application of these techniques, and the creativity, imagination, determination, and ingenuity with which they are applied.

To prepare yourself for sparring, you must first master the basic blocking and striking techniques until you are very proficient at them and until they become second nature. This can be accomplished only by constant practice. There is no time in sparring—or in combat—to think about how to execute a technique. The action must be instinctive and reflexive to be effective. Each strike and block must be totally efficient, with no wasted motion. Wasted motion is wasted time. It robs speed. Worst of all, wasted motion telegraphs what you are about to do and sets you up for your opponent.

In Taekwondo, there are four stages of training which lead to good sparring technique. The first is Three-Step Sparring. This develops speed and defensive blocking techniques. It develops a level of confidence in the beginning student.

The second stage is One-Step Sparring. It leaves much less time to think about counterattack, so it develops more advanced counterattacking techniques. It, too, must be practiced until it is as natural as walking or punching. One-Step Sparring techniques should be practiced continually, in a totally random order, until you can confidently counter the attack without knowing what kind of attack is coming.

A subcategory of One-Step Sparring is One-Step Sparring make-ups. Here, the student combines and applies all of the techniques he or she has learned in an infinite number of combinations. Each black belt student should have hundreds of these make-up techniques in his or her repertoire, and they, too, must be second nature. This eliminates the need for thinking about technique during actual sparring.

The third stage is Prearranged Free Sparring. In this stage, techniques of attack and defense are applied in continuous sequence, in prescribed combinations. This develops balance, coordination, reflexes, and endurance. It allows you to practice your techniques and combinations in a dynamic, fluid situation. As one great master has said, "Flexibility is life. Rigidity is death." In Prearranged Free Sparring, the two partners apply their techniques, rearrange the patterns of attack and response, and choose techniques to suit themselves and the situation. They practice blocking, moving swiftly to avoid attacks, and counterattacking.

The fourth stage is Free Sparring. This is the ultimate dynamic fluid situation. It builds endurance and trains perception in anticipating offensive moves. Practiced diligently, it develops the ability to understand patterns of attack and to overcome them with confidence.

Eye contact is critical in Free Sparring. The gaze should be large and broad, so that it can take in everything from the tip of the opponent's toe to the top of his head. The student must train to see without moving his eyes. Eye movement is a giveaway of intent. Watching the opponent's eyes tells you what he is about to do. Not moving yours prevents him from anticipating you. The masters have said, "Perception is strong, but sight is weak." It is important to learn to use your eyes in a sixth-sense sort of way. Thus, you instinctively perceive and react, eliminating the middleman of conscious thought.

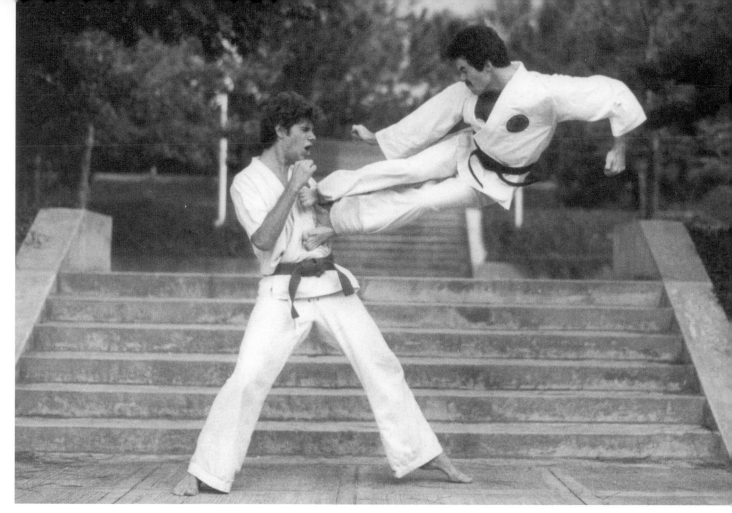

In addition, Taekwondo teaches us that to fix an opponent's eyes is to gaze into his heart. This can be disquieting, to say the least.

As you spar, assess you opponent. Judge his likely reactions to a given attack. Use your imagination to vary your methods and keep him guessing. This keeps him off balance and vulnerable. Shift your weight in a feint. When he moves in defense, strike in another place.

Do not allow yourself to become excited. Discipline yourself into serene impassivity. Use your judgment and timing, and move decisively and deliberately. Feint, parry, and thrust. Build your judgment and psyche out your opponent. Use hard and soft techniques to throw your opponent off balance. For instance, if he is attacking, dodge him, evade him, and block him softly, then suddenly strike out with a powerful kick as he lunges in at you.

Judge your distances accurately. Your speed, strength, and precision will depend on this. Determine your target before you attack. When you feint an attack, be prepared to follow it through if the opponent fails to respond defensively. Focus your attack with speed, precision, and strength.

Before you attack, take your time. Study your opponent's reflexes and rhythms. Be defensive in the beginning, and be on the alert for an opportunity to strike. When you do strike, strike with swift, economical moves. Don't allow your eyes or a shift in your stance to telegraph your intentions. Keep your body low, so you don't have to coil up for a leap. Keep your head level. Resist the temptation to move it up or down. It, too, will give you away.

Use your feints creatively. Appear to strike one target and swiftly turn your attack toward another that becomes undefended in response to your feint. Develop the ability to combine two, three, or four techniques in rapid fluid sequence. Deliver two techniques simultaneously. But don't grow overly dependent on one or two combinations. To be too familiar with one technique is as bad as not knowing it well enough. You don't want your opponent to be able to predict your moves. You must lead him around, keeping him off balance and on the defensive.

When you are defending, use your dodges and blocks to frustrate and confuse your opponent. Keep your rhythm unpredictable and avoid repetition, depriving your opponent of the opportunity to practice on you. Remember, Free Sparring approximates the kinds of conditions you are likely to encounter in a real attack situation. You must train yourself to be calm, observant, and decisive; disregarding the distractions present in your environment and in yourself.

In combat, your inner spirit will not be different from your normal, relaxed state. You can be determined but calm. You should be able to pay attention to tiny details, without losing sight of the overall picture. And you must not stray into doing things that are of no use.

You must also learn to make use of your opponent's fighting rhythm and to lead him around toward awkward places and positions, causing loss of essential balance. Use your *kiyup!* (yell) suddenly and unexpectedly. It shows energy, and it is the voice of your Ki. It startles your opponent momentarily, making him vulnerable. Then you strike, and you *cling to the attack*, pursuing without letting the opportunity get away, so your opponent can't recover. Once you have closed with your assailant, you can hit as directly and quickly as possible through a gap in his guard, while he is still undecided.

Your purpose in Taekwondo is not to fight but rather to end the fight.

But the real prize of our art and our philosophy is personal. Just knowing that we could physically hold our own if a situation were to require it provides the confidence we need to avoid intimidation. As a great master of the martial arts said over three hundred years ago, "To think only of the practical benefit of wisdom and technology is vulgar."

Numerous examples of Three-Step, One-Step, and Free Sparring techniques have been covered in my previous book, *Tae Kwon Do: The Korean Martial Art*. Because of the limitations of space, I will not repeat them here but will give several further examples of more advanced techniques.

ONE-STEP SPARRING TECHNIQUES

1. Middle Punch Attack

a. Attacker slides his left foot forward into a Left Front Stance and simultaneously executes a Left-Hand Low Block with a yell, indicating that he is ready to attack. Defender, waiting at attention, yells to indicate that he is ready to defend himself.

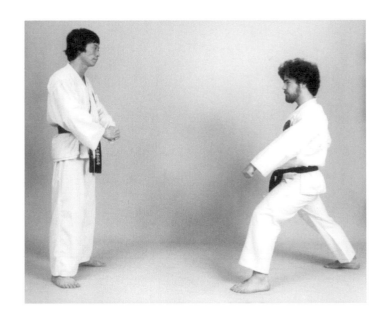

b. Attacker executes a Right-Hand Middle Punch. Defender blocks the punch by executing an Inward Crescent Kick with his right foot (Crescent Kick Block).

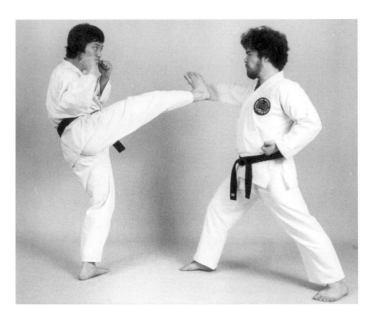

c. Defender brings his kicking leg into a Side Kick Position.

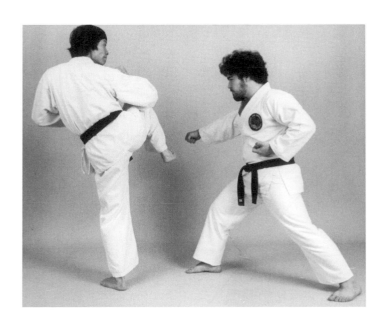

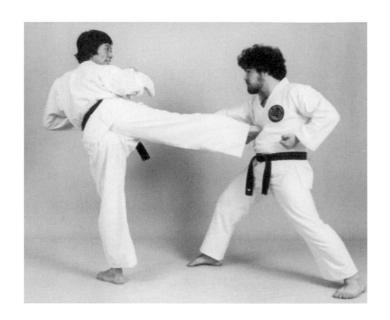

d. Defender executes a Right Side Kick to the midsection.

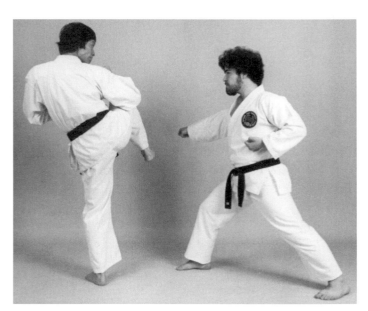

e. Defender brings the same foot into the Side Kick Position.

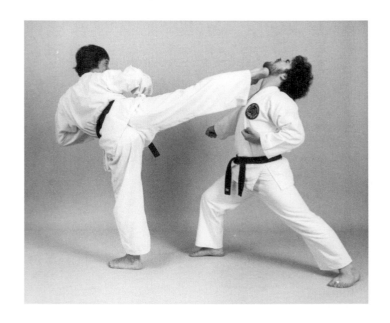

f. Defender executes a second Right Side Kick to the attacker's face or chin.

2. Middle Punch Attack

a. Attacking and defending position.

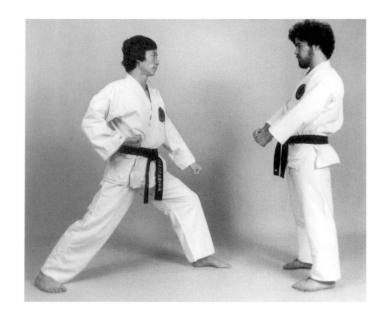

b. Defender blocks the Right-Hand Middle Punch by executing a Left Inside Knife-Hand Middle Block.

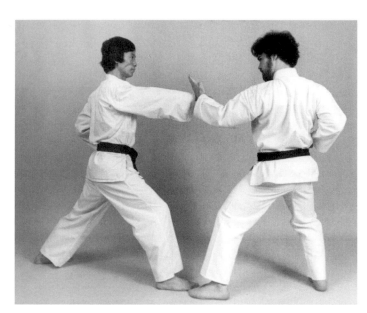

c. Grabbing the attacker's fist, the defender executes a sweep with his front foot.

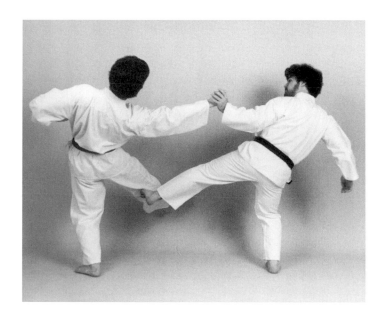

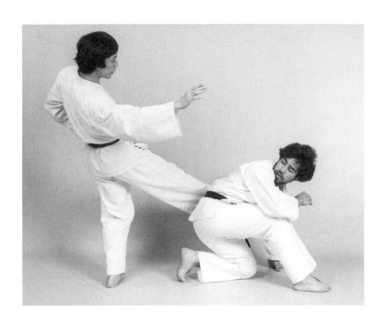

d. Placing his sweeping foot on the floor, the defender prepares to execute a Stooping Turning Kick with his front foot.

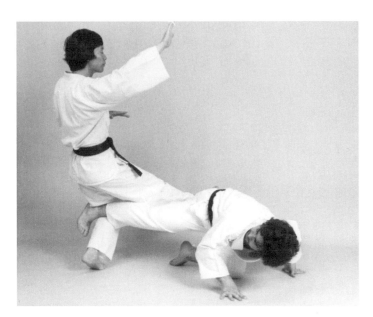

e. Defender executes a Stooping Turning Kick, throwing his opponent to the ground.

f. Defender turns into Front Kneeling Position.

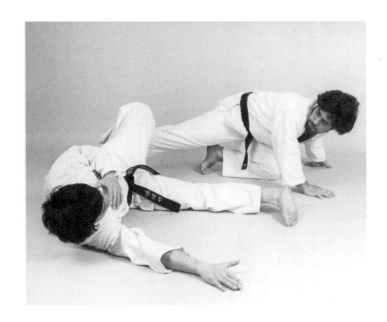

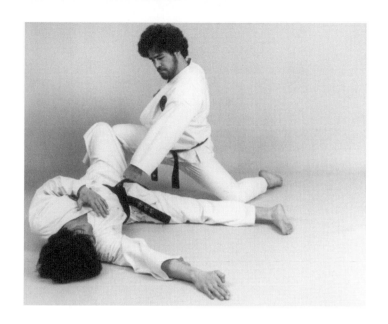

g. Defender executes a Left Reverse Punch to the groin.

3. Middle Punch Attack

a. Starting position.

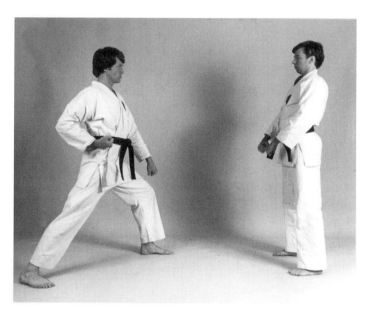

b. Defender blocks a Middle Punch with an Inward Crescent Kick.

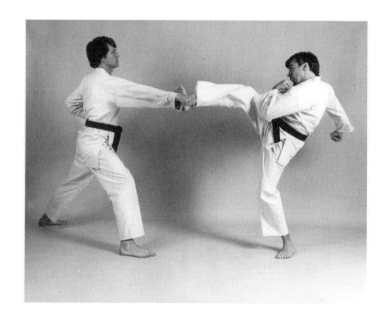

c. Defender places his kicking foot on the floor and turns to the left in preparation for a Turning Side Kick with his left foot.

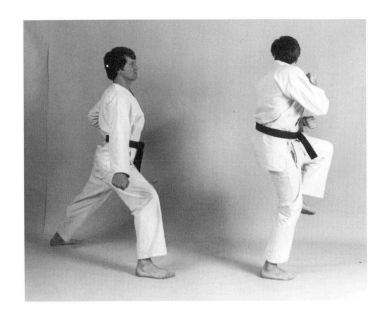

d. Defender executes the Turning Left Side Kick.

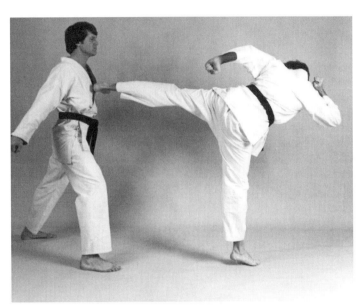

e. Defender returns his kicking leg to the floor, ready to execute a Right Front Kick.

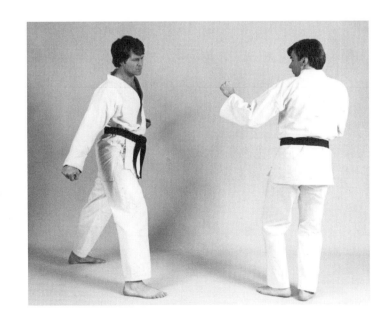

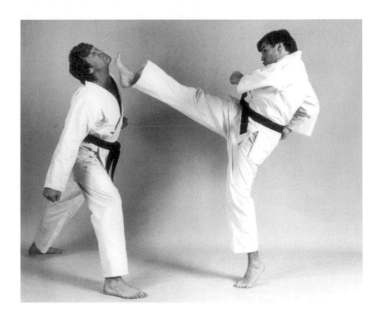

f. Defender executes a Front Kick to the face.

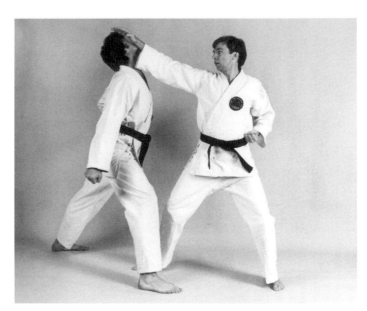

g. Defender steps down into a Back Stance and simultaneously executes a Right Knife Hand Strike to the temple.

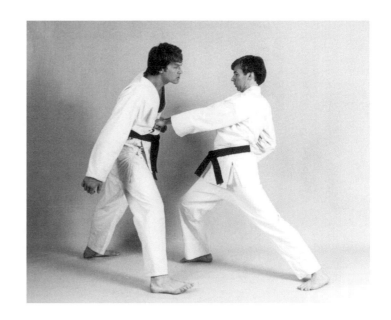

h. Shifting to a Right Front Stance, the defender executes a Left-Hand Reverse Punch to the midsection.

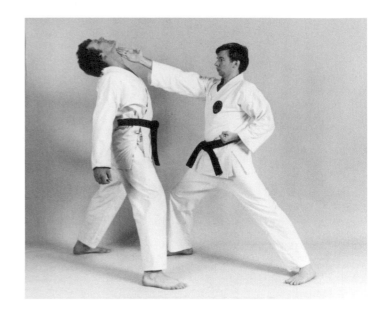

i. He then executes a Right Spear-Hand Thrust to the throat.

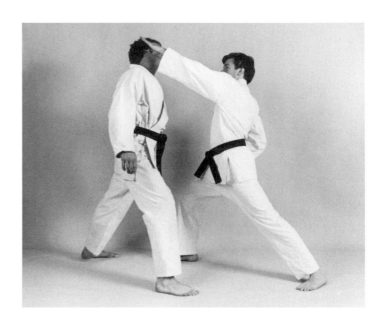

j. From the same position, he executes a Left Ridge-Hand Strike to the temple.

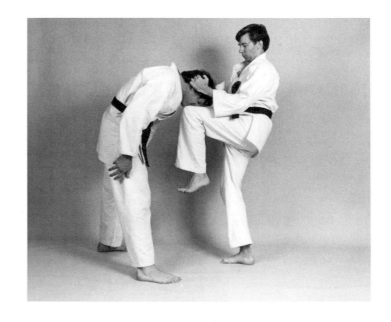

k. Defender grabs attacker's head and executes a Left Knee Attack to the face.

4. High Punch Attack

a. Starting position.

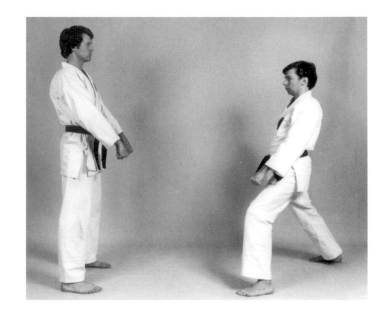

b. Defender leaps up, lifting his right foot.

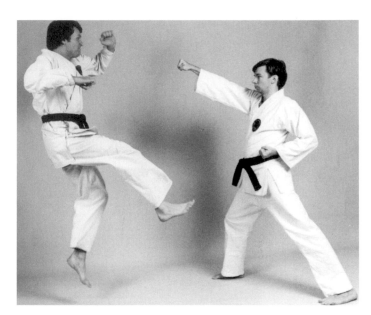

c. Raising his left knee in the air, the defender prepares to execute a Left Jumping Front Kick.

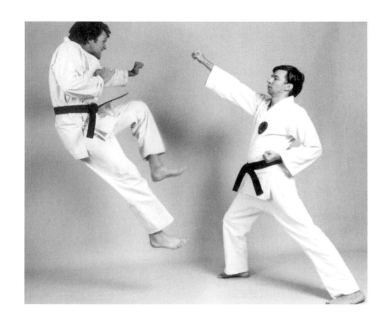

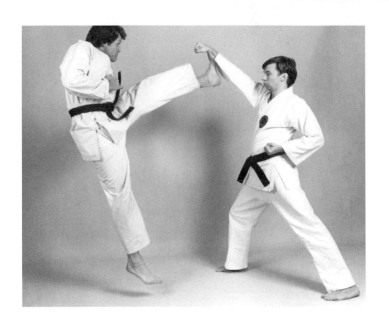

d. Defender blocks the High Punch with a Jumping Front Kick.

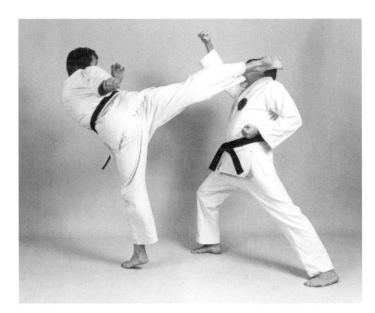

e. Immediately as his kicking leg touches the floor, the defender executes a Right Instep Round Kick to the face.

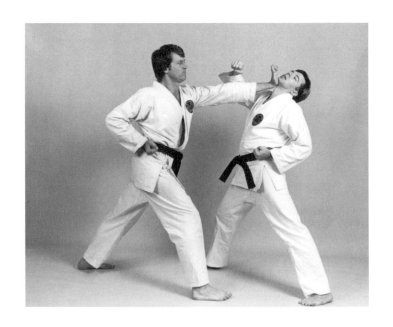

f. Bringing his right foot down into Front Stance, the defender executes a Reverse Palm-Heel strike with his left hand to the attacker's chin.

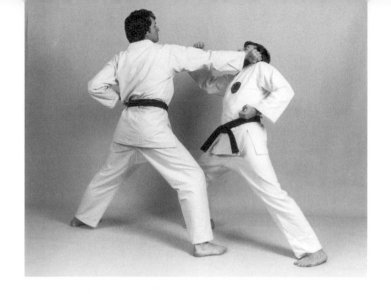

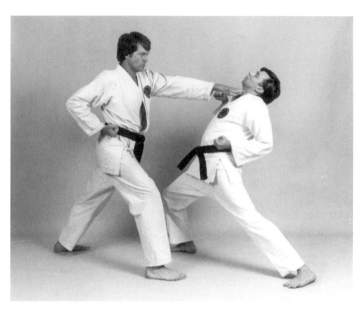

i. Defender then sweeps with an Inside Crescent Kick under the attacker's knee with his right foot.

j. Defender executes a Right Side Kick to the head.

g. From the same stance, defender executes an Ox-Jaw Wrist Strike to the attacker's jaw with his right hand.

h. From the same stance, defender executes a Left Reverse Spear-Hand Strike, palm down, to the throat.

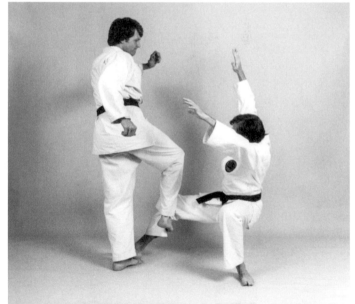

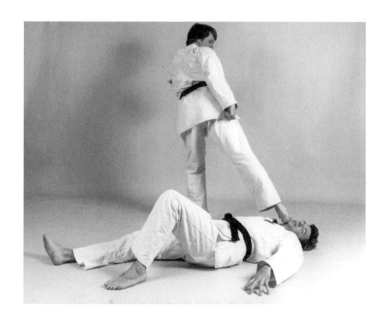

FREE SPARRING TECHNIQUES

1. Axe Kick Response to Front Kick Attack

a. b. c. Free Sparring procedures.

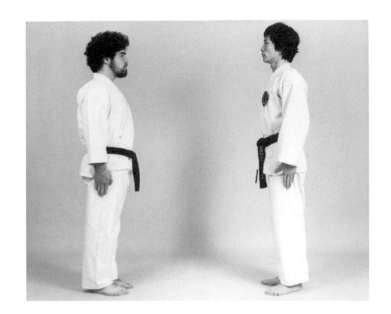

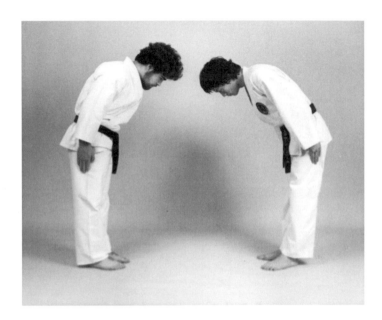

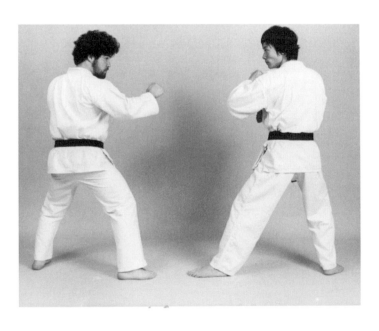

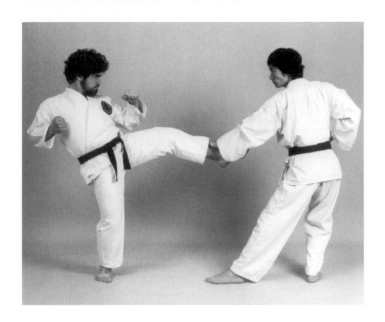

d. Execute a Left Palm-Heel Block.

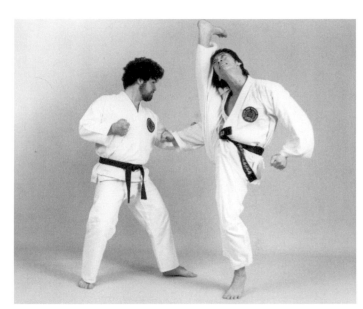

e. Raise your kicking leg as high as possible as in a Front Straight Kick.

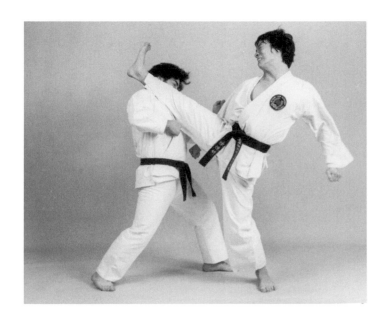

f. Forcefully bring down your heel with your leg locked, striking the opponent's head, face, or collarbone with the back of our heel.

2. Combination Attack

Ready.

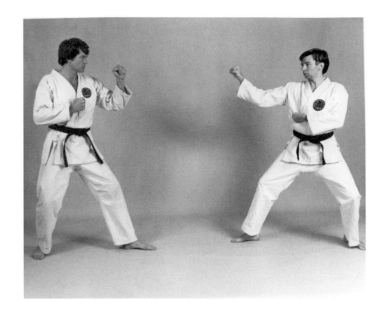

a. Execute an Axe Kick to the face with your left foot.

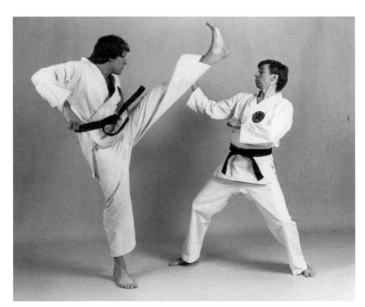

b. Step down with your left foot.

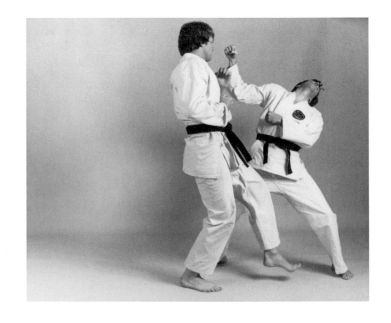

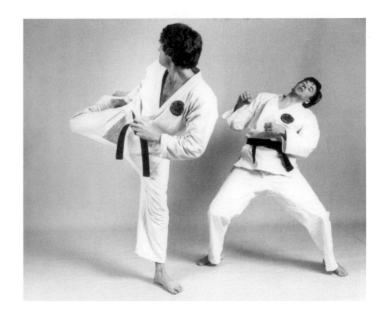

c. Turn to the right.

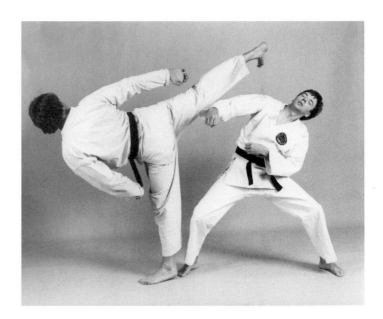

d. Execute a Turning Hook Kick to the face with your right foot.

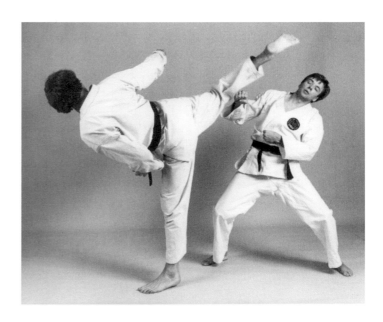

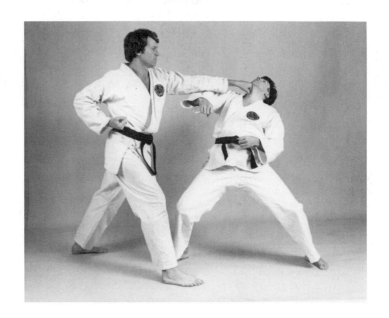

e. Step down with your right foot and execute a Left-Hand Reverse Punch to the face.

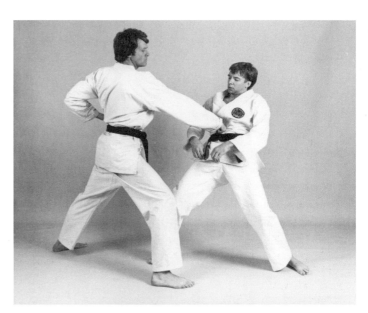

f. Right-Hand Middle Punch to the solar plexus.

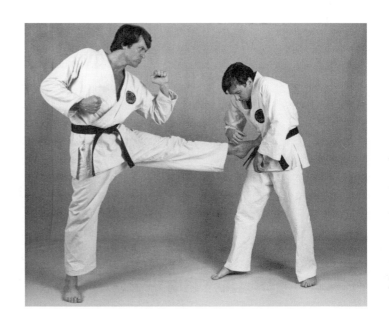

g. Follow up with a Front Kick to the midsection.

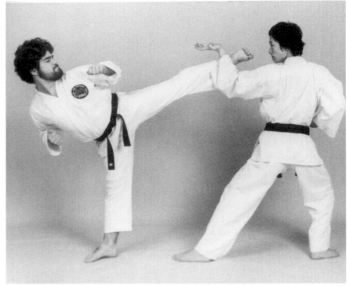

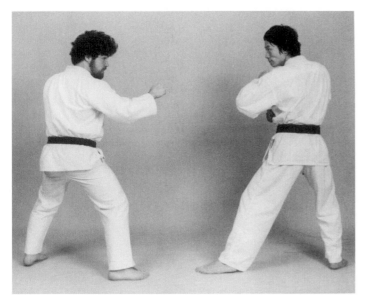

3. Combination Response to the Round Kick

Ready.

a. Execute an Inside Middle Block with open left hand.

b. Turn to the right, raise your right foot, and execute a Turning Right Hook Kick to the face.

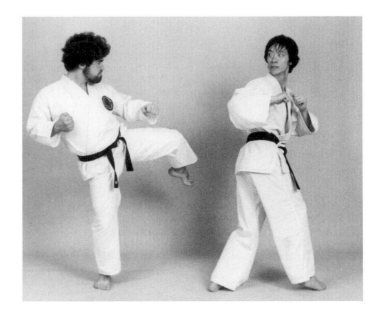

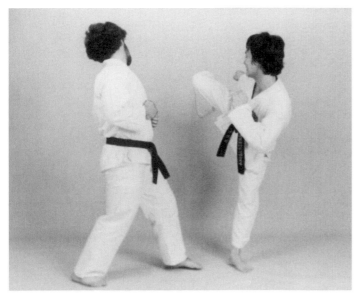

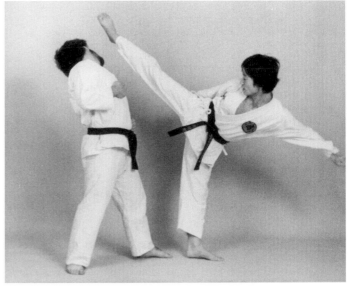

c. Immediately execute an Instep Round Kick to the face with the same foot.

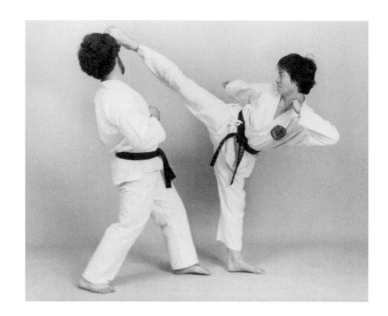

d. Step down with your right foot.

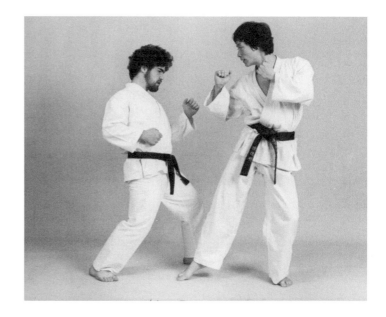

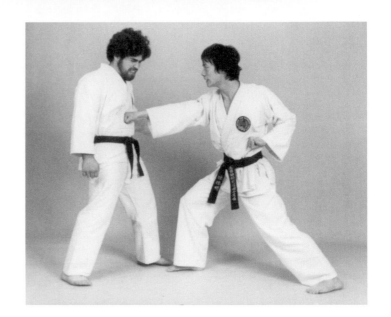

e. Execute a Double Punch to the midsection.

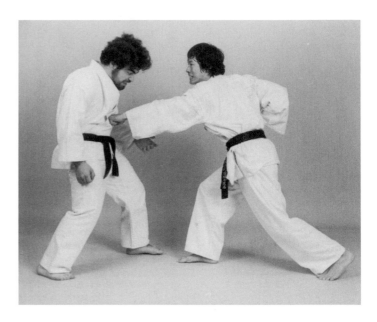

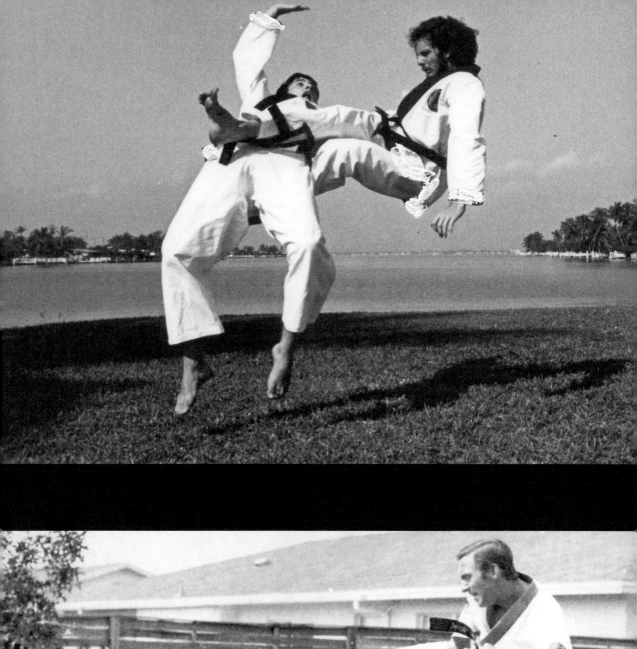

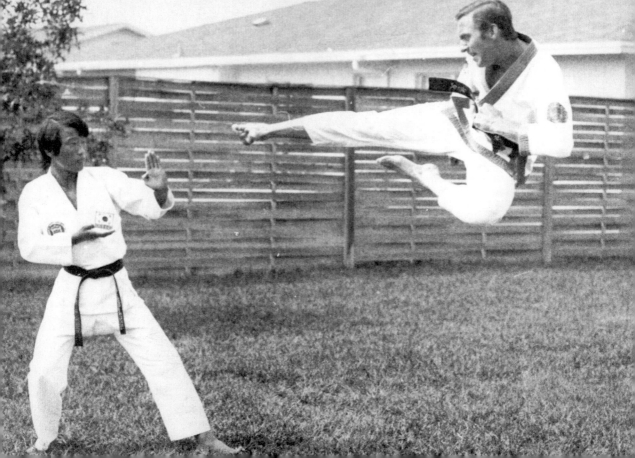

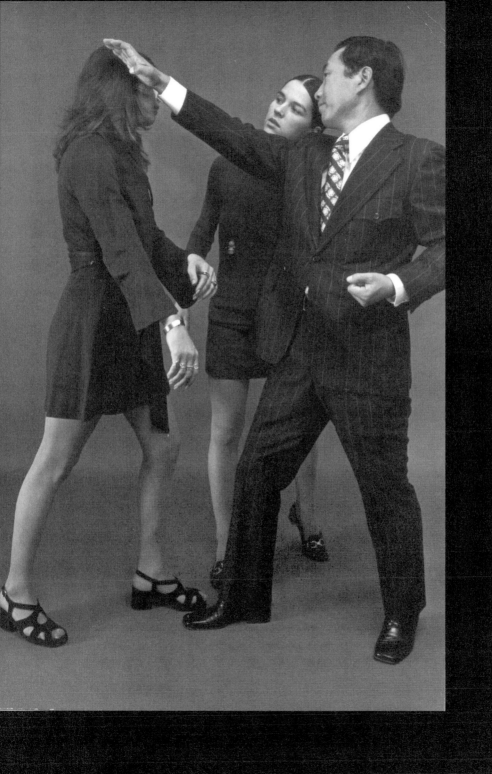

Self-Defense Techniques

TAEKWONDO is the art of kicking and punching. It relies for its power on shock or impact force, rather than on throwing techniques, as in judo, or on holds, as in aiki-do. However, situations do arise in which the student of Taekwondo would be well served to know some of these techniques. So we address them here, recognizing that they are only a part of your training, not its mainstream.

You should know how to fall without getting hurt. You could be thrown off-balance or tripped during training in class or on the street. Knowing how to fall can keep you from injuring your head, your elbow, or your hip. Knowing how to recover from the fall can often allow you to deliver a devastating kicking attack from the ground.

Or suppose someone grabs you from behind and you can't use your hands or feet. Your punching and kicking techniques would then be of minimal use. In such a case, it is helpful to know how to properly apply throwing techniques. After you throw the assailant, you can then use basic Taekwondo techniques.

Hold-breaking techniques are valuable when an opponent grabs your shoulder, arm, or other part of your body, and you want to break loose without injuring the opponent because you judge that your life is not in danger. Such situations can occur at a dance, in a bar, or when you come in contact with a drunk on the street. At such times, the principle of least force to do a job should apply. You are not interested in permanently injuring the person but in defending yourself.

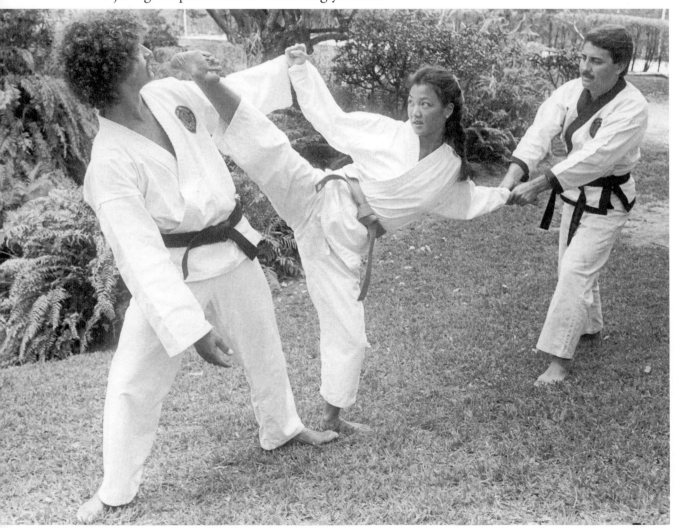

Of course, you must be ready to attack after breaking a hold, just in case. Or you can decide to disappear quietly and unobtrusively. That is a judgment decision which you can make in the light of our philosophy and your own sense of well-being and control over the situation.

In my book *Tae Kwon Do: The Korean Martial Art,* I included eight sections on self-defense: basic self-defense techniques, basic falling practice, basic throwing practice, defenses in lying-down positions, miscellaneous grabs and holds, defenses against assault with weapons, defenses in sitting positions, and defenses against two assailants. Space considerations preclude my repeating all of that information here, but I recommend that you review all of these techniques and practice them until you are quite proficient at them. Then you can combine them with advance punching and kicking combinations to develop your skills as formidable fighting machine.

In this section, we will examine five advanced self-defense techniques, including three that are effective against an assailant with a knife.

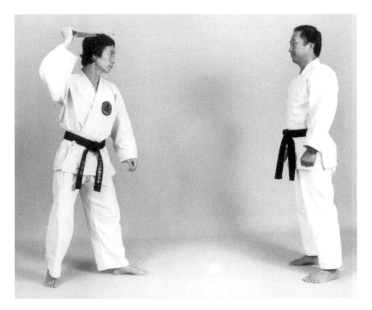

1. Defense Against Overhead Knife Attack
a. Starting position.

b. Slide your right foot back into a Left Front Stance, simultaneously executing a Left-Hand High Block.

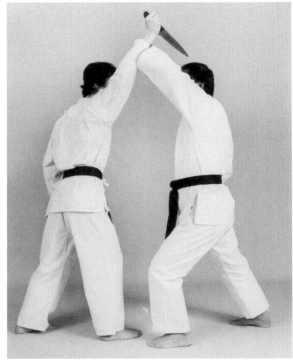

c. Pivot slightly to the left on the balls of both feet, grabbing the inside of the assailant's wrist, pulling it to the left.

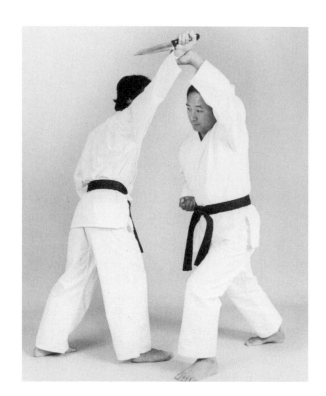

d. Slide your right foot forward and to the outside of the opponent's front foot. Then, turn your body under the attacking arm by sliding your right foot to the left, pivoting on the ball of your right foot and moving your left foot behind it.

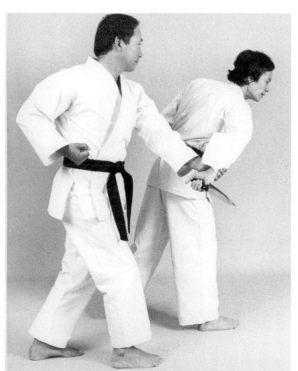

e. Twist the opponent's attacking arm up, sliding your left foot forward.

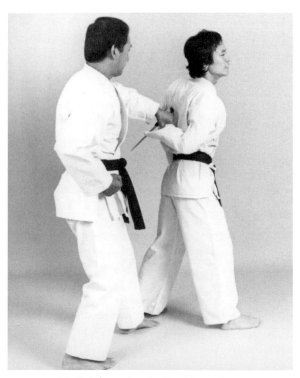

f. Slip your right arm up through the attacker's arm under his elbow, grabbing his collar.

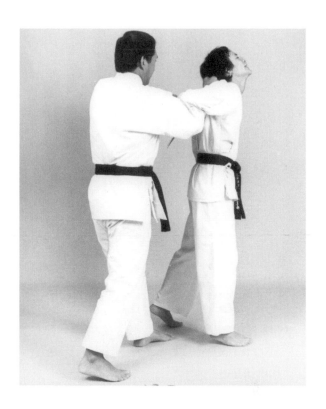

g. Pull your right hand down while simultaneously pushing the opponent's arm up with your left hand, breaking the assailant's arm and shoulder.

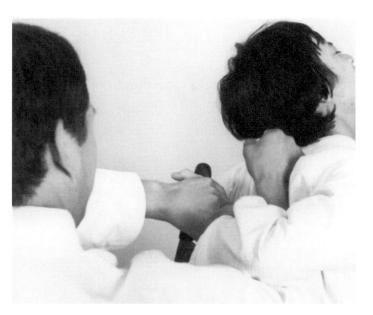

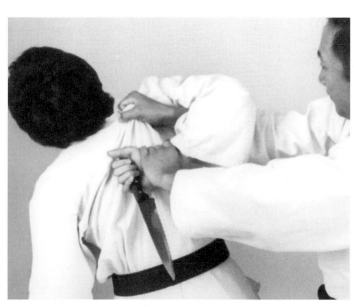

2. Defense Against Overhead Knife Attack

a. Starting position

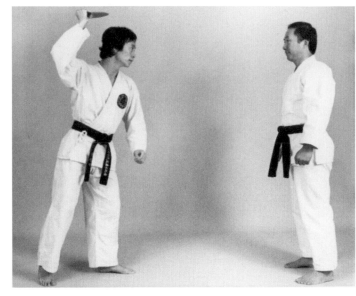

b. Slide your right foot back into a Left Front Stance and simultaneously execute a Left-Hand High Block.

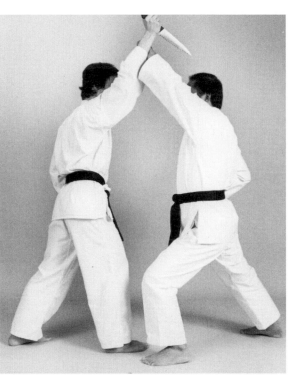

c. Grab the inside of the opponent's wrist, swinging it out and down in a circular motion.

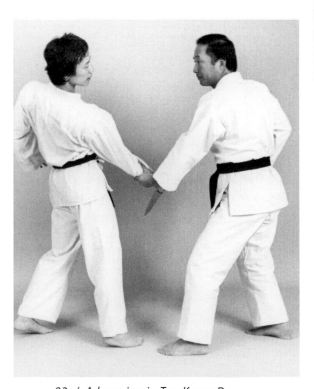

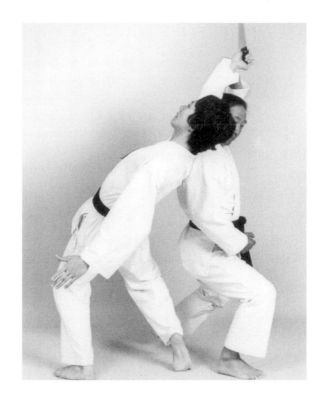

d. Continue the circle upward with the opponent's palm facing up, pivoting to the right on the balls of both feet, and slide your left foot to the left, moving your body under the opponent's attacking arm.

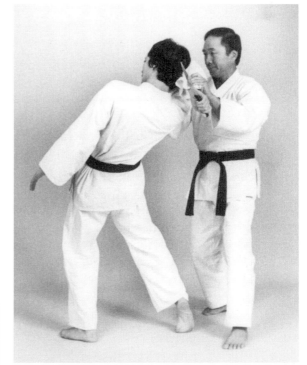

e. Continue turning your body to the right, until you are facing the opponent's right side. Stepping forward with your left foot, force the opponent's wrist to his shoulder with your left hand, locking his elbow. Simultaneously push his elbow up with a forward thrust of your right palm.

f. This will throw the opponent off-balance and cause him to fall on his back. Extend the opponent's arm and break his elbow with a downward thrust of your right palm.

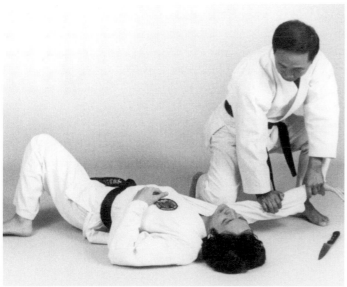

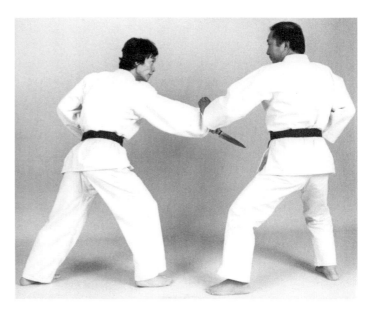

3. Defense Against Stabbing Attack to the Midsection

a. Step back with your right foot into Back Stance, simultaneously executing a Left-Hand Inside Middle Block, and grab the opponent's wrist.

b. Turn to the right, and step forward with your left foot, simultaneously pulling the opponent's attacking arm forward, throwing him off-balance.

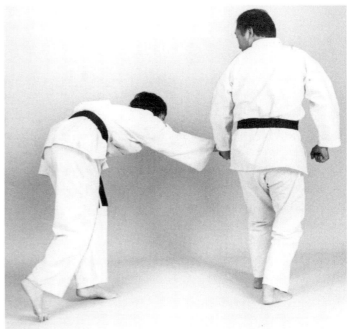

c. Pivoting to the left on the ball of you right foot, move your left foot to the outside, simultaneously twisting the opponent's wrist inward with your left hand, locking the wrist.

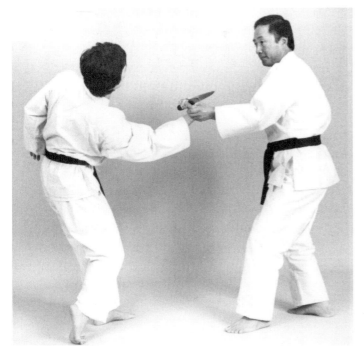

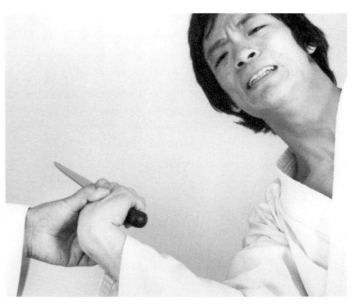

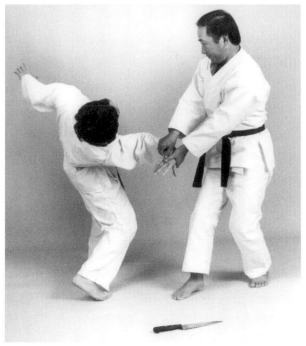

d. Moving your right foot forward and to the outside, use both hands to twist the attacking wrist. This will cause the attacker to fall.

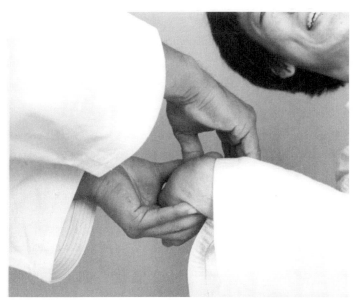

e. Extend the attacker's arm, break his elbow with your right knee, and break his wrist by twisting it all the way.

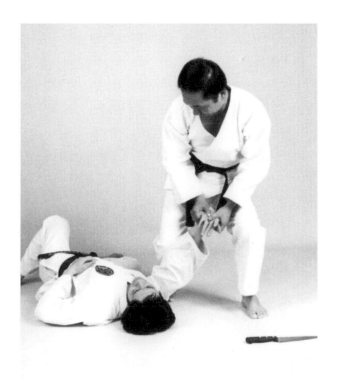

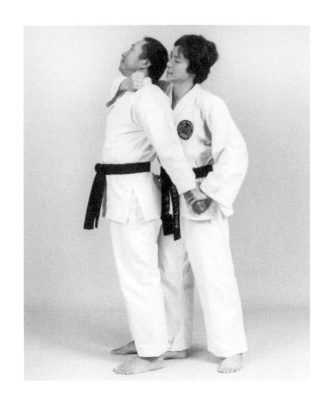

4. Defense Against a Choking Hold and Arm Lock from Behind

a. Starting position.

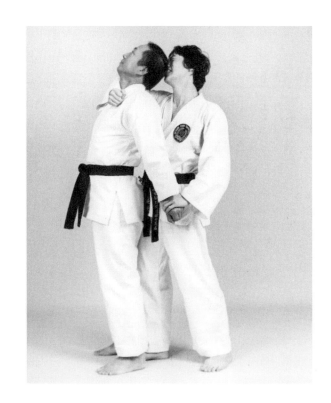

b. Thrust your head back, breaking the opponent's nose.

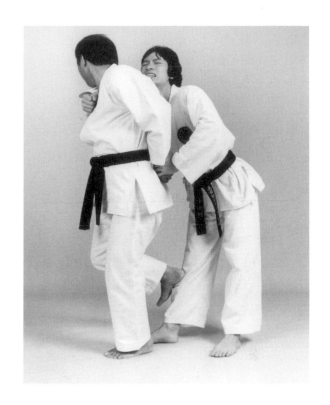

c. With your right foot, execute a Back Kick to the assailant's shin.

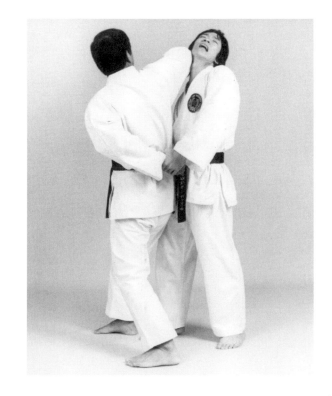

d. Turning to the right, execute a Right Elbow Attack to the opponent's face.

e. Pivoting to the left on the ball of your left foot, bring your right foot forward and face the opponent's left side. Simultaneously grab the opponent's wrist with your right hand.

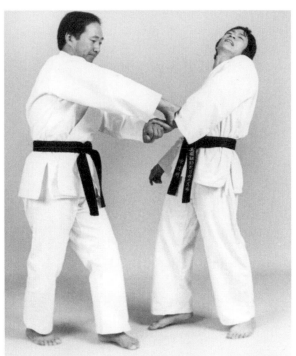

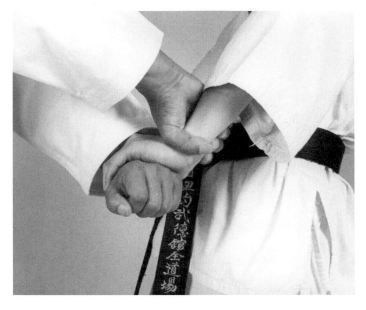

f. While holding the opponent's wrist with your right hand, open your left hand and twist it palm up, grabbing the opponent's palm and fingers. Twist his hand clockwise and upward with your left hand.

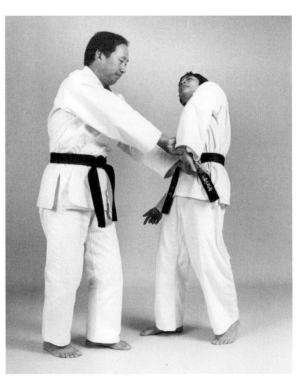

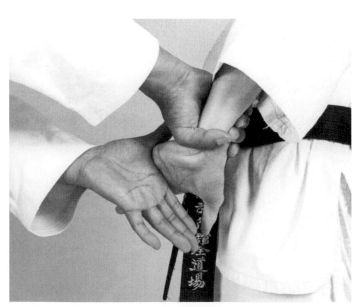

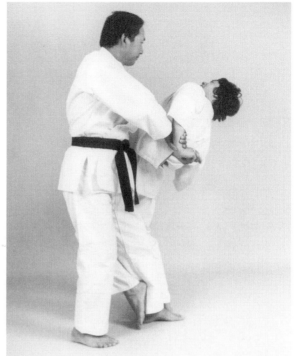

g. Slide your right foot forward and step behind the opponent's left leg with your left foot, keeping the opponent's arm extended and locked.

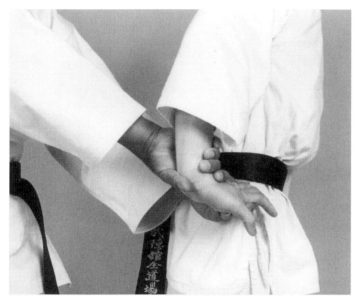

h. Throw your opponent onto his back, forcing his left hand behind him and push it up toward his neck, breaking his elbow and shoulder.

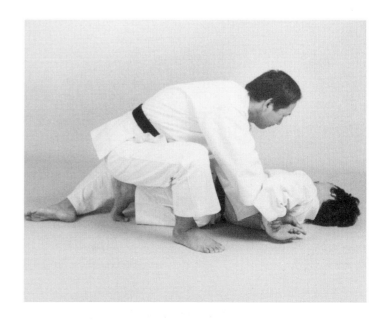

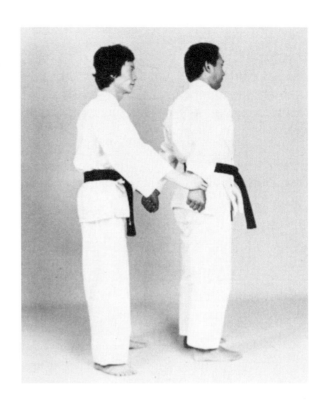

5. Defense Against an Assailant Who Grabs Both of Your Wrists from Behind.

a. Starting position.

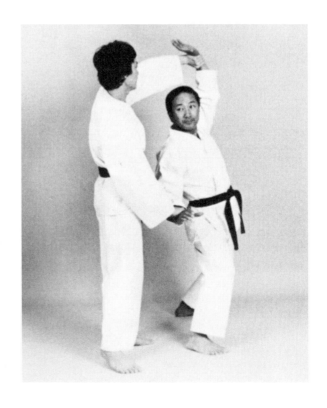

b. Twist your body to the right, pivoting on the balls of both feet. Open both hands, and swing your left hand upward and your right hand down.

c. Continue the swing, simultaneously stepping back with your foot. Then, step forward with your right foot, and grab the opponent's right wrist from below with your right hand (palm up) and his left wrist from above with your left hand, palm down. Push his right arm up, locking it over his left elbow.

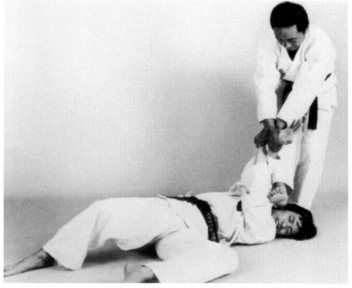

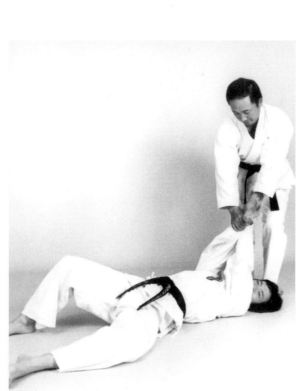

d. Slide your left foot forward, simultaneously thrusting forward with your right hand, throwing your opponent to the ground on his back.

e. Execute a Right Heel Kick to the assailant's face.

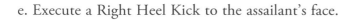

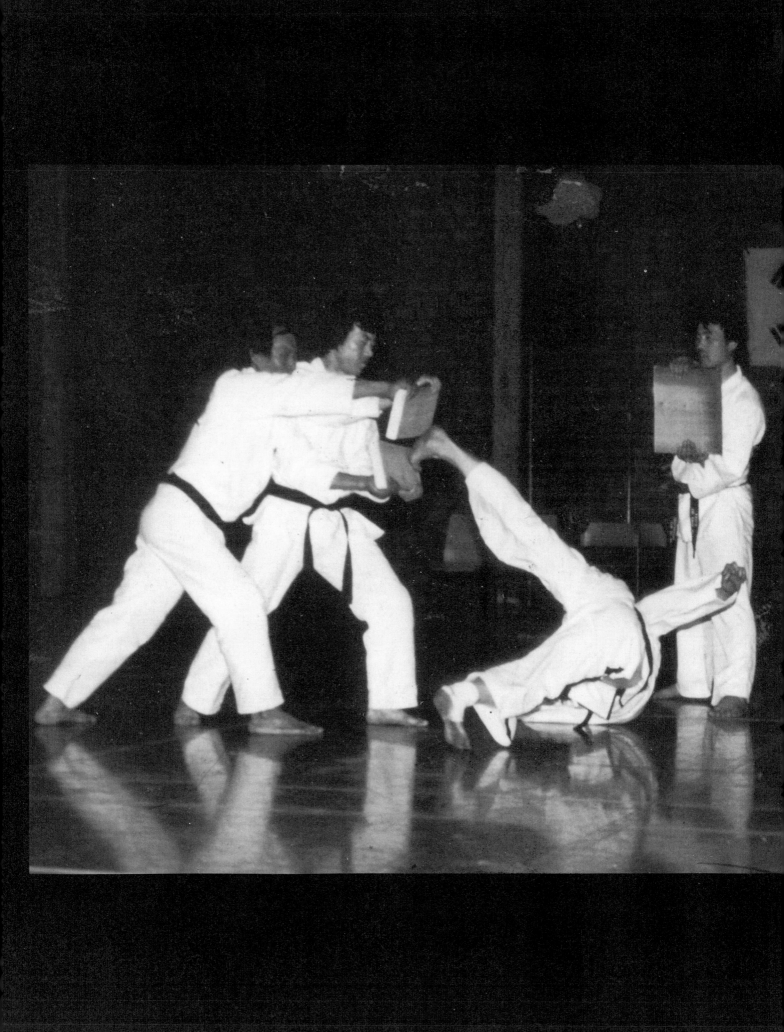

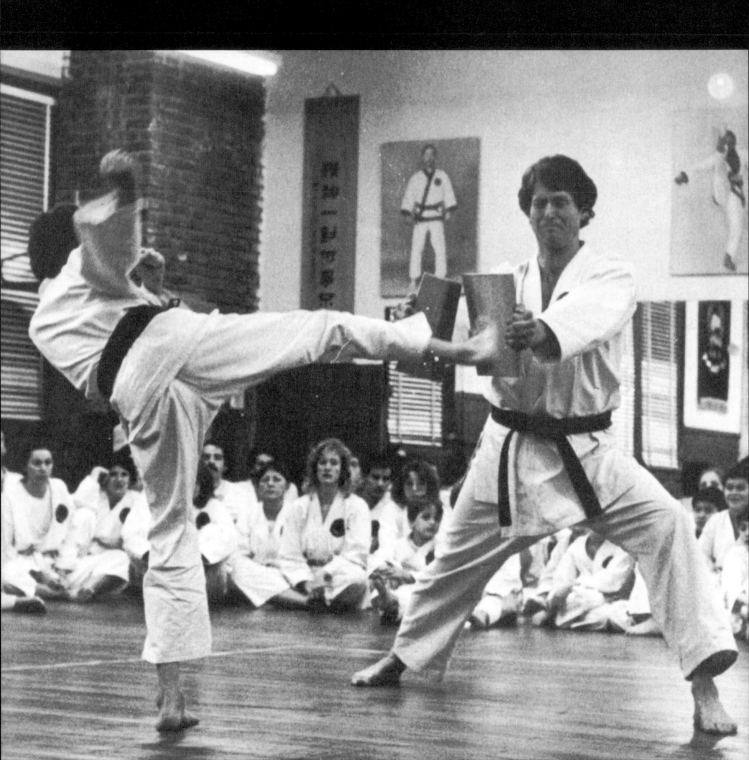

CHAPTER 8

AS FAR AS the uninitiated public is concerned, the most dramatic thing about Taekwondo is the sight of a human hand or foot breaking through a board, a stack of roofing tiles, or a brick, and coming away unscathed.

In fact, however, breaking techniques are not the aim but the practical result of Taekwondo training in strength, speed, and accuracy. Of the three, strength is the least important, because power is the product of speed and accuracy.

In Chapter 3, we discussed the scientific reasons why seemingly strong objects can be broken by seemingly weak objects. In this section, we will concentrate on the practical applications and scientific knowledge.

The first thing to recognize is that some objects are easier to break than others. A ¾-inch pine board that is dry is not too difficult to break if you hit with the grain. An oak or hickory board is another matter. So as you begin to work on breaking techniques, whether they be speed breaks, flying jump breaks, spear-hand breaks, or whatever, consider the material first. If you fail to break the object because you have misjudged your material, you can hurt yourself, and, even more importantly, you can destroy your confidence. And that will take you a lot of time and courage to regain.

Start with easy boards until you gain confidence. Have them held by an instructor, so you will strike with the grain, not against it. Then you can work your way up to more difficult boards and materials. Rocks, bricks, and cinder blocks have their grains and weak points. Study them, and learn where and how to strike for maximum effect.

It helps to toughen your hands and knuckles before you attempt breaking techniques with them. Knuckle and fingertip push-ups will help you develop strength, rigidity, and tolerance for a minor amount of pain. If you perform your first breaking technique perfectly, you will feel absolutely no pain. But if you are a bit off on your speed, distance, or timing, you can feel pain, and it is better for your confidence if your hands can tolerate the discomfort.

The second thing to develop is perfect technique. Your punch or kick should make your tobok snap like a flag in a brisk wind. It should be precise in its placement, so the punch or kick lands where you intended it to, not an inch or two away from your intended target. Practice hitting a spot on the board no bigger than a dime. That will make the whole board look ridiculously large to you, will focus your aim on the board's center.

Judge your distance accurately. Remember, you are aiming at a spot several centimeters *inside* the board, not just at the surface. If you strike at the surface, the power you have developed will be spent before it reaches the critical point in the board. If you aim too far beyond the board, your punch or kick will not have developed its full velocity when it makes contact, and the board may fail to break. You can hurt yourself in the attempt. Practice judging distances. It will help you in sparring as well. After a while, you will find that you can strike with great precision and confidence.

Breaking force is shock or impact force. It must not be interrupted at the last instant by a failure of will or a slight flinch. You must keep your spirit stable and recognize that the board has *no choice* but to break under your attack. Again, if you waver, you can hurt yourself. If you are confident, you will be break the board without feeling anything.

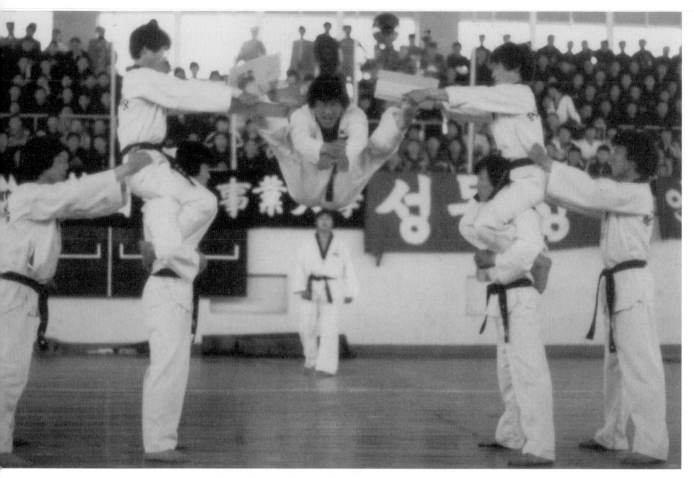

In speed breaking, the trick is to hit the board with such velocity that it will not have the split second to be thrust out of the way on contact. You can practice developing this speed by punch a piece of paper suspended from the ceiling by two threads, or at a piece of paper floating in a tub of water. As you gain speed, float a board in the tub and strike it. Once you develop the speed, you can break boards in the air.

Here are several examples of dramatic advanced breaking techniques which should not be attempted until you have mastered the most basic techniques, discussed and illustrated in my previous book.

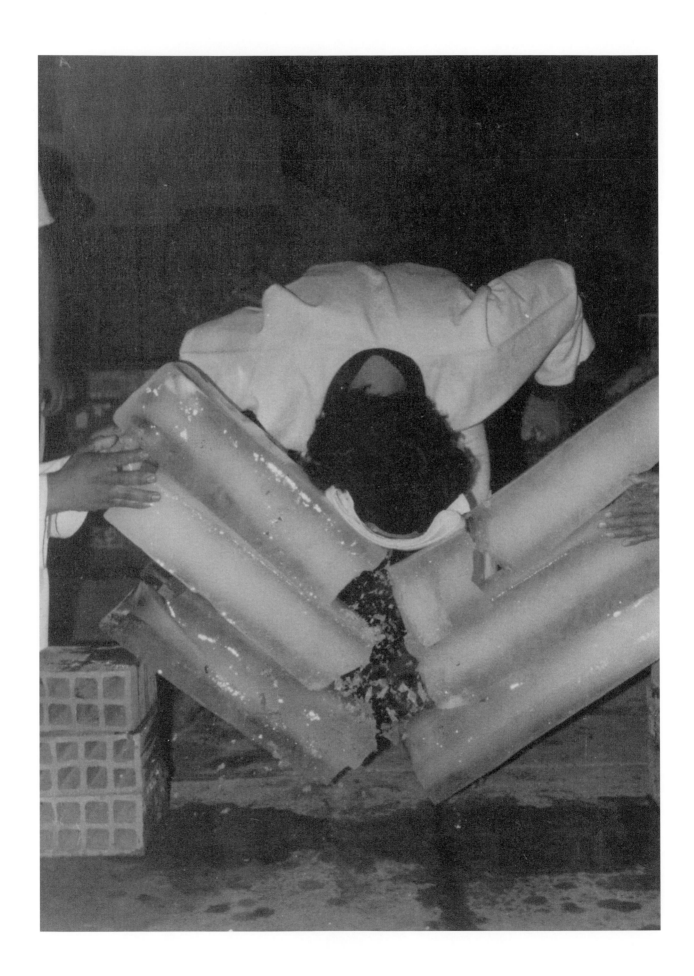

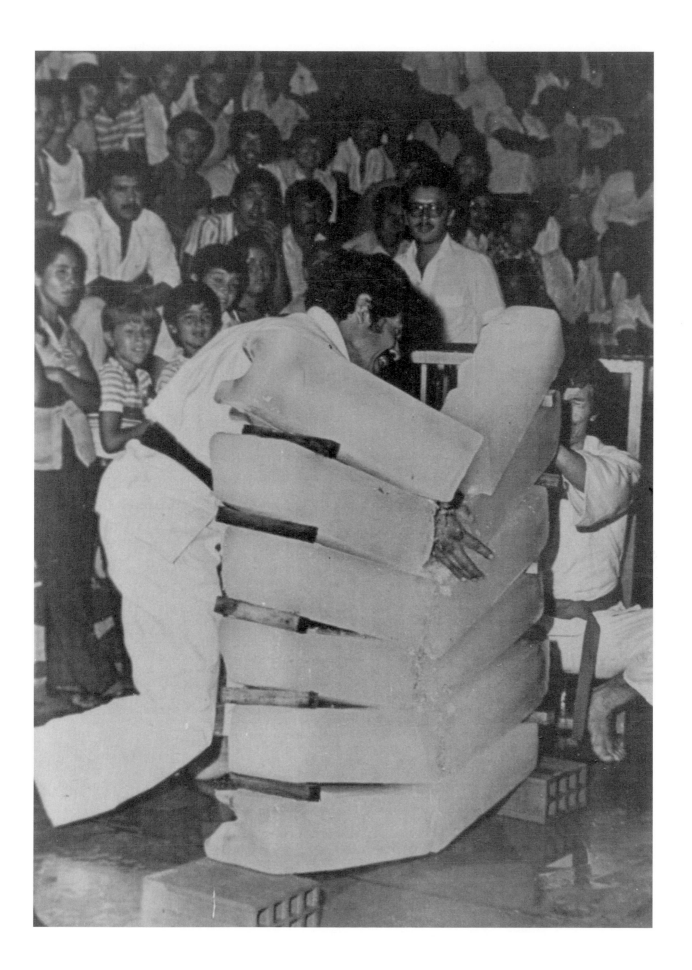

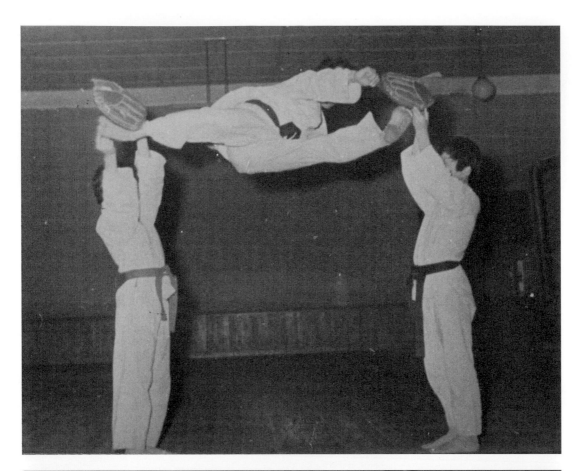

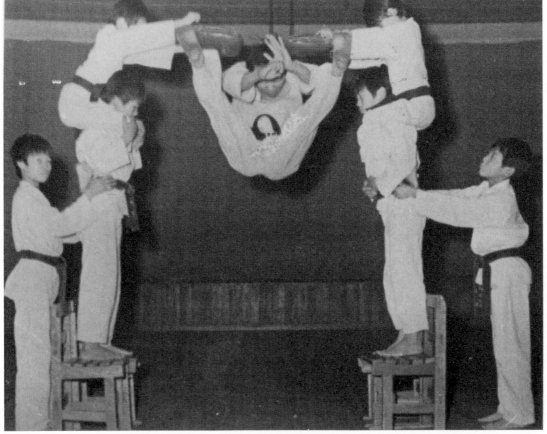

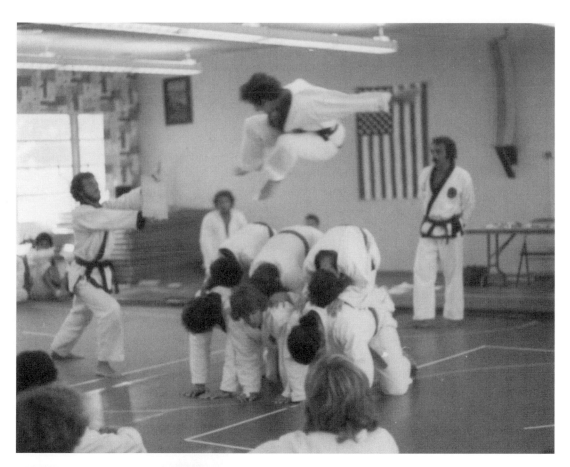

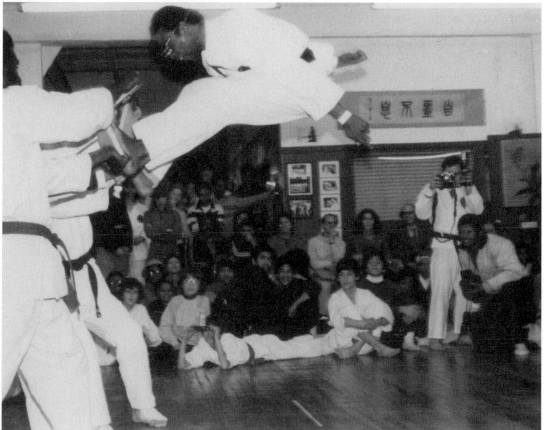

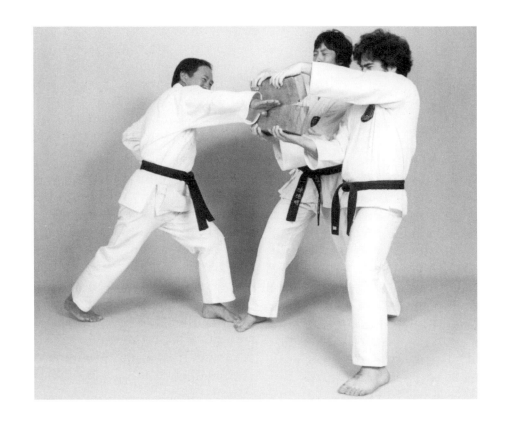

1. Breaking Technique with Ridge Hand Strike

(*Sohn-Nal-Doong-Chi-Ki*)

2. Breaking Technique with Wrist (Ox-Jaw) Strike

(*Sohn-Mok-Chi-Ki*)

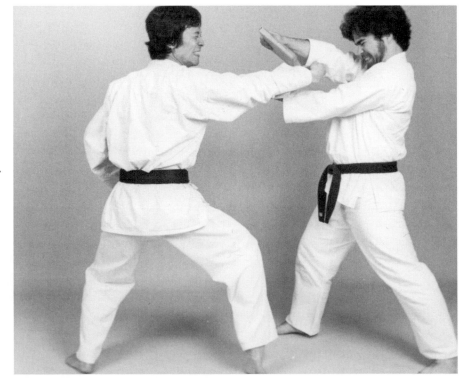

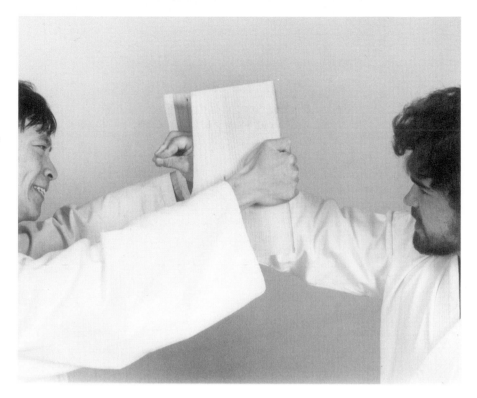

3. Breaking Technique with Chicken-Beak Strike)

(Sohn-Koot-Jo-Ki)

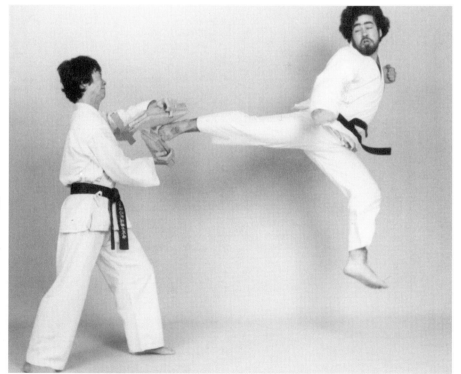

4. Breaking Technique with Turning Back Kick

(Tdwi-Yo-Mom-Dol-Rio-Dwi-Cha-Ki)

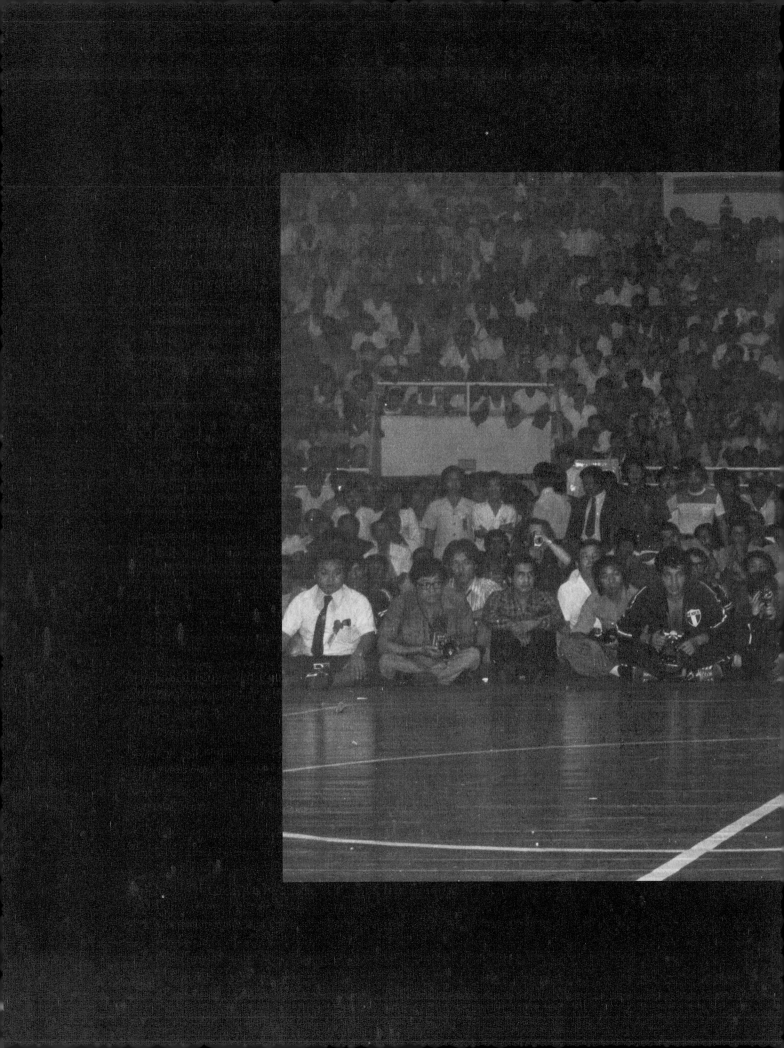

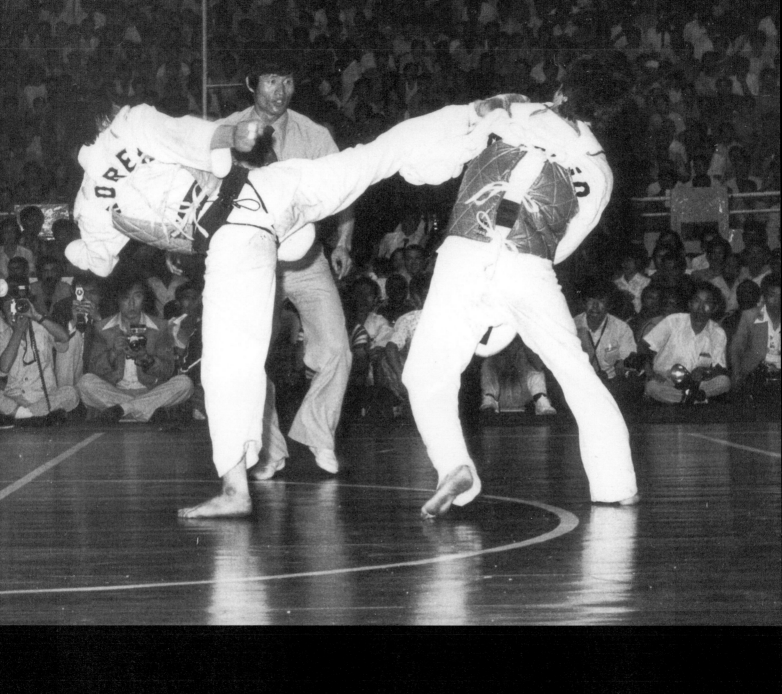

Taekwondo as a Sport

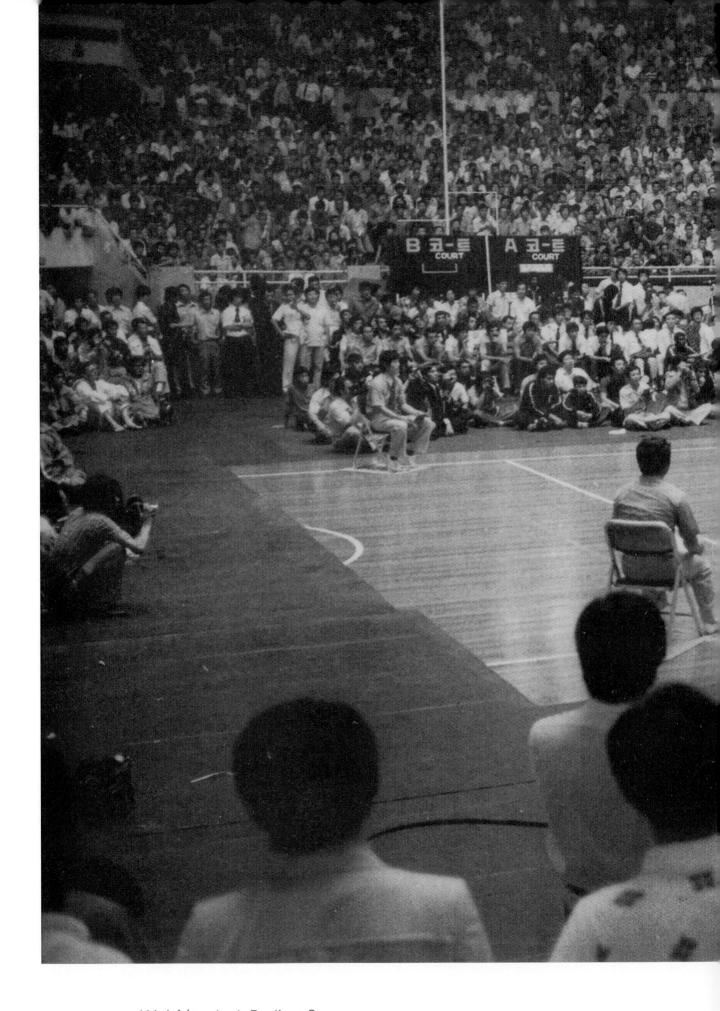

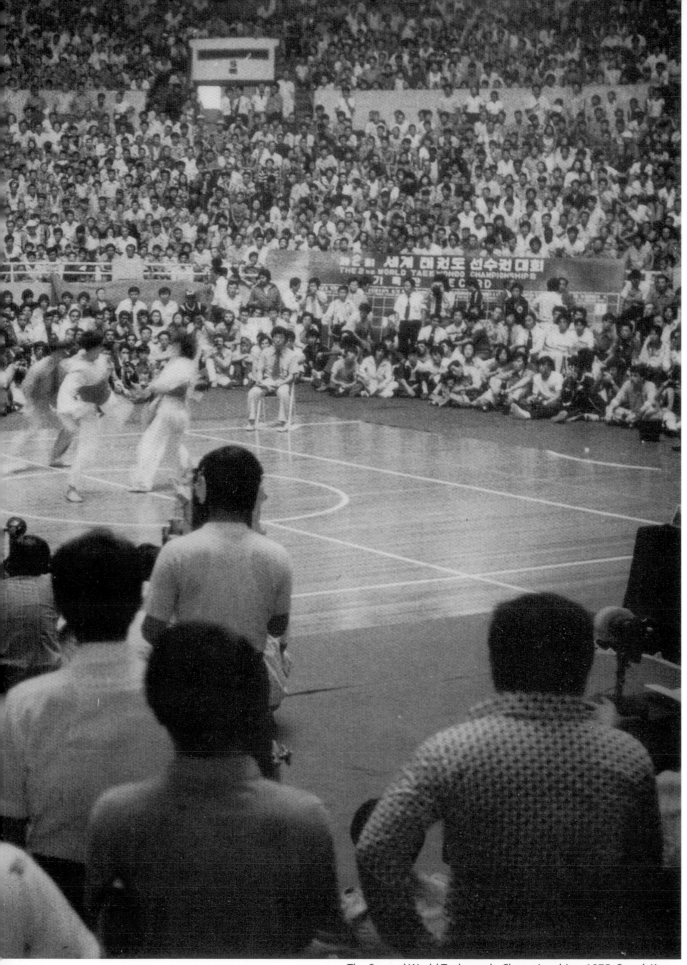

The Second World Taekwondo Championships, 1975, Seoul, Korea.

IN ADDITION to being an incomparable system of self-defense, Taekwondo has become an international amateur sport—the second martial art to have been adopted as an Olympic Sport by the International Olympic Committee after judo.

In addition to sparring, tournaments often provide competition in the performance of formal exercises, which gives full recognition to the most nearly perfect demonstration of technique, similar to an Olympic gymnastics competition.

Levels of competition are fixed to correspond with the levels of achievement of the participants. Beginners compete with beginners, intermediates with those of their own class, and the more advanced, such as brown and black belt holders, within their respective categories. Sometimes categories are further divided according to body weight.

In sparring competition, the rules and scoring systems vary among the different localities and sponsors of the events, although certain conditions are standard. In the United States, for example, sparring competition is generally restricted to no-contact scoring. The competitor is given a score for techniques executed as close to the vulnera-

Highlight of the First Taekwondo Championships, 1973, Seoul, Korea.

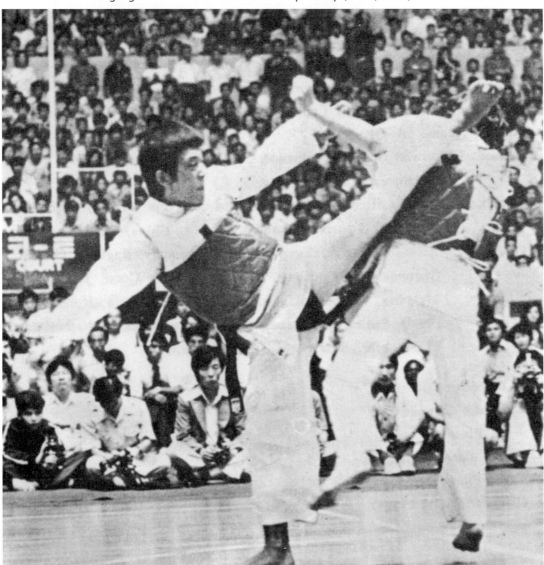

ble points of his opponent as possible without actually touching him. Actual contact is given no score, or even a negative score.

In Korea, on the other hand, full-contact competition is the rule. For this purpose, participants wear a cushioned pad, protecting chest, ribs, and abdomen. Therefore, American practitioners who plan to compete in Korea should practice full-contact sparring—with a chest protector.

Scoring methods are fairly standardized according to a point system in which the competitors score a point for every attacking technique—such as a punch, kick, knifehand strike, etc.—accurately execut-

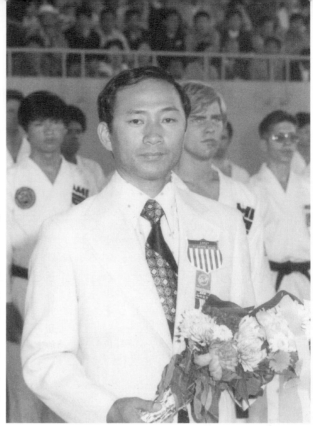

Richard Chun, Head Coach of the U.S.A. Taekwondo Team at the First Taekwondo Championships, 1973, Seoul, Korea.

ed and not blocked by an arm or leg interposed in defense. An injurious strike to certain vital points are generally not permitted, such as Spear-Hand attacks to the eyes, choking attacks to the throat, and punches or kicks to the back or groin. A knock-down is scored as a point, but more than one technique of attack against a fallen participant while he is down is normally forbidden.

The participants are required to control their tempers as well as their techniques. Violent or vicious attacks executed in rage are not permitted and may result in disqualification. Negative scores are given to infractions of the rules, such as stepping outside the prescribed area of combat, executing attacks after the time limit is called, or executing illegal attacks. The time limit set for sparring matches also varies. Three minutes is common. If the competitors do not score or if their scores are tied at the end of the initial time limit, a sudden-death match is usually called, in which they are enjoined to spar until one scores the first point and is proclaimed the winner.

For study by the serious student who wishes to compete in world championships, the competition rules of World Taekwondo Federation (member of the Olympic Committee) are introduced. In order to familiarize you with the World Taekwondo Federation, a brief description of the rules and regulations is also included.

Rules and Regulations of World Taekwondo Federation

General Regulations

Article 1. Objects and Name

1. Taekwondo is a product of traditional Korean culture. The purpose of organizing the Federation is to propagate and standardize Taekwondo along with its traditional Taekwondo spirit throughout the world.

2. The Federation shall be called the World Taekwondo Federation (abbreviated as the WTF).

3. The Federation seeks to realize the ideals, "Swiftly, Powerfully, and Accurately" through the medium of Taekwondo competition.

4. The WTF, recognized by the International Olympic Committee, shall observe the general and fundamental principles of the Olympic Charter.

5. The WTF shall promote the principles that the Kukkiwon, center of traditional Taekwondo, has adopted in respect to Taekwondo philosophy, development of techniques and Dan certification.

Article 2. Operations

1. To attain the objects of Article 1, the WTF shall conduct the following operations.

    A. World Taekwondo Championships

    B. World Taekwondo Poomsae Championships

    C. Regional Taekwondo Championships

    D. World University Taekwondo Championships, Women's World Taekwondo Championships, and World Junior Taekwondo Championships

    E. Various International Championships

    F. International Referee Seminar

    G. International Coach Training Course

    H. Concerted effort to continuously incorporate Taekwondo into the Olympic Games

    I. Research for propagation and development of Taekwondo techniques

    J. Publication of necessary materials

    K. Other operations necessary to attain the objects of Article 1

2. The Operations shall be conducted as follows.

    A. The World Championships and the World Junior Championships shall be held every two years under the auspices of the WTF and organized by the host member national Association. However, the World Junior Championships shall not be held in the same year when the World Championships are held.

    B. The Regional Championships shall be held every two years with the approval, and under the supervision of the WTF and shall be organized by the host member National Association selected at the General Assembly of each Regional Union. However, the Regional Championships shall not be held in the same year when the World Championships are held.

    C. Other international championships, such as invitational and goodwill ones, may be held by any of the member Nations provided that these championships are not named "World" or "Regional" championships.

    D. The results of each championship shall be reported to the WTF within one month of the conclusion of the championships.

    E. The WTF Competition Rules shall be applied to all the championships listed above.

    F. The International Referee Seminar and the International Coach Training Course shall be conducted by the WTF only apart from member National Associations, no other organization shall be authorized to organize or execute referee seminars or coach training courses nor issue certificates therein. World Championships, each Regional Championships and other international championships shall be officiated only by the International Referees sanctioned by the WTF.

    G. The President shall grant qualification of International Referee to those who have successfully completed the International Referee Seminar and who have passed the test.

H. The President shall grant qualification of International Coach to those who have successfully completed the International Coach Training Course and who have passed the test.

3. The rules for organizing the championships and regulations for the International Referee and International Coach shall be enacted by the Executive Council.

4. Amateurism—to be eligible for participation in international competition under the patronage of the World Taekwondo Federation, a competitor must not have received any financial rewards or material benefit in connection with his or her sports participation. All competitors, men or women, who conform to the criteria set out in this code, may participate in international competition except those who have:

   A. been registered as professional athletes or professional coaches;

   B. accepted without the knowledge of the WTF, or the National Association and/or of the NOC, material advantages for their preparation or participation in sports competition;

   C. allowed their person, name, or pictures of sports performances to be used for advertising, except when the WTF or their National Association has entered into a contract for sponsorship or equipment. All payment must be made to the WTF or National Association and not to the athlete;

   D. carried advertising material on their person or clothing in competition under the patronage of the WTF, other than trademarks on technical equipment or clothing as agreed to by the WTF and the respective National Association;

   E. manifestly contravened the spirit of fair play in the exercise of sport, particularly through doping or violence.

Article 3. Headquarters and Official Language

1. The headquarters of the WTF shall be located permanently in Seoul, Korea.

2. The official languages of the WTF shall be English, French, German, Spanish, and Korean.

3. In case of disagreement over interpretation or translation, the English version shall prevail. In case of disagreement over interpretation of technical matters of Taekwondo, the Korean original version shall prevail.

4. Any member National Association shall have the right to speak in its mother tongue, but the speech shall be translated into the five official languages.

Article 4. Organization and Membership

1. The WTF membership shall consist of National Taekwondo Associations representing their respective nations or self-governing territories with the recognition of the WTF.

2. Admittance into the WTF shall require the approval of the Executive Council and the General Assembly of the WTF. The National Association applying for the membership of the WTF are required to present designated application documents to the WTF together with a letter of recognition from the pertinent National Olympic Committee. In addition to that, they are also needed to hand in a letter pledging to dispatch at least three or more competitors to the World Taekwondo Championships and the World Junior Taekwondo Championships of the WTF. Those considered to have met the requirements for membership status, are admitted as provisional members until their admittance are finally approved. The provisional members have no voting right, but are able to participate in all international Taekwondo competitions approved or promoted by the WTF.

3. The WTF shall approve only one association for each nation or each self-governing territory on the condition that its NOC having recognition from the IOC has recognized the association.

4. In case more than one organization claim to represent a nation or self-governing territory, the dispute shall be resolved by the WTF with consideration of the opinions of the NOC.

5. All the affiliated member National Associations and regional organizations shall constitute their respective statutes strictly in conformity with the principles of the WTF Rules and Regulations so as not to contravene any provisions therein.

6. A member National Association shall neither be affiliated to any other international Taekwondo organization not recognized by the WTF, nor participate in any Taekwondo events organized by such an organization.

7. All the member National Associations shall be equal before the WTF Rules and Regulations, and shall be free from any political, religious, racial, or other forms of prejudices.

8. Any member National Association may withdraw its membership from the WTF.

9. All member National Associations are obliged to dispatch at least three or more competitors to the World Taekwondo Championships and the World Junior Taekwondo Championships. The membership status of those who fail to take part in those competitions for two consecutive years without justifiable reasons including natural calamities are set to be demoted as provisional members.

The demoted members will no longer be able to exercise voting rights in official meetings, though they still retain the right to compete in all official competitions of the WTF. However, their full membership status can be restored when they present a document to the WTF confirming their impending participation in one of the two Championships together with a letter pledging to dispatch at least three or more competitors to the both Championships in the days to come.

Competition Rules (effective as of May, 2006)

Article 1. Purpose

The purpose of the Competition Rules is to manage fairly and smoothly all matters pertaining to competitions of all levels to be promoted and/or organized by the WTF, Regional Unions and member National Associations, ensuring the application of standardized rules.

Article 2. Application

The Competition Rules shall apply to all the competitions to be promoted and/or organized by the WTF, each Regional Union and member National Association. However, any member National Association wishing to modify some part of the Competition Rules must first gain the approval of the WTF.

Article 3. Competition Area

The Competition Area shall measure 10m by 10m using the metric system. The Competition Area shall have a flat surface without any obstructing projections, and be covered with an elastic mat.

The Competition Area may also be installed on a platform 0.5m to 0.6m high from the base, if necessary, and the outer part of the Boundary Line shall be inclined with a gradient of less than 30 degrees, for the safety of the contestants

1. Demarcation of the Competition Area

   The 10m by 10m area shall be called the Competition Area, and the marginal line of the Competition Area shall be called the Boundary Line. The front Boundary Line adjacent to the Recorder's Desk and the Commission Doctor's Desk shall be deemed Boundary Line #1. Clockwise from Boundary Line #1, the other lines shall be called Boundary Lines #2, #3, and #4.

2. Indication of Positions

   1) Position of the Referee

      The position of the Referee shall be marked at a point 1.5m back from the center point of the Contest Area to the 3rd Boundary Line and designated as the Referee's Mark.

   2) Position of the Judges

      The position of the 1st Judge shall be marked at a point 0.5m from the corner of Boundary Line #1 and Boundary Line #2. The position of the 2nd Judge shall be marked at a point 0.5m from the corner of Boundary Line #2 and Boundary Line #3. The position of the 3rd Judge shall be marked at a point 0.5m from the corner of Boundary Line #3 and Boundary Line #4. The position of the 4th Judge shall be marked at a point 0.5m from the corner of Boundary Line #4 and Boundary Line #1.

   3) Position of the Recorder

      The position of the Recorder shall be marked at a point 2m back from Boundary Line #1 facing the Competition Area 2m adjacent to the corner of Boundary Line #1 and Boundary Line #2.

   4) Position of the Commission Doctor

      The position of the Commission Doctor shall be marked at a point more than 3m to the right side from the Boundary Line.

   5) Position of the Contestants

      The position of the Contestants shall be marked at two opposing points, 1m from the center point of the Competition Area, 5m from Boundary Line #1 (red Contestant toward Boundary Line #2 and blue Contestant toward #4).

   6) Position of the Coaches

      The position of the Coaches shall be marked at a point 1m away from the center point of the Boundary Line of each contestant's side.

   7) Position of the Inspection Desk

      The position of the Inspection Desk shall be near the entrance of the Competition Area for inspection of the contestants' protective equipment.

Article 4. Contestants

1. Qualification of Contestants

    1) Holder of the nationality of the participating team

    2) One recommended by the national Taekwondo Association

    3) Holder of Taekwondo Dan certificate issued by the Kukkiwon, and in case of the World Junior Taekwondo Championships, holder of Kukkiwon Poom/Dan certificate aged 14 through 17 years old based on the year when the Championships are held.

2. Contestant Uniform and Protective Equipment

    1) The contestant shall wear the trunk protector, head protector, groin guard, forearm guards, shin guards, gloves, and a mouthpiece before entering the contest area.

    2) The groin guard, forearm guards, and shin guards shall be worn beneath the Taekwondo uniform. The contestant shall bring this WTF-approved protective equipment, as well as gloves and the mouthpiece, for his/her personal use. Wearing any item on the head other than the head protector shall not be permitted.

3. Medical Control

    1) At the Taekwondo events promoted or sanctioned by the WTF, the use or administration of drugs or chemical subtances described in the WTF anti-doping by-laws is prohibited. However, IOC doping by-laws shall be applied to the Olympic Games and other multi-sport games.

    2) The WTF may carry out any medical testing deemed necessary to ascertain if a contestant has committed a breach of this rule, and any winner who refuses to undergo this testing or who proves to have committed such a breach shall be removed from the final standings, and the record shall be transferred to the contestant next in line in the competition standings.

    3) The organizing committee shall be liable for arrangements to carry out medical testing.

    4) The details of the WTF anti-doping regulation shall be enacted by the by-laws.

Article 5. Weight Divisions

1. Weights are divided into male and female divisions.

2. Weight divisions are divided as follows:

Weight Category	Male Division	Female Division
Fin	Not exceeding 45kg	Not exceeding 42kg
Fly	Over 45kg & not exceeding 48kg	Over 42kg & not exceeding 44kg
Bantam	Over 48kg & not exceeding 51kg	Over 44kg & not exceeding 46kg
Feather	Over 51kg & not exceeding 55kg	Over 46kg & not exceeding 49kg
Light	Over 55kg & not exceeding 59kg	Over 49kg & not exceeding 52kg
Welter	Over 59kg & not exceeding 63kg	Over 52kg & not exceeding 55kg
Light Middle	Over 63kg & not exceeding 68kg	Over 55kg & not exceeding 59kg
Middle	Over 68kg & not exceeding 73kg	Over 59kg & not exceeding 63kg
Light Heavy	Over 73kg & not exceeding 78kg	Over 63kg & not exceeding 68kg
Heavy	Over 78kg	Over 68kg

3. Weight divisions for the Olympic Games are divided as follows:

Weight Category (Male Division)	Weight Category (Female Division)
Not exceeding 58kg	Not exceeding 49kg
Over 58kg & not exceeding 68kg	Over 49kg & not exceeding 57kg
Over 68kg & not exceeding 80kg	Over 57kg & not exceeding 67kg
Over 80kg	Over 67kg

4. Weight divisions for the World Junior Championships are divided as follows;

Weight category	Male division	Female division
Fin	Not exceeding 45kg	Not exceeding 42kg
Fly	Over 45kg & not exceeding 48kg	Over 42kg & not exceeding 44kg
Bantam	Over 48kg & not exceeding 51kg	Over 44kg & not exceeding 46kg
Feather	Over 51kg & not exceeding 55kg	Over 46kg & not exceeding 49kg
Light	Over 55kg & not exceeding 59kg	Over 49kg & not exceeding 52kg
Welter	Over 59kg & not exceeding 63kg	Over 52kg & not exceeding 55kg
Light Middle	Over 63kg & not exceeding 68kg	Over 55kg & not exceeding 59kg
Middle	Over 68kg & not exceeding 73kg	Over 59kg & not exceeding 63kg
Light Heavy	Over 73kg & not exceeding 78kg	Over 63kg & not exceeding 68kg
Heavy	Over 78kg	Over 68kg

Article 6. Classifications and Methods of Competition

1. Competitions are divided as follows

1) Individual competition shall normally be between contestants in the same weight class. When necessary, adjoining weight class may be combined to create a single classification. No contestant is allowed to participate in more than one (1) weight category in one event.

2) Team Competition: Systems of Competition

(1) Five (5) contestants by weight classification with the following category:

Weight Category (Male Division)	Weight Category (Female Division)
Not exceeding 54kg	Not exceeding 47kg
Over 54kg & not exceeding 63kg	Over 47kg & not exceeding 54kg
Over 63kg & not exceeding 72kg	Over 54kg & not exceeding 68kg
Over 72kg	Over 68kg

(2) Eight (8) contestants by weight classification

(3) Four (4) contestants by weight classification (Consolidation of the eight weight classifications into four weight categories by combining two adjoining weight classes)

2. Systems of competition are divided as follows.

1) Single elimination tournament system

2) Round robin system

3. Taekwondo competition of the Olympic Games shall be conducted in individual competition system between contestants.

4. All International-level competitions recognized by the WTF shall be formed with participation of at least 4 countries with no less than 4 contestants in each weight class, and any weight class with less than 4 contestants cannot be recognized in the official results.

Point System

Team ranking shall be decided by the total points based on the following guidelines:

- Basic one (1) point per each contestant who entered the competition area after passing the official weigh-in

- One (1) point per each win (win by a bye included)

- Additional seven (7) points per one gold medal

- Additional three (3) points per one silver medal

- Additional one (1) point per one bronze medal

In case more than two (2) teams are in tie score, the rank shall be decided by 1) number of gold, silver and bronze medals won by the team in order, 2) number of participating contestants and 3) higher points in heavier weight category.

Article 7. Duration of Contest

The duration of the contest shall be three rounds of two minutes each, with a one-minute rest period between rounds.

In case of a tie score after the completion of the 3rd round, a 4th round of two minutes will be conducted as the sudden death overtime round, after a one-minute rest period following the 3rd round.

Article 8. Drawing Lots

1. The drawing of lots shall be conducted one day prior to the first competition in the presence of the WTF officials and the representatives of the participating nations, and the drawing of lots shall be done from Fin weight up in the English alphabetical order of the official names of the participating nations.

2. Officials shall be designated to draw lots on behalf of the officials of participating nations not present at the drawing.

3. The order of the draw may be changed according to the decision of the Head of Team meeting.

Article 9. Weigh-In

1. Weigh-in of the contestants on the day of competition shall be completed on the previous day of the pertinent competition.

2. During weigh-in, the male contestant shall wear underpants and the female contestant shall wear underpants and brassiere. However, weigh-in may be conducted in the nude in the case that the contestant wishes to do so.

3. Weigh-in shall be made once, however, one more weigh-in is granted within the time limit for official weigh-in to the contestant who did not qualify the first time.

4. So as not to be disqualified during official weigh-in a scale, the same as the official one, shall be provided at the contestants' place of accommodation or at the arena for pre-weigh-in.

Article 10. Procedure of theContest

1. Call for Contestants
   The name of the contestants shall be announced three times beginning three minutes prior to the scheduled start of the contest. The contestant who fails to appear in the contest area within one minute after the scheduled start of the competition shall be regarded as withdrawn.

2. Physical and Costume Inspection
   After being called, the contestants shall undergo physical and costume inspection at the designated inspection desk by the inspector designated by the WTF, and the contestant shall not show any signs of aversion, and also shall not bear any materials which could cause harm to the other contestant.

3. Entering the Competition Area
   After inspection, the contestant shall enter into the waiting position with one coach.

4. Start and End of the Contest
   The contest in each round shall begin with the declaration of "Shi-jak" (start) by the referee and shall end with the declaration of "Keu-man" (stop) by the referee. Although the referee has not declared "Keu-man," the contest shall be regarded as having ended when the prescribed time is over.

5. Procedure Before the Beginning and After the End of the Contest
   1) The contestants shall face each other and make a standing bow at the referee's command of "Cha-ryeot" (attention) and "Kyeong-rye" (bow). A standing bow shall be made from the natural standing posture of "Cha-ryeot" by inclining forward at the waist to an angle of more than 30° degrees with the head inclined to an angle more than 45° degrees and the fists clenched at the sides of the legs.

   2) The referee shall start the contest by commanding "Joon-bi" (ready) and "Shi-jak" (start).

   3) After the end of the last round, the contestants shall stand at their respective positions facing each other and exchange a standing bow at the referee's command of "Cha-ryeot," "Kyeong-rye," and then wait for the referee's declaration of the decision in a standing posture.

   4) The referee shall declare the winner by raising his/her own hand to the winner's side.

   5) Retirement of the contestants

6. Contest Procedure in Team Competition
   Both teams shall stand facing each other in line in submitted team order towards the 1st Boundary Line from the Contestants' Marks.

Article 11. Permitted Techniques and Areas

1. Permitted Techniques
   1) Fist techniques: Delivering techniques by using the front parts of the forefinger and middle finger of the tightly clenched fist.

   2) Foot techniques: Delivering techniques by using the parts of the foot below the ankle bone.

2. Permitted Areas

    1) Trunk: Attack by fist and foot techniques on the areas covered by the trunk protector are permitted. However, such attacks shall not be made on the part of the back not covered by the trunk protector.

    2) Face: This area is the face excluding the back of the head, and attack by foot techniques only is permitted.

Article 12. Valid Points

1. Legal Scoring Areas

    1) Mid-section of the trunk: The part covered by the trunk protector

    2) Face: The whole part of the face including both ears

2. Points shall be awarded when permitted techniques are delivered accurately and powerfully to the legal scoring areas of the body.

3. The valid points are divided as follows.

    1) One (1) point for attack on trunk protector

    2) Two (2) points for attack on face.

    3) One (1) additional point shall be awarded in the event that the contestant is knocked down and the referee counts.

4. Match score shall be the sum of points of the three rounds.

5. Invalidation of points: When a contestant performs an attack to score through the use of the prohibited acts, the points scored shall be annulled.

Article 13. Scoring and Publication

1. Valid points shall be immediately recorded and publicized

2. In the use of body protectors not equipped with electronics, valid points shall be immediately marked by each judge by using the electronic scoring instrument or judge's scoring sheet.

3. In the use of electronic trunk protectors

    A. Valid points scored on the mid-section of the trunk shall be recorded automatically by the transmitter in the electronic trunk protector.

    B. Valid points scored to the face shall be marked by each judge by using the electronic scoring instrument or judge's scoring sheet.

4. In the case of scoring with an electronic scoring instrument or on a judge's scoring sheet, valid points shall be those recognized by at least three or more judges.

Article 14. Prohibited Acts and Penalties

1. Penalties on any prohibited acts shall be declared by the referee.

2. Penalties are divided into "Kyong-go" (warning penalty) and "Gam-jeom" (deduction penalty).

3. Two "Kyong-gos" shall be counted as deduction of one (1) point. However, the odd "Kyong-go" shall not be counted in the grand total.

4. A "Gam-jeom" shall be counted as minus one (-1) point.

5. Prohibited acts: "Kyong-go" penalty

    1) The following acts shall be classified as prohibited acts, and "Kyong-go" shall be declared.

        a. Crossing the Boundary Line

        b. Evading by turning the back to the opponent

        c. Falling down

        d. Avoiding the match

        e. Grabbing, holding, or pushing the opponent

        f. Attacking below the waist

        g. Pretending injury

        h. Butting or attacking with knee

        i. Hitting the opponent's face with the hand

        j. Uttering undesirable remarks or any misconduct on the part of a contestant or a coach

2) The following acts shall be classified as prohibited acts, and "Gam-jeom" shall de declared.

    a. Attacking the opponent after "Kal-yeo"

    b. Attacking the fallen opponent

    c. Throwing down the opponent by grappling the opponent's attacking foot in the air with the arm or by pushing the opponent with the hand

    d. Intentionally attacking the opponent's face with the hand

    e. Interrupting the progress of the match on the part of a contestant or a coach

    f. Violent or extreme remarks or behavior on the part of a contestant or a coach

6. When a contestant intentionally refuses to comply with the Competition Rules or the referee's order, the referee may declare the contestant loser by penalty after one (1) minute.

7. When a contestant receives minus four (-4) points, the referee shall declare him/her loser by penalties.

8. "Kyong-go" and " Gam-jeom" shall be counted in the total score of the three rounds.

Article 15. Sudden Death and Decision of Superiority

1. In the event of a tied score after the completion of the 4th round, the winner shall be decided by superiority of all refereeing officials. The final decision shall be based on the initiative shown during the 4th round.

Article 16. Decisions

1. Win by K.O.

2. Win by Referee Stop Contest (RSC)

3. Win by score or superiority

    1) Win by final score

    2) Win by Point Gap: when there is a 7-point gap, the match will be stopped and a winner declared.

    3) Win by Point Ceiling: when a competitor scores a maximum of 12 points, the match shall be stopped and a winner declared.

4. Win by withdrawal

5. Win by disqualification

6. Win by referee's punitive declaration

Article 17. Knock Down

1. When any part of the body other than the sole of the foot touches the floor due to the force of the opponent's delivered technique.

2. When a contestant is staggered showing no intention or ability to pursue the match.

3. When the referee judges that the contest cannot continue as the result of any power technique having been delivered.

Article 18. Procedure in the Event of a Knock Down

1. When a contestant is knocked down as the result of the opponent's legitimate attack, the referee shall take the following measures:

    A. The referee shall keep the attacker away from downed contestant by declaration of "Kal-yeo" (break).

    B. The referee shall count aloud from "Hanah" (one) up to "Yeol" (ten) at one-second interval towards the downed contestant, making hand signals indicating the passage of time.

    C. In case the downed contestant stands up during the referee's count and desires to continue the fight, the referee shall continue the count up to " Yeodul" (eight) for recovery of the downed contestant. The referee shall then determine if the contestant is recovered and, if so, continue the contest by declaration of "Kye-sok" (continue).

    D. When a contestant who has been knocked down cannot demonstrate the will to resume the contest by the count of "Yeodul," the referee shall announce the other contestant winner by K.O.

    E. The count shall be continued even after the end of the round or the expiration of the match time.

    F. In case both of the contestants are knocked down, the referee shall continue counting as long as one of the contestants has not sufficiently recovered.

G. When both of the contestants fail to recover by the count of "Yeol," the winner shall be decided upon the match score before the occurrence of knock down.

H. When it is judged by the referee that a contestant is unable to continue, the referee may decide the winner either without counting or during the counting.

2. Procedures to be followed after the contest:

A. Any contestant suffering a knock-out as the result of a blow to the head will not be allowed to compete for the next 30 days.

B. Before entering a new contest after 30 days, the contestant must be examined by a medical doctor designated by the National Taekwondo Association, who must certify that the contestant is recovered and able to compete.

Article 19. Procedures for Suspending the Match

1. When a contestant is to be stopped due to the injury of one or both of contestants, the referee shall take the following measures:

2. The referee shall suspend the contest by declaration of "Kal-yeo" and order the Recorder to suspend the time keeping by announcing "Kye-shi" (suspend).

3. The referee shall allow the contestant to receive first aid within one minute.

4. The contestant who does not demonstrate the will to continue the contest after one minute, even in the case of a slight injury, shall be declared loser by the referee.

5. In case resumption of the contest is impossible after one minute the contestant causing the injury by a prohibited act to be penalized by "Gam-jeom" shall be declared loser.

6. In case both of the contestants are knocked down and are unable to continue the contest after one minute, the winner shall be decided upon points scored before the injuries occurred.

7. When it is judged that a contestant's health is at risk due to losing consciousness of falling in an apparently dangerous condition, the referee shall suspend the contest immediately and order first aid to be administered. The referee shall declare as loser, the contestant causing the injury if it is deemed to have resulted from a prohibited attack to be penalized by "Gam-jeom," or in the case the attack was not deemed to be penalized by "Gam-jeom," shall decide the winner on the basis of the score of the match before suspension of the time.
In case of the situation which warrants suspending the match beyond the above prescribed procedure, the referee shall declare "Shi-gan" (time) to stop the match and continue the match by declaring "Kye-sok" (continue).

Article 20. Refereeing Officials

1. Qualifications
   Holders of International Referee Certificate registered by the WTF

2. Duties

   1) Referee

      (1) The referee shall have control over the match)

      (2) The referee shall declare "Shi-jak," "Keu-man," "Kal-yeo," "Kye-sok," and "Kye-shi," winner and loser, deduction of points, warnings and retiring. All the referees' declarations shall be made when the results are confirmed.

      (3) The referee shall have the right to make decisions independently in accordance with the prescribed rules.

      (4) The referee shall not award points.

      (5) In case of a tie or scoreless match the decision of superiority shall be made by all refereeing officials after the end of the fourth round.

   2) Judges

      (1) The judges shall mark the valid points immediately.

      (2) The judges shall sate their opinions forthrightly when requested by the referee.

3. Responsibility for Judgement
   Decisions made by the referees and judges shall be conclusive and they shall be responsible to the Competition Supervisory Board for those decisions.

4. Uniform of the Refereeing Officials

    1) The referees and judges shall wear the uniform designated by the WTF.

    2) The refereeing officials shall not carry or take any materials to the arena which might interfere with the contest.

Article 21. Recorder

The recorder shall time the contest and periods of time-out, suspension, and also shall record and publicize the awarded points, and/or deduction of points.

Article 22. Assignment of Officials

1. Composition of Refereeing Officials' Squad

    1) With the use of a non-electronic trunk protector, the officials' squad is composed of one (1) referee and four (4) judges.

    2) With the use of an electronic trunk protector, the officials' squad is composed of one (1) referee and two (2) judges

2. Assignment of Refereeing Officials

    1) The assignment of the referees and judges shall be made after the contest schedule is fixed.

    2) Referees and judges with the same nationality as that of either contestant shall not be assigned to such a contest. However, an exception shall be made for the judges when the number of refereeing officials is insufficient as the case may be.

Article 23. Other Matters Not Specified in the Rules

In the case that any matters not specified in the Rules occur, they shall be dealt with as follows:

1. Matters related to the competition shall be decided through consensus by the refereeing officials of the pertinent contest.

2. Matters that are not related to a specific contest, shall be decided by the Executive Council or its proxy.

3. The organizing committee shall prepare for a video tape recorder at each court for recording and preservation of the match process.

Article 24. Arbitration

1. Composition of the Competition Supervisory Board

    1) Qualification of members: Qualified Competition Supervisory Board members shall be members of the WTF Executive Council or persons with sufficient Taekwondo experience and who are recommended by the WTF President or Secretary General. One Technical Delegate shall be the ex-officio member.

    2) Composition of the Competition Supervisory Board: one Chairman and fewer than six members plus the Technical Delegate

    3) The President, on the recommendation of the Secretary General, shall appoint the Chairman and members of the Competition Supervisory Board.

2. Responsibility: The Board of Arbitration shall make corrections of misjudgments according to their decision regarding protests and take disciplinary action against the officials committing the misjudgment or any illegal behavior and the results of which shall be sent to the Secretariat of the WTF.

3. Procedure of Protest

    1) In case there is an objection to a referee judgment, an official delegate must submit an application for re-evaluation of decision (protest application) together with the prescribed fee to the Board of Arbitration within 10 minutes after the pertinent contest.

    2) Deliberation of re-evaluation shall be carried out excluding those members with the same nationality as that of either contestant concerned, and resolution on deliberation shall be made by majority.

    3) The members of the Board of Arbitration may summon the refereeing officials for confirmation of events.

    4) The resolution made by the Board of Arbitration will be final and no further means of appeal will be applied.

4. Procedure of Sanction

    1) The WTF President of Secretary General (in case of their absence, the Technical Delegate) may request the Extraordinary Committee of Sanction for deliberation when any of the following behaviors are committed by a coach or a contestant

        a. Interfering with the management of contest

        b. Stirring up the spectators or spreading false rumor.

    2) When judged reasonable, the Extraordinary Committee of Sanction shall deliberate over the matter and take disciplinary action immediately. The result of deliberation shall be announced to the public and reported to the WTF Secretariat afterwards.

    3) The Extraordinary Committee of Sanction may summon the person concerned for confirmation of events.

Poomsae (Form) Rules (effective as of April, 2006)

Article 1. Purpose

The purpose of the Competition Rules is to manage fairly and smoothly all matters pertaining to competitions of all levels to be promoted and/or organized by the WTF, Regional Unions and member National Associations, ensuring the application of standardized rules.

(Interpretation)

The objective of Article 1 is to ensure the standardization of all Taekwondo Poomsae competitions worldwide. Any competition not following the fundamental principles of these rules cannot be recognized as a Taekwondo Poomsae competition

Article 2. Application

The Competition Rules shall apply to all competitions promoted and/or organized by the WTF, each Regional Union and a member National Association. However, any member National Association wishing to modify some part of the Competition Rules must first gain the approval of the WTF.

(Explanation #1)

Amendment approval:

Any organization desiring to make a change in some portion of the existing rules must submit to the WTF the contents of the desired amendment along with the reasons for the desired change. Approval for any change in these rules must be received from WTF one month prior to the scheduled competition.

(Explanation #2)

Change in category, increase or decrease in the number of International Referees, change of the courtside position of the inspector, recorder and/or commission doctor, etc., are subjects which may be included in the category of Poomsae competition aspects which may be modified after first gaining the approval of the WTF however, such germane matters as scoring, are not to be changed under any circumstances whatsoever.

Article 3. Competition Area

The Competition Area shall comprise Contest Area measuring 14m by 14m in metric system and have a flat surface without any obstructing projections. The Contest Area shall be covered with an elastic mat. However the Contest Area may be installed on a platform 0.5cm-0.6cm high from the base, if necessary, and the outer part of the Boundary Line shall be inclined with a gradient of less than 30 degrees for the safety of the contestants.

1. Demarcation of the Contest Area

    1) The 14m by 14m area shall be called the Contest Area.

    2) The demarcation of the contest area shall be distinguished by a white line with 5cm wide in case of wooden competition area

2. Indication of Positions

    1) Position of the Judges: Seven judges' tables shall be positioned 2m in front of the contest area, with 1m between the judges. The adjacent boundary line shall be deemed Boundary Line #1. Clockwise from Boundary Line #1 will be Boundary Lines #2, #3, and #4.

    2) The position of the Referee shall be at a point 1m inward from the corner of Boundary Lines #1 and #2.

3) The positions of the contestants shall be marked at 1m back from the center of the contest area, toward Boundary Line #3.

4) The recorder's desk shall be positioned at 2m in front of the contest area and 2m from judge #1's table, outside the corner of Boundary Line #1 and #4.

5) The competition coordinators shall be positioned 2m outside of Boundary Lines #4, one coordinator adjacent to the corner of Boundary Lines #3 and #4, and one coordinator adjacent to the corner of Boundary Lines #1 and #4.

6) The position of the coach shall be at a point 2m outwards from Boundary Line #2 adjacent to the corner of Boundary Lines #2 and #3.

7) The inspection desk shall be positioned at the entrance of the contest area outside the corner of Boundary Lines #3 and #4.

Article 4. Contestant

1. Qualifications of contestants

    1) Holder of the nationality of the participating team

    2) One recommended by the National Taekwondo Association

    3) Holder of Taekwondo Dan certificate issued by Kukkiwon or WTF

    4) Junior Division (14-17 years old)

    5) 1st Senior Division (18-30 years old)

    6) 2nd Senior Division (31-40 years old)

    7) Masters Division (Over age of 41)

(Interpretation)

The age limits for the Junior, Senior, and Masters division are based on the year, not on the date, when the Championships are held. For example, in the junior division, contestants shall be between 14 and 17 year old. E.g., were the Junior Poomsae Championships to be held on September 9, 2005, those contestants born between January 1, 1988, and December 31, 1991 is eligible to participate

2. Contestants' uniforms

    1) Contestants shall wear only a WTF-approved uniform at WTF-sanctioned Poomsae Championships.

    2) Those contestants who wish to participate in the 1st and 2nd Creative Poomsae competition may wear Taekwondo uniform designed by participating team. However, the dress must be similar with the official Taekwondo uniform. Contestants who wish to wear Taekwondo uniform must wear those duly recognized by the WTF.

3. Medical control

    1) At the Taekwondo events promoted or sanctioned by the WTF, any use or administration of drugs or chemical substances described in the WTF anti-doping laws is prohibited.

    2) The WTF may carry out all medical testing deemed necessary to ascertain if a contestant has committed a breach of WTF Anti-Doping Rules, and any winner who refuses to undergo this testing or who proves to have committed such a breach shall be removed from the final standings, and the win must be transferred to the contestant next in line in the competition standings.

    3) The Organizing Committee shall be liable for arrangements to carry out medical testing.

    4) All details regarding doping matters shall be handled according to WTF Anti-Doping Rules.

Article 5. Classifications of Competition

1. Men's Individual Compulsory

2. Women's Individual Compulsory

3. Men's Team Compulsory

4. Women's Team Compulsory

5. Mixed Team Compulsory

6. Mixed Team 1st Creative

7. Mixed Team 2nd Creative (Taekwon rhythm)

Article 6. Divisions

1. Men, women, and mixed divisions shall be divided according to age

2. There is no specific limitation to Poom, Dan for group competition.

3. The percentage of one gender shall be over 30% in the Mixed Team competition.

4. The divisions shall be grouped as follows:

> **Junior Division** (14-17 years old)
> J/M/I/Compulsory, J/M/T/Compulsory, J/Mi/T/Compulsory
> J/F/I/Compulsory, J/F/T/Compulsory, J/Mi/T/Creative
>
> **1st Senior Division** (18-30 years old)
> 1st S/M/I/Compulsory, 1st S/M/T/Compulsory, 1st S/Mi/T/Compulsory
> 1st S/F/I/Compulsory, 1st S/F/T/Compulsory, 1st S/Mi/T/Creative
>
> **2nd Senior Division** (31-40 years old)
> 2nd S/M/I/Compulsory, 2nd S/M/T/Compulsory, 2nd S/Mi/T/Compulsory
> 2nd S/F/I/Compulsory, 2nd S/F/T/Compulsory, 2nd S/Mi/T/Creative
>
> **Master Division** (Over age of 41)
> M/M/I/Compulsory, M/M/T/Compulsory, M/Mi/T/Compulsory
> M/F/I/Compulsory, M/F/T/Compulsory, M/Mi/T/Creative

Article 7. Methods of Competition

1. All international-level competitions recognized by the WTF shall be formed with the participation of at least five (5) countries with no fewer than five (5) contestants in each division.

2. The systems of competition are divided as follows:

    1) Single elimination tournament system

    2) Round robin system

3. Competitions are divided as follows.

    1) Individual Division: Individual participating contestants shall conduct two compulsory Poomsae, Contestants participating in the individual competition may also participate in the team competition.

    2) Team Division: Participating teams shall conduct two compulsory Poomsae. Contestants participating in the team competition may also participate in the individual competition.

Article 8. Recognized Poomsae (1st and 2nd Compulsory Poomsae)

Division	1st Compulsory Poomsae	2nd Compulsory Poomsae
Junior Division (14-17 years old)	Taeguek 5, 6, 7, 8 Jang	Koryo, Keumgang, Taeback
Senior Division (18-30 years old)	Taeguek 6, 7, 8 Jang, Koryo	Keumgang, Taeback, Pyongwon, Shipjin
Senior Division (31-40 years old)	Taeguek 6, 7, 8 Jang, Koryo	Keumgang, Taeback, Pyongwon, Shipjin
Masters Division (Over age of 41)	Taeguek 6, 7, 8 Jang, Koryo, Keumgang, Taeback	Pyingwon, Shipjin, Jitae, Hansu

Article 9. 1st Creative Poomsae, 2nd Creative Poomsae (Taekwon rhythm)

1. 1st Creative Poomsae

    1) Contestants who wish to participate in the 1st Creative Poomsae Competition must submit a detailed program in advance. Each performance shall be presented once.

    2) The detailed program shall be submitted prior to the designated deadline.

    3) The number of participating contestants per team shall be limited to five (5).

    4) All patterns and movements of the 1st Creative Poomsae shall be exclusively Taekwondo techniques.

5) The movements to be included in the 1st Creative Poomsae are:

Junior Division (14-17 years old)

    1. Ap Chagi (Front Kick)

    2. Yop Chagi (Side Kick)

    3. Arae Makki (Low Block)

    4. Momtong Makki (Body Block)

    5. Momtong Jireugi (Body Punch)

    6. Deungjumeok Ap Chigi (Back Fist Front Strike)

    7. Jupm Chagi (Jump Kick)

1st Senior Division (18-30 years old)

2nd Senior Division (31-40 years old)

    1. Ap Chagi (Front Kick)

    2. Yop Chagi (Side Kick)

    3. Momtong Makki (Body Block)

    4. Olgul Makki (Face Block)

    5. Momtong Jireugi (Body Punch)

    6. Hansonnal Makki (Hand-Blade Block)

    7. Jump Chagi (Jump Kick)

Masters Division (Over age of 41)

    1. Ap Chagi (Front Kick)

    2. Dwidora Yop Chagi (Turning Side Kick)

    3. Momtong Makki (Body Block)

    4. Olgul Macki (Face Block)

    5. Momtong Chagi (Body Kick)

    6. Jump Chagi (Jump Kick)

(Interpretation)

All movements in the 1st Creative Poomsae shall be composed of Taekwondo techniques recognized by Kukkiwon.

2. 2nd Creative Poomsae (Taekwon rhythm)

1) Contestants who wish to participate in the 2nd Creative poomsae must submit a detailed program in advance each performance shall be presented once.

2) Music may be used for the 2nd Creative Poomsae competition.

3) A detailed program and a music cassette tape or CD shall be submitted prior to the designated deadline.

4) The number of participants contestants per team shall be limited to five (5).

5) 70% of the patterns and movements shall be Taekwondo techniques.

6) No religious or ideological music may be played by the participating teams.

Article 10. Duration of Contest

1. Duration of Contest by Division

1) Individual competition: From 1 minute to 2 minutes

2) Team competition: From 1 minute to 2 minutes

3) 1st Creative Poomsae: From 1 minute to 3 minutes

4) 2nd Creative Poomsae (Taekwon rhythm): From 2 minutes to 4 minutes

5) The time between the end of the 1st Compulsory Poomsae and the start of the 2nd Compulsory Poomsae shall be 1 minute.

Article 15. Scoring Criteria

1. Individual

   1) Accuracy of Poomsae Technique
      Contestants' technical accuracy of (Jirgi (Punch), Makki (Block), Chagi (Kick), Seogi (Stance)) in accordance with WTF standards shall be observed.

   2) Presentation
      Judges will observe connection of movements, distribution of power, breathing, and spirit, etc.

2. Team

   1) Accuracy of Poomsae Technique
      Contestants' technical accuracy of (Jirgi (Punch), Makki (Block), Chagi (Kick), Seogi (Stance)) in accordance with WTF standards shall be observed.

   2) Presentation
      Judges will observe connection of movements, distribution of power, breathing, and spirit, etc.

   3) Cohesion
      The judges will observe contestants' accomplishment of designated techniques, technical organization, and technical abilities. Should discrepancies be noted, point deductions shall be assessed.

3. 1st Creative Poomsae

   1) Accuracy of Poomsae Technique
      Contestants' technical accuracy of (Jirgi (Punch), Makki (Block), Chagi (Kick), Seogi (Stance)) in accordance with WTF standards shall be observed.

   2) Presentation
      Judges will observe connection of movements, distribution of power, breathing, and spirit, etc.

   3) Cohesion
      The judges will observe contestants' accomplishment of designated techniques, technical organization, and technical abilities. Should discrepancies be noted, point deductions shall be assessed.

   4) Degree of Difficulty
      Points shall be awarded considering the degree of difficulty, i.e., performance of difficult movements and techniques, including jumping and spinning techniques and a high rate of innovative performance shall be noted.

4. 2nd Creative Poomsae

   1) Accuracy of Poomsae Technique
      Contestants' technical accuracy of (Jirgi (Punch), Makki (Block), Chagi (Kick), Seogi (Stance)) in accordance with WTF standards shall be observed.

   2) Presentation
      Judges will observe connection of movements, distribution of power, breathing, and spirit, etc.

   3) Cohesion
      The judges will observe contestants' accomplishment of designated techniques, technical organization, and technical abilities. Should discrepancies be noted, point deductions shall be assessed.

   4) Degree of Difficulty
      Points shall be awarded considering the degree of difficulty, i.e., performance of difficult movements and techniques, including jumping and spinning techniques and a high rate of innovative performance shall be noted.

   5) Coordination
      The coordination of movements and music shall be observed.

Article 16. Methods of Scoring

1. For each item in technical accuracy, a maximum of 10 points can be given. The score shall be the average of the total sum.

2. For presentation category, a maximum of 10 points can be given.

3. In scoring the cohesion category, 0.5 points shall be deducted for each error.

4. In scoring the degree of difficulty category, a maximum of 10 points can be given.

5. In scoring the coordination category, a maximum of 10 points can be give.

6. The final score shall be the average of five (5) judges, following the deletion of the highest and lowest scores among the seven (7) judges.

7. Deduction of points

   1) Should a contestant exceed the time limit, 0.5 points shall be deducted from final score.

   2) Should a contestant cross the boundary line, 0.5 points shall be deducted from the final score.

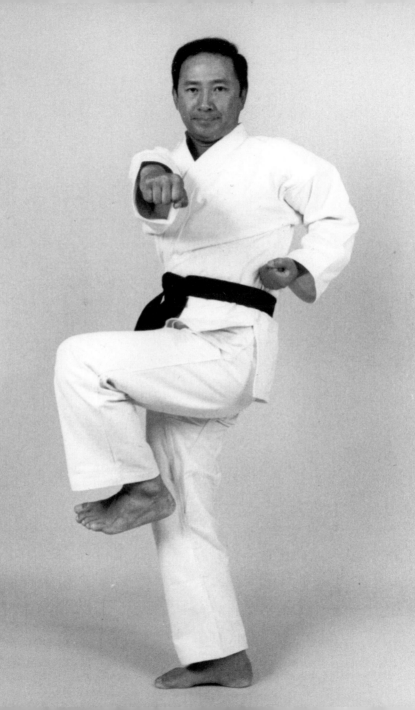

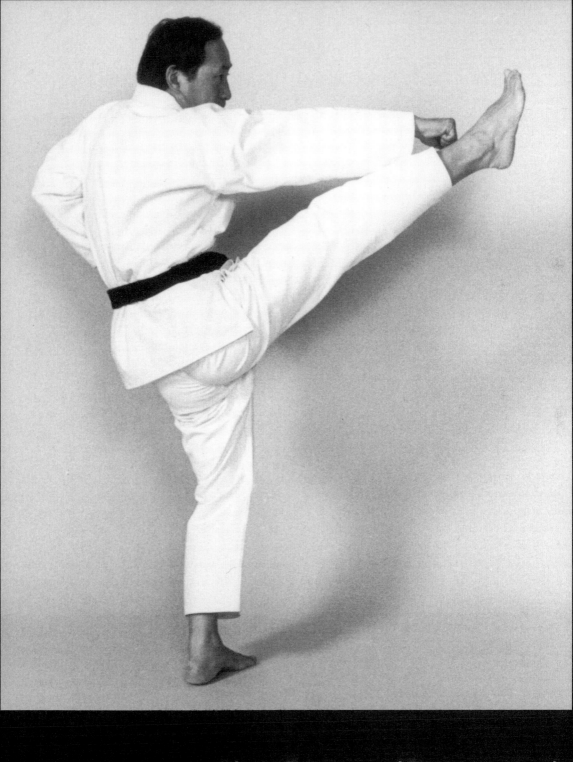

The Forms (Poomsae):
Formal Exercises

INDIVIDUAL FUNDAMENTAL TECHNIQUES are the alphabet of Taekwondo. The forms are its grammar.

The formal exercises of Taekwondo have evolved over many hundreds of years, and they serve many practical purposes. It is a basic principle of Taekwondo that the body and the spirit are one and indivisible, and that purification of the spirit can be achieved by disciplining, tempering, and training the body. Developed in these formal exercises are three elements of training the body: *movement,* which requires stretching for flexibility; *speed,* which requires the perfection of precise techniques; and *power,* which requires training for strength and coordination.

The diligent practice of the formal exercises helps to develop these important characteristics in a variety of ways:

1. The formal exercises develop physical and spiritual concentration, and train you to concentrate your soul in each given instant of life, so that you can borrow from your life force and mobilize it at the critical instant.

2. Practiced conscientiously, the Poomsae are a type of active meditation, which provides both spiritual and physical experience.

3. They help to perfect individual fundamental techniques.

4. They develop rhythm and timing, and thus create smooth and efficient motion.

5. They help to perfect individual fundamental techniques.

6. The forms train you to combine those techniques so that they work effectively together in combination.

7. They develop balance, accuracy, and endurance.

8. They help weave defensive and offensive techniques into one coordinated whole.

9. They develop patience, passivity, and an understanding of the deep meaning of the art.

10. They develop confidence and speed.

11. They help develop a "sixth sense" of perception and intuition.

12. They simulate active combat, enabling you to fight more than one assailant from any direction for as long as necessary without tiring.

Each of the formal exercises in this book has a purpose and a philosophy of its own. We will examine each of these forms with this in mind.

In learning the forms, it is important to keep in mind that it is far better to master one form and be able to apply it properly than to learn great numbers of forms imperfectly.

There are two types of forms practices at the beginning and intermediate levels: eight Palgwe forms and eight Taegeuk forms. The *Palgwe* forms are conservative

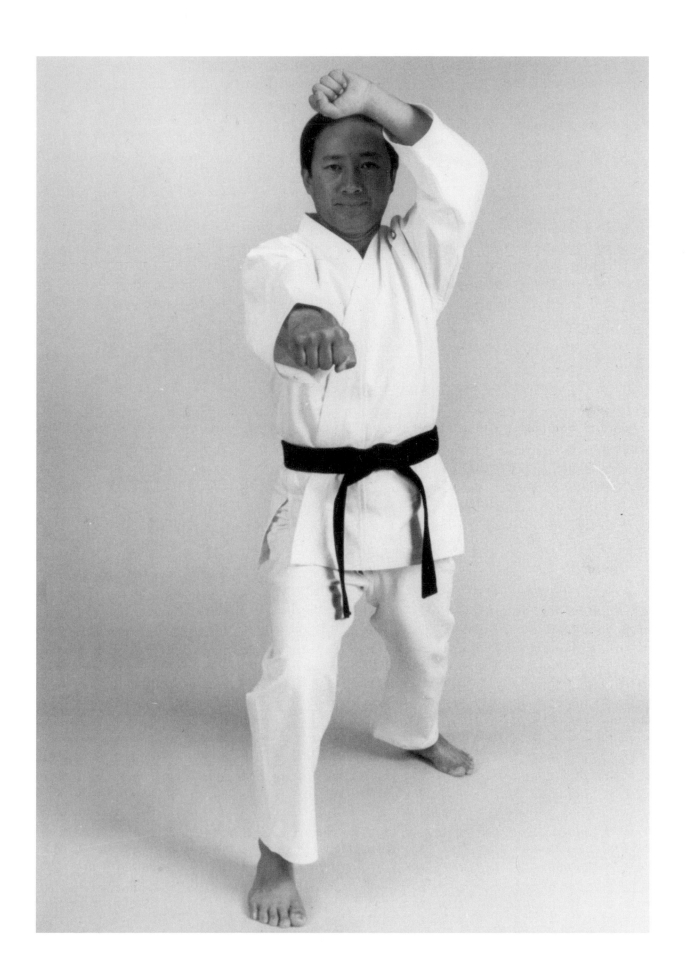

because they emphasize fundamental techniques of Taekwondo movements. *Taegeuk* forms stress techniques that are more applicable to sparring situations by teaching students combinations of defensive and offensive techniques and coordination of speed and power.

Palgwe forms are explained in *Tae Kwon Do: The Korean Martial Art;* the Taegeuk forms are being introduced here so that practitioners of Taekwondo may have an opportunity to learn them.

At the advanced level there are two types of forms. One group consists of more traditional forms (about 50, to be discussed in a future publication) that are practiced in many different styles of martial arts, including advanced Taekwondo. The origins of some of the traditional forms are lost in antiquity, but their spontaneity, speed, economy of motion, and effectiveness seem to be borrowed from nature and the way animals fight—blocking, turning, and striking instinctively.

The other group consists of advanced Taekwondo forms which are required by the World Taekwondo Federation to improve your techniques and also to test for the purpose of degree promotion. This chapter explains these nine advanced forms in detail.

Note: the following points should be observed in the performance of all formal exercises:

1. Execute each position cleanly and completely before going on to the next; do not run any two positions together.
2. Breathe regularly throughout the form, using the diaphragm rather than the chest, and exhale simultaneously with the last action in each position.
3. Keep your fists tight and your body relaxed, except at the instant you complete each block, punch, strike, and kick, when your whole body should be locked into tense focus on that action.
4. While standing at attention, before beginning the form, take a *deep* breath, using the diaphragm, not the chest, and concentrate on what you are about to do.

KORYO (KOREA)

The word "Korea" derives from *Koryo*, the name of an ancient dynasty (A.D. 918-1392). The Koryo men were people of strong convictions and will, which they demonstrated in battle. They persistently resisted the aggressions of the Mongolians, who were sweeping the world at the time. Their firm resolution and intrepid spirit, born of wisdom rather than brute strength or numbers, earned them the title "men of conviction."

The form Koryo can be a way of cultivating the strength that arises from firm conviction. With every motion, you must demonstrate confidence and a strong will.

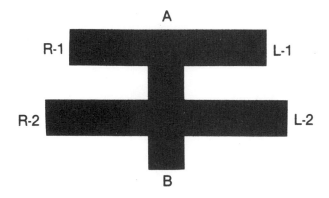

Koryo

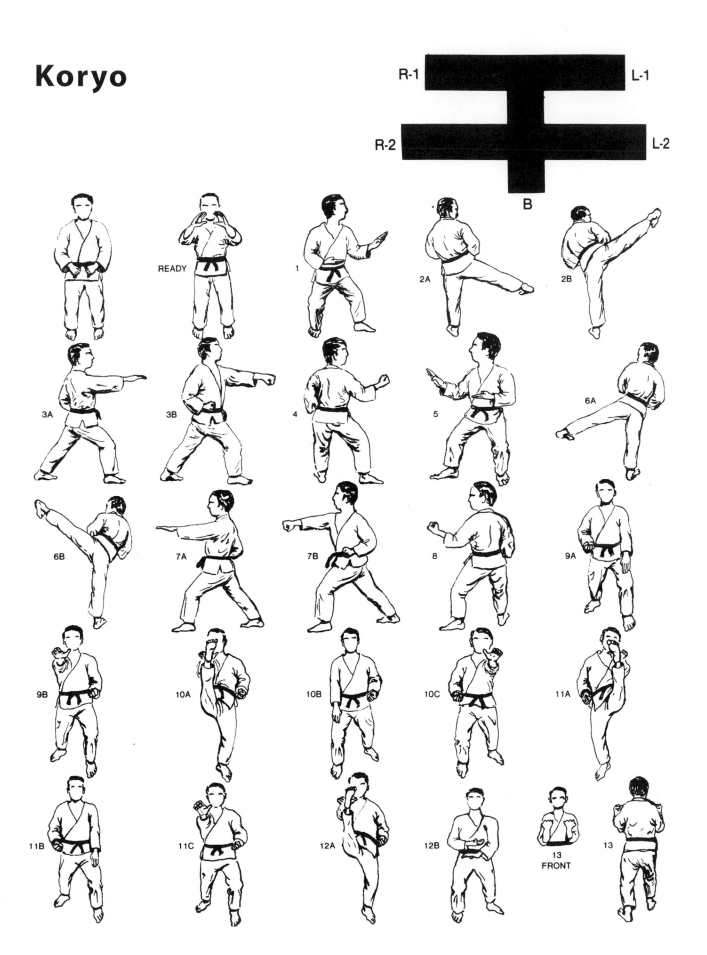

R-1   L-1

R-2   L-2

B

READY

1

2A

2B

3A

3B

4

5

6A

6B

7A

7B

8

9A

9B

10A

10B

10C

11A

11B

11C

12A

12B

13 FRONT

13

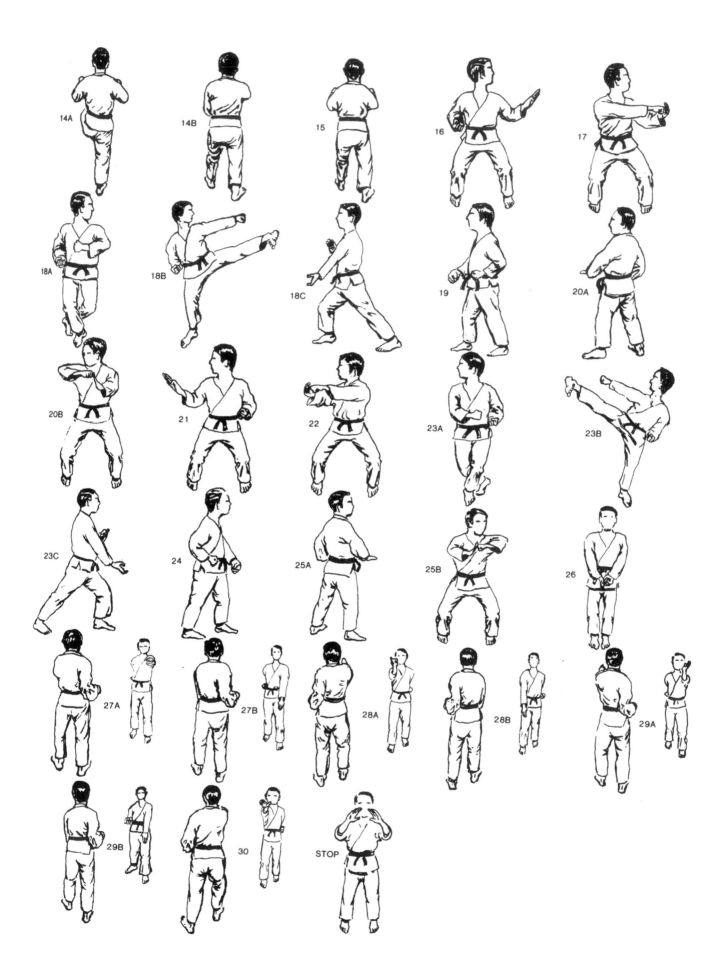

14A 14B 15 16 17

18A 18B 18C 19 20A

20B 21 22 23A 23B

23C 24 25A 25B 26

27A 27B 28A 28B 29A

29B 30 STOP

Ready (Barrel Pushing Ready), (Tong-Milgi-Choonbi)

Maintain ready stance, facing **B** at point **A**, eyes focused straight ahead. At the same time raise both open hands to neck and push forward, palms out, with arms and hands tensed, as if pushing a heavy barrel.

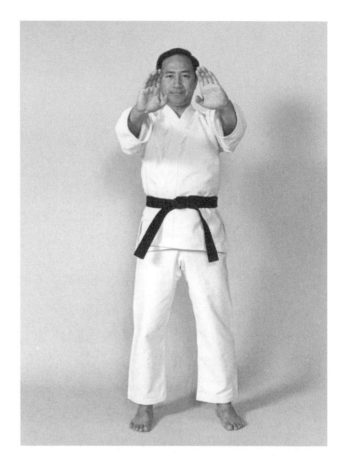

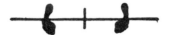

First Position:
Knife-Hand Middle Block

a. Slide your left foot 90° to the left (toward **L-1**).

b. Assume Left Back Stance.

c. Simultaneously execute a Left Knife-Hand Middle Block.

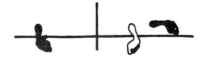

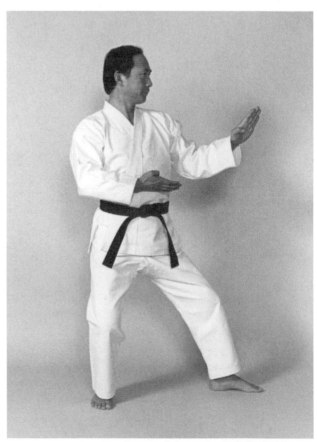

Second Position:
  Low Side Kick, High Side Kick, Outside
  Knife-Hand Strike *(Sonnal-Bakat-Chiki)*

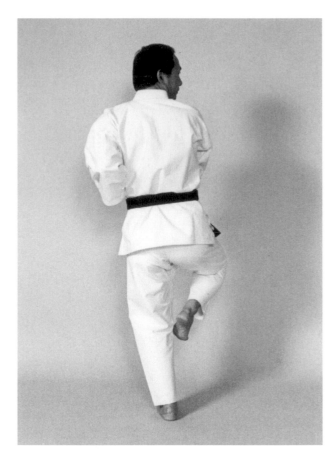

1. Low Side Kick

a. Place your left fist at waist level, palm up, and place your right fist over your left fist, palm in.

b. Simultaneously execute a Side Kick with your right foot to knee level (toward **L-1**).

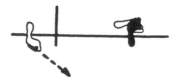

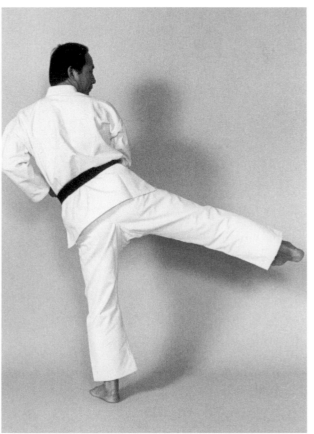

2. High Side Kick

a. Keep fist in same position as in Low Side Kick.

b. Consecutively, without placing your foot on the floor, execute a Side Kick with your Right foot to the face.

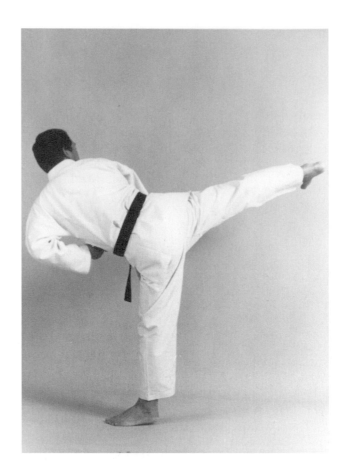

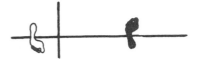

3. Knife-Hand Strike

a. Immediately bring your right foot down one step forward.

b. Assume Right Front Stance.

c. Simultaneously, execute a Right Outside Knife-Hand Strike to the neck, palm down.

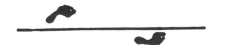

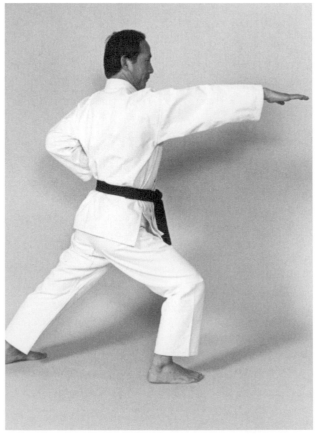

Third Position:
  Reverse Middle Punch

  a. Maintain the same stance

  b. Execute a Left-Hand Reverse Middle Punch.

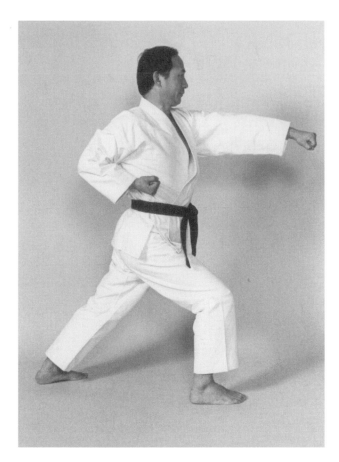

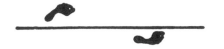

Fourth Position:
  Inside Middle Block

  a. Slide your right foot slightly backward.

  b. Assume Right Back Stance.

  c. Simultaneously execute a Right-Hand Inside Middle Block.

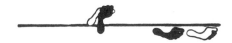

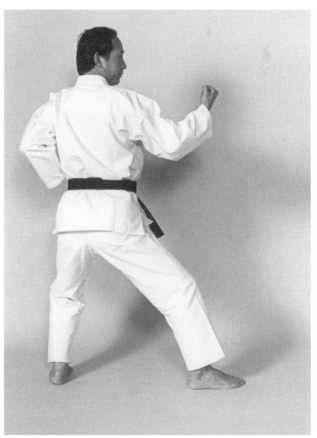

Fifth Position:
Knife-Hand Middle Block

    a. Pivoting to the right on the ball of your foot, slide your right foot out and back in a wide arc, turning 180˚ to the right (toward **R-1**).

    b. Assume Right Back Stance.

    c. Simultaneously execute a Right Knife-Hand Middle Block.

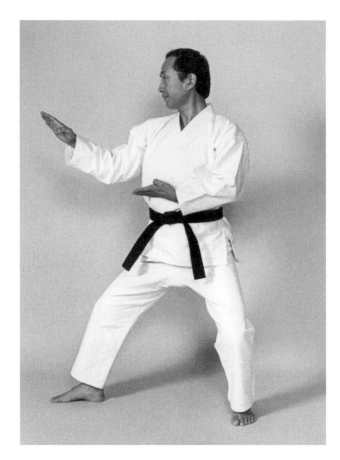

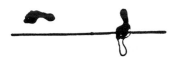

Sixth Position:
Low Side Kick, High Side Kick, Outside Knife-Hand Strike

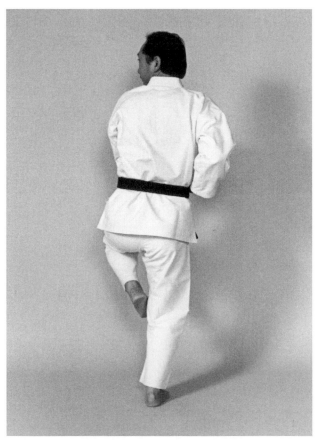

1. Low Side Kick

a. Place your right fist at waist level, palm up, and place left fist over your right fist, palm in.

b. Simultaneously execute a Side Kick with your left foot to knee level (toward **R-1**).

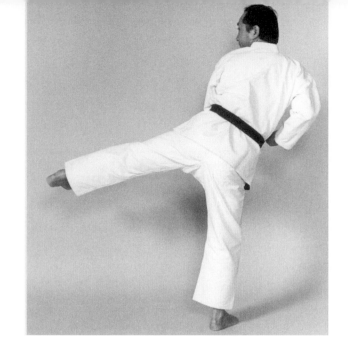

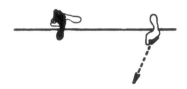

2. High Side Kick

a. Keep fists in the same position as in Low Side Kick.

b. Consecutively, without placing your foot on the floor, execute a Side Kick with your left foot to the face.

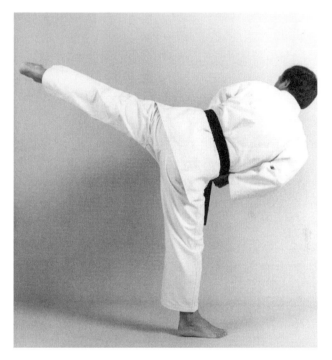

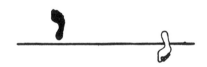

3. Knife-Hand Strike

a. Immediately bring your left foot down one step forward (toward **R-1**).

b. Assume Left Front Stance.

c. Simultaneously execute a Left Outside Knife-Hand Strike to the neck, palm down.

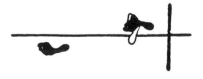

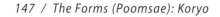

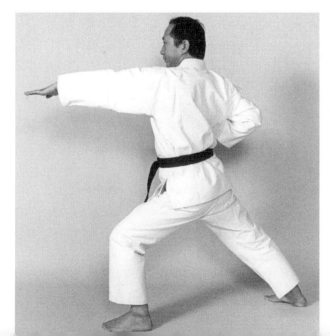

Seventh Position:
Reverse Middle Punch

a. Maintain the same position. Execute a Right-Hand Reverse Middle Punch.

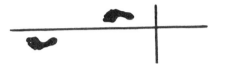

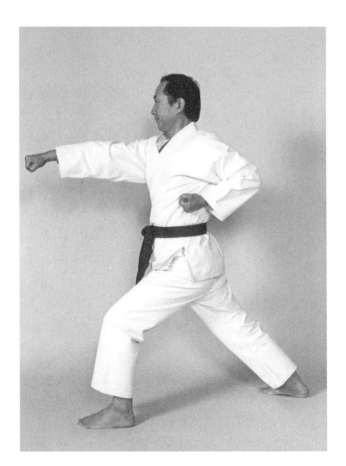

Eighth Position:
Inside Middle Block

a. Slide your left foot slightly backward.

b. Assume Left Back Stance.

c. Simultaneously execute a Left-Hand inside Middle Block.

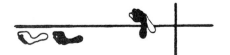

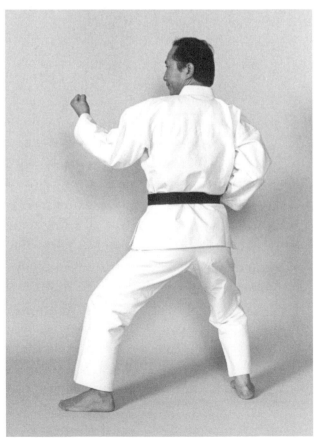

Ninth Position:
Single Knife-Hand Low Block (Hansonnal-Are-Makki), Tiger-Mouth Thrust (Hanson-Kaljaebi)

1. **Single Knife-Hand Low Block**

a. Pivoting to the left on the ball of your right foot, slide your left out to the left, turning 90° (toward **B**).

b. Assume Left Back Stance.

c. Simultaneously execute a Single Left Knife-Hand Low Block, and at the same time bring your right fist to waist level, palm up.

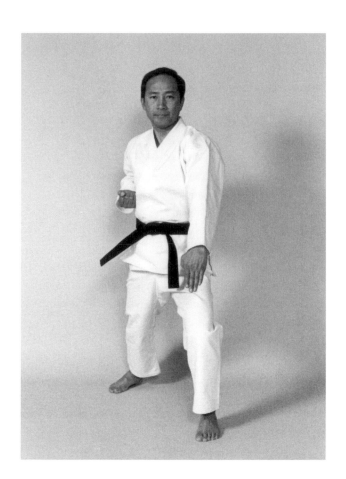

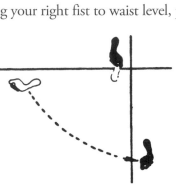

2. **Tiger Mouth Thrust**

a. Maintain the same stance

b. Execute a Right Tiger-Mouth Thrust to the throat and at the same time bring your left fist to waist level, palm up.

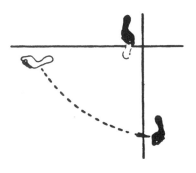

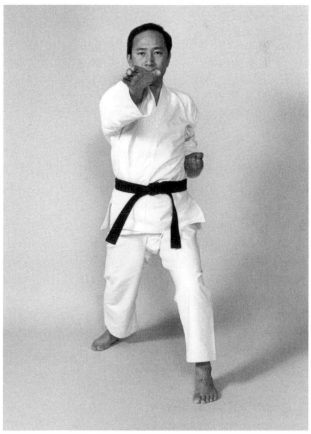

Tenth Position:
  Front-Kick, Single Knife-Hand Low Block,
  Tiger-Mouth Thrust

1. Front Kick

a. Execute a Front Kick with your right foot to the face.

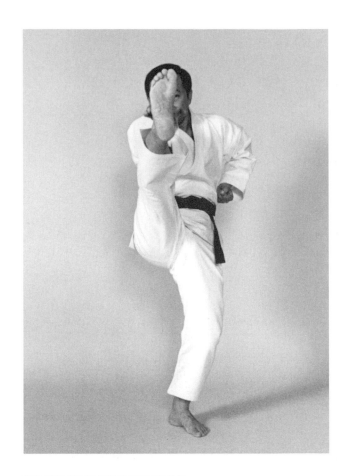

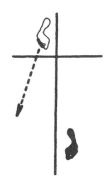

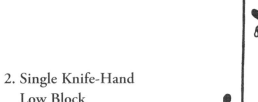

2. Single Knife-Hand Low Block

a. Step forward with your right foot.

b. Assume Right Front Stance.

c. Simultaneously execute a Single Right Knife-Hand Low Block and at the same time bring your left fist to waist level, palm up.

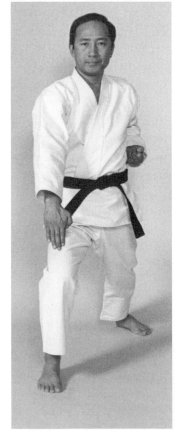

3. Tiger-Mouth Thrust

a. Maintain the same stance

b. Execute a Left Tiger-Mouth Thrust to the throat and at the same time bring right fist to waist level, palm up.

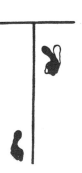

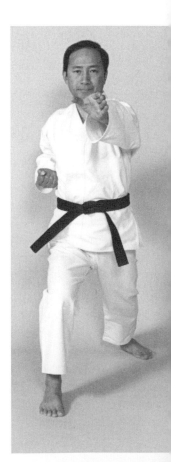

Eleventh Position:
Front Kick, Single Knife-Hand Low Block,
Tiger-Mouth Thrust

1. Front Kick
a. Execute a Front Kick with your left foot to the face.

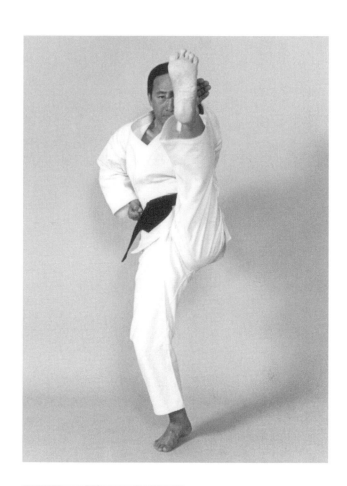

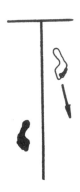

2. Single Knife-Hand Low Block
a. Step forward with your left foot.

b. Assume Left Front Stance.

c. Simultaneously execute a Single Left Knife-Hand Low Block and at the same time bring your right fist to waist level, palm up.

3. Tiger-Mouth Thrust
a. Maintain the same stance.

b. Execute a Right Tiger-Mouth Thrust to the throat and at the same time bring your left fist to the waist, palm up.

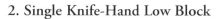

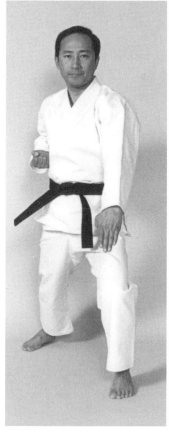

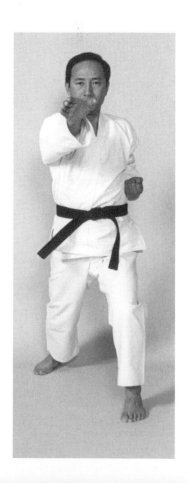

Twelfth Position:
Front Kick, Knee Break (*Mooreup-keokki*),
and Yell

1. Front Kick

a. Execute a Front Kick with your right foot to the face.

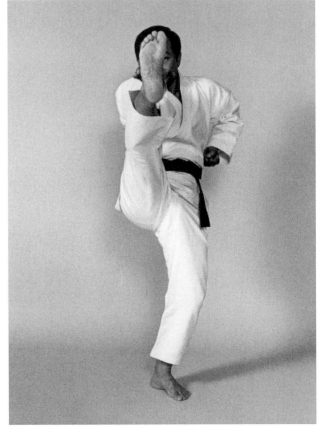

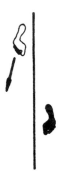

2. Knee Break

a. Step forward with your right foot.

b. Assume Right Front Stance.

c. Simultaneously, in front of body, bring your right open hand, palm up and tensed, from the thigh area to the stomach area and at the same time bring your left open hand, palm down and tensed, to the neck area and thrust downward, extending arm and yell! (This is a motion to grab your opponent's heel with your right open hand and break his knee by thrusting down your left open palm.)

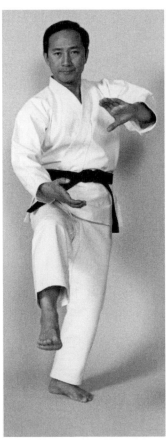

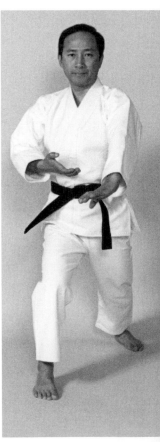

Thirteenth Position:
Spread Middle Block (Palm in) *(Anpalmok-Momtong-Hechyo-Makki)*

a. Pivoting to the right on the ball of your right foot, slide your left foot forward and slightly out in an arc (toward **B**), turning 180° to face **B**.

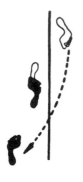

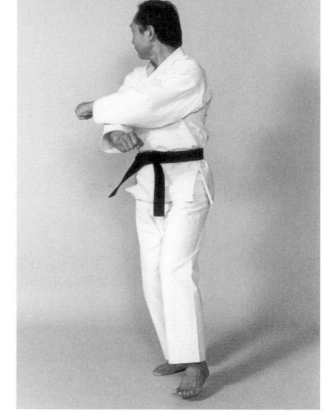

b. Assume Right Front Stance.

c. Simultaneously execute a Spread Middle Block, inner edges of forearms palms in.

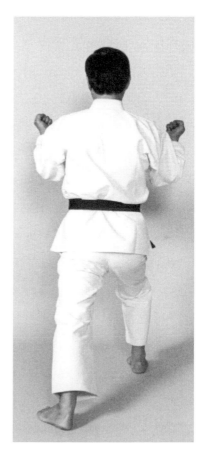

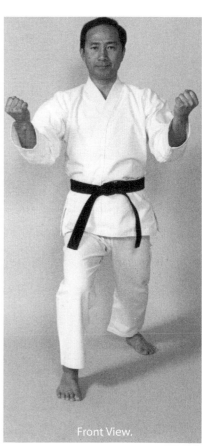

Front View.

153 / The Forms (Poomsae): Koryo

Fourteenth Position:
Front Kick, Knee Break

1. Front Kick

a. Execute a Front Kick with your left foot to the face.

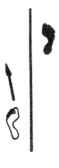

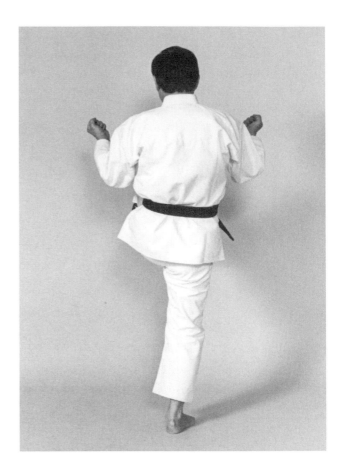

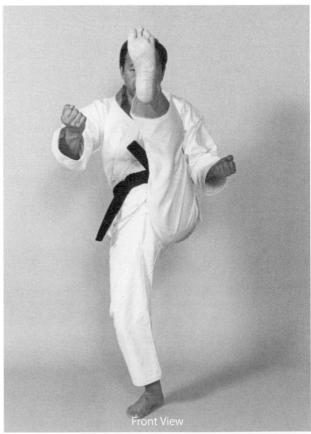

Front View

2. Knee Break

a. Step forward with your left foot.

b. Assume left Front Stance.

c. Simultaneously, in front of body, bring your left open hand, palm up and tensed, from the thigh area to the stomach area and at the same time bring your right open hand, palm down and tensed, to the neck area and thrust downward, extending arm.

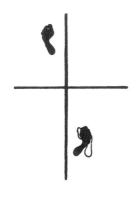

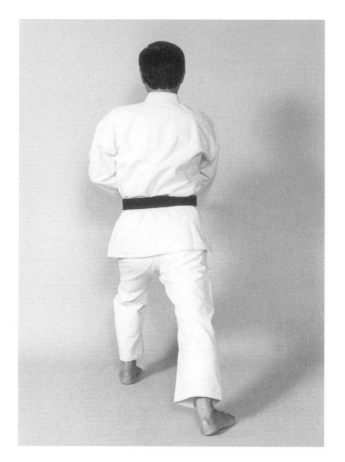

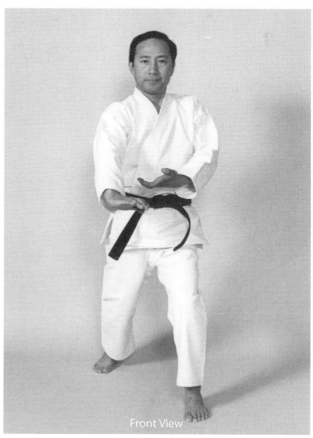

Front View

Fifteenth Position:
Spread Middle Block

a. Slide your left foot slightly backward.

b. Assume Left High-Front Stance.

c. Simultaneously execute a Spread Middle Block, palms in.

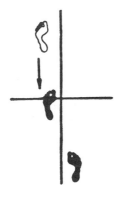

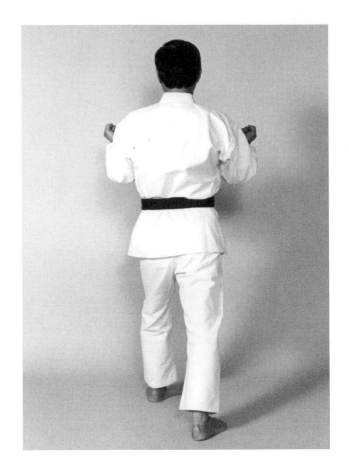

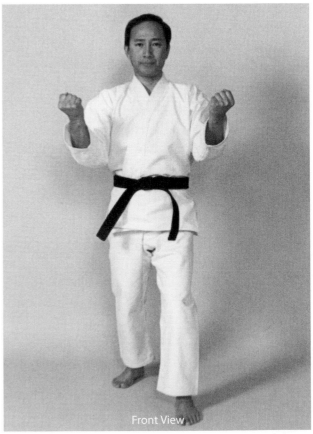

Front View

Sixteenth Position:
Single Knife-Hand Middle Block

a. Pivoting on the ball of your left foot to the right, slide your right foot out to the right and back in an arc (toward **R-2**), turning 180° to the right.

b. Assume Horseback Stance, body facing **B** with face turned toward **L-2**.

c. Simultaneously execute a Single Left Knife-Hand Middle Block and at the same time bring right fist to the waist, palm up.

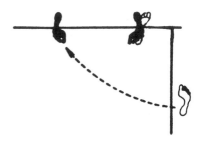

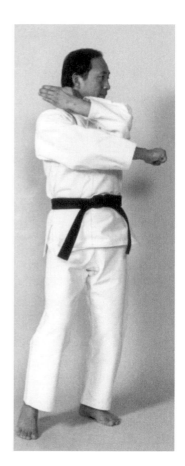

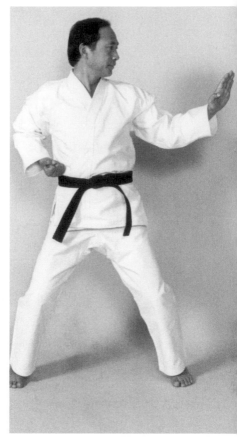

Seventeenth Position:
Target Hook Punch (*Joomeok-Pyojeok-Cihki*)

a. Maintain the same stance.

b. Execute a Target Hook Punch to the midsection with your right fist, hitting left open palm area. (Twist left hand, palm in, so that palm becomes target for punch.)

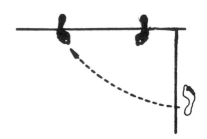

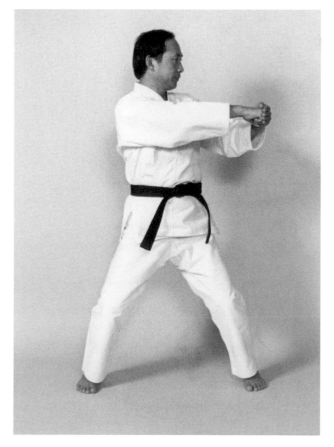

Eighteenth Position:
 Cross Stance, Side Kick, Spear-Hand Strike
 (Palm Up) (Pyeonsonkeut-Jecheo-Jiluki)

1. Cross Stance

a. Move your right foot to the left and cross over your left foot. At the same time bring you right fist to the waist, palm up, and bring your left fist over your right fist, palm in.

b. Assume Right Cross Stance.

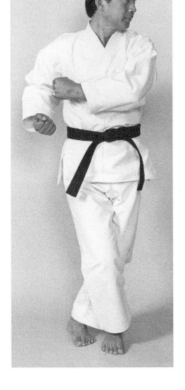

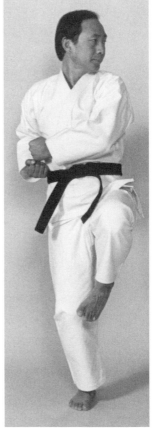

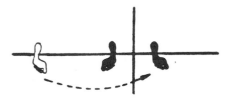

2. Side Kick

a. Execute a Side Kick with your left foot and at the same time execute a left side punch.

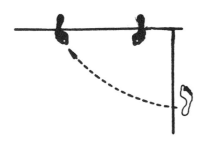

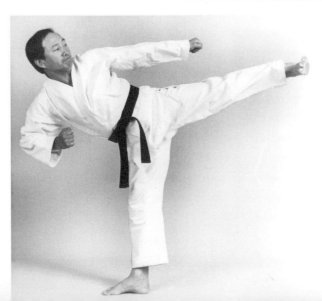

3. Spear-Hand Strike (Horizontal)

a. Step forward with your left foot toward **L-1** and at the same time turn your body toward **R-2** and move your right foot slightly to the right.

b. Assume Right Front Stance.

c. Simultaneously execute a Left Spear-Hand Strike toward **R-2**, palm up, and at the same time bring your right open hand to the left shoulder area, palm up.

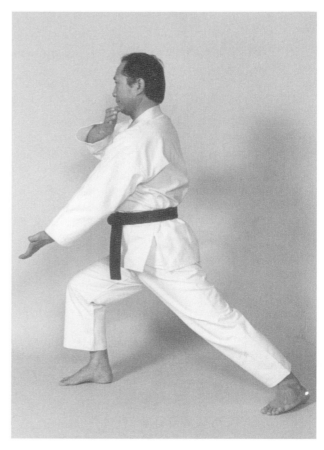

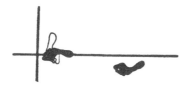

Nineteenth Position:
Low Block

a. Slide your right foot slightly backward

b. Assume Right High Front Stance.

c. Simultaneously execute a Right-Hand Low Block.

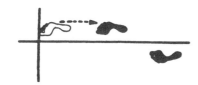

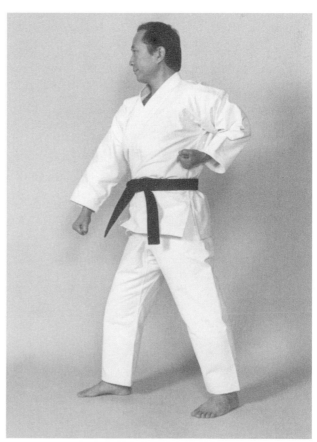

Twentieth Position:
Palm Heel Block (Batangson-Noolleo-Makki), Elbow Attack

1. Palm Heel Block

a. Slide your left foot forward.

b. Assume Left High Front Stance.

c. Simultaneously execute a Left Palm Heel Block to the midsection, palm down.

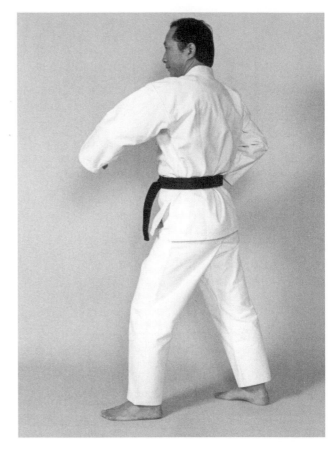

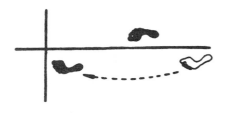

2. Elbow Attack

a. Slide your right foot forward, body turning. Head continues to face **R-2** direction.

b. Assume Horseback Stance.

c. Simultaneously execute a Right Elbow Attack toward **R-2**, with the left hand supporting and pushing right fist.

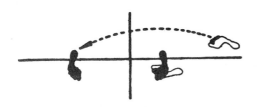

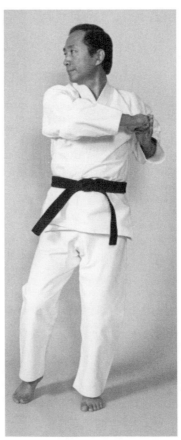

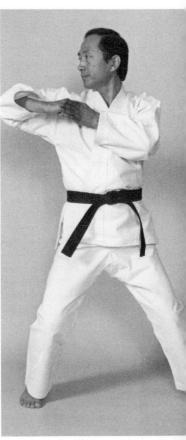

Twenty-First Position: Single Knife-Hand Middle Block

a. Maintain the same stance.

b. Execute a Single Right Knife-Hand Middle Block toward **R-2**, left fist at waist level, palm up.

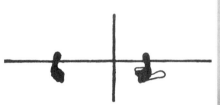

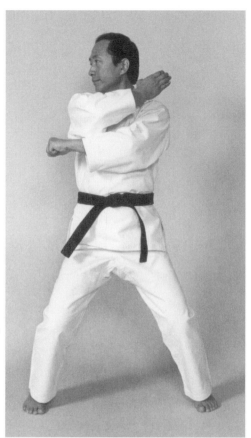

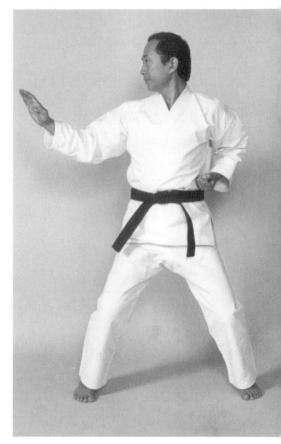

Twenty-Second Position: Target Hook Punch

a. Maintain the same stance.

b. Execute a Target Hook Punch to the Middle section with your left fist hitting right open palm area. (Twist right hand, palm in, so that palm becomes target for punch.)

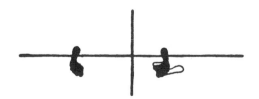

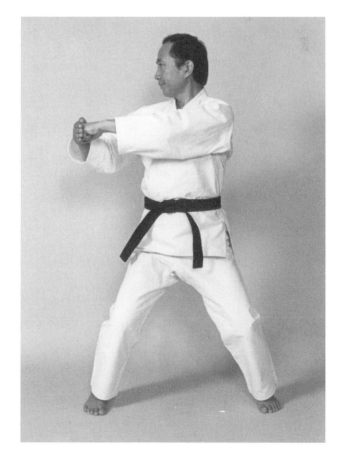

Twenty-Third Position:
(Cross Stance, Side Kick, Spear-Hand Strike)

1. Cross Stance

a. Move your left foot to the right and cross over your right foot. At the same time, bring your fist to the waist, palm up, and bring your right fist over your left fist, palm in.

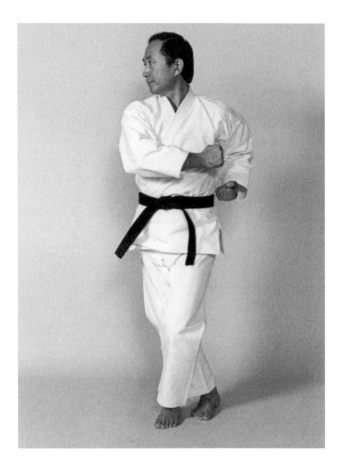

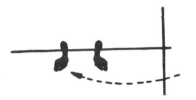

2. Side Kick

a. Execute a Side Kick with your right foot and at the same time execute a Right Side Punch.

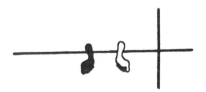

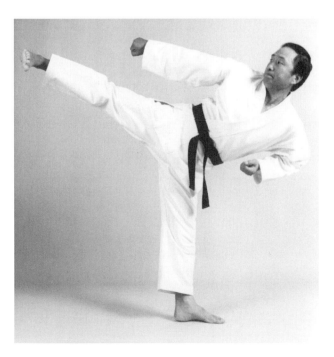

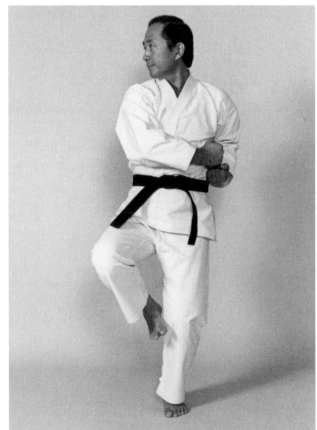

3. Spear-Hand Strike (Horizontal)

a. Step forward with your right foot toward **R-2** and at the same time turn your body toward **L-2**, moving your left foot slightly to the left.

b. Assume Left Front Stance (facing **L-2**).

c. Simultaneously execute a Right Spear-Hand Strike toward **L-1**, palm up, and at the same time bring your left open hand to the right shoulder area.

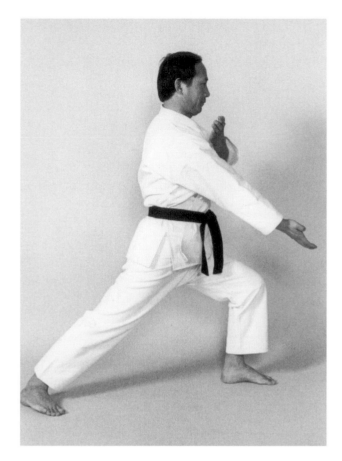

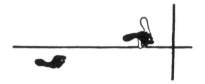

Twenty-Fourth Position:
Low Block

a. Slide your left foot slightly backward.

b. Assume Left High Front Stance.

c. Simultaneously execute a Left-Hand Low Block.

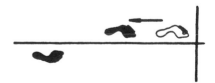

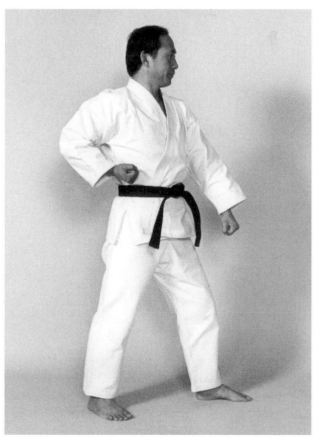

Twenty-Fifth Position:
   Palm Heel Block, Elbow Attack

1. Palm Heel Block

a. Slide your right foot forward.

b. Assume Right High Front Stance.

c. Simultaneously execute a Right Palm Heel Block to the midsection, palm down.

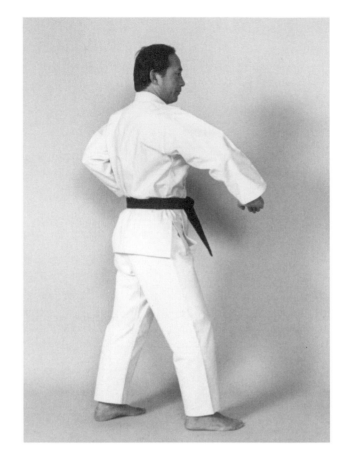

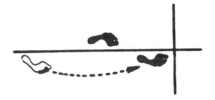

2. Elbow Attack

a. Slide left foot forward (body turning toward **B**), and head continues to face **L-2** direction.

b. Assume Horseback Stance.

c. Simultaneously execute a Left Elbow Attack toward **L-2**, with right hand supporting and pushing left fist.

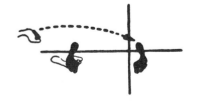

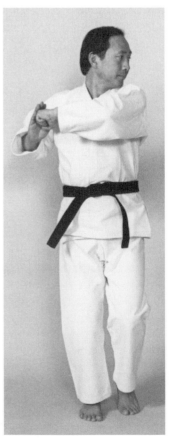

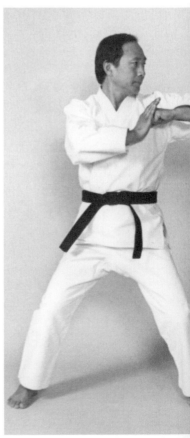

Twenty-Sixth Position:
Hammer Fist Target Strike *(Mejoomeok Pyojeok Chiki)*

a. Slide your right foot next to the left foot.

b. Assume Informal Stance, feet together.

c. Simultaneously lift both hands above the head in slow motion. Then, making a wide circle, execute a Left Hammer Fist Strike, palm out, to the right open palm in front of the abdomen. The above movements should be performed in slow motion with Breathing Control.

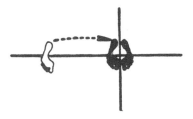

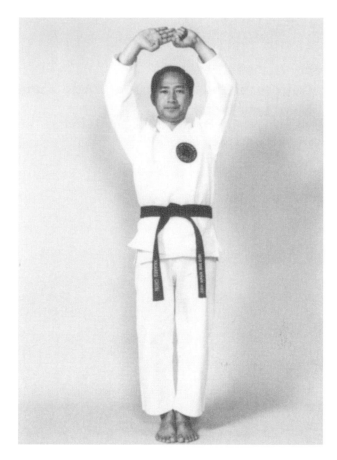

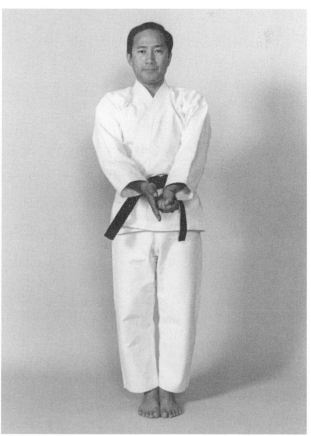

Twenty-Seventh Position:
Outside Knife-Hand Strike, Single Knife-Hand Low Block

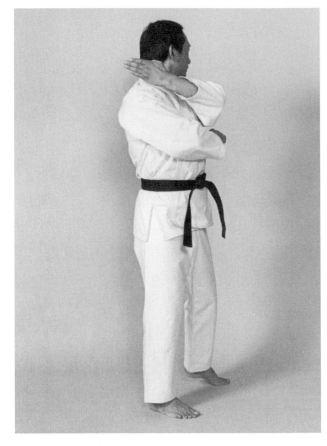

1. Outside Knife-Hand Strike

a. Pivoting to the left on the ball of your right foot and making a 180° turn facing **A**, slide your left foot out to the left and forward one step toward **A**.

b. Assume Left Front Stance

c. Simultaneously execute an Outside Left Knife-Hand Strike, palm down.

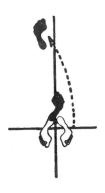

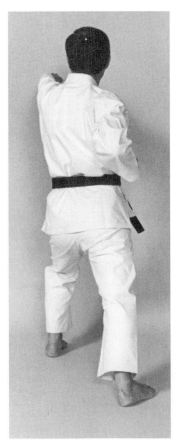

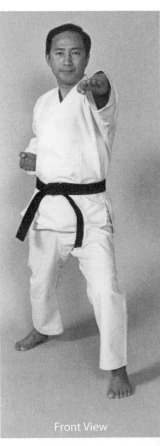

Front View

2. Single Knife-Hand Low Block

a. Maintain the same stance.

b. Execute a Single Left Knife-Hand Low Block.

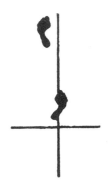

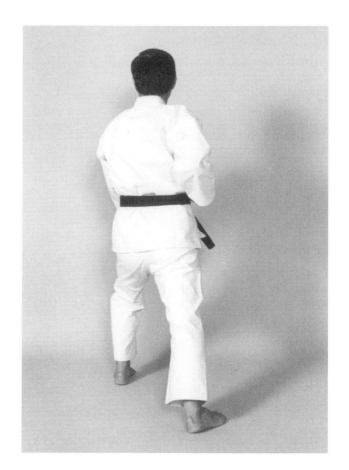

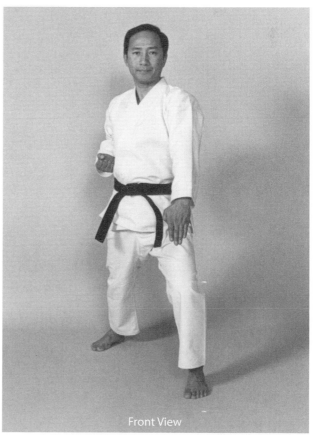

Front View

Twenty-Eighth Position:
Inside Knife-Hand Strike, Single Knife-Hand
Low Block

1. Inside Knife-Hand Strike

a. Slide your right foot forward.

b. Assume Right Front Stance.

c. Simultaneously execute an Inside Right Knife-Hand Strike to the neck, palm up.

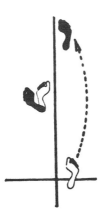

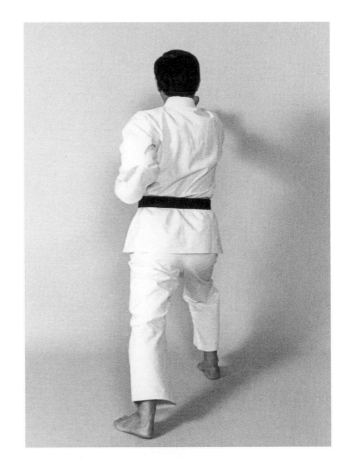

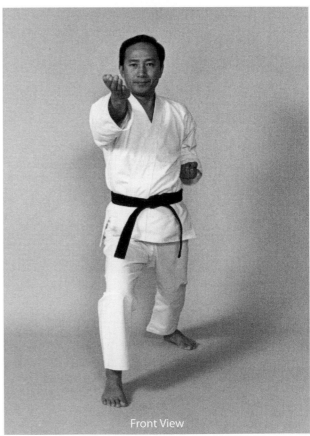

Front View

2. Single Knife-Hand Low Block

a. Maintain the same stance.

b. Execute a single Right Knife-Hand Low Block.

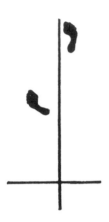

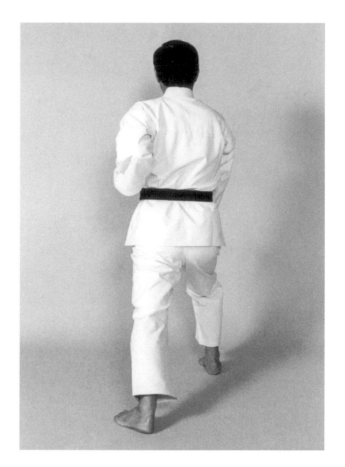

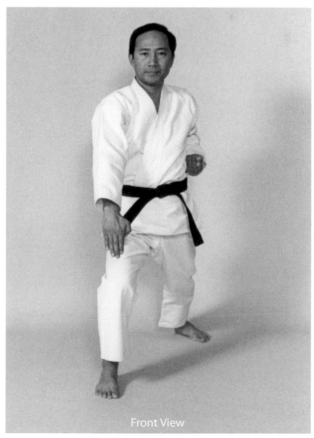

Front View

Twenty-Ninth Position:
Inside Knife-Hand Strike, Single Knife-Hand Low Block

1. Inside Knife-Hand Strike

a. Slide your left foot forward.

b. Assume Left Front Stance.

c. Simultaneously execute an Inside Left Knife-Hand Strike to the neck, palm up.

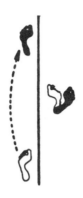

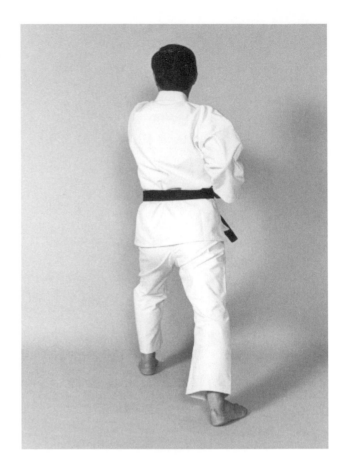

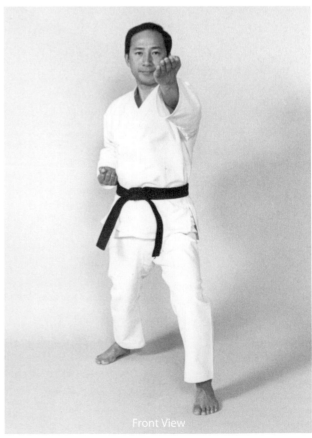

Front View

2. Single Knife-Hand Low Block

a. Maintain the same stance.

b. Execute a Single Left Knife-Hand Low Block.

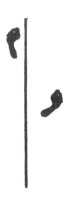

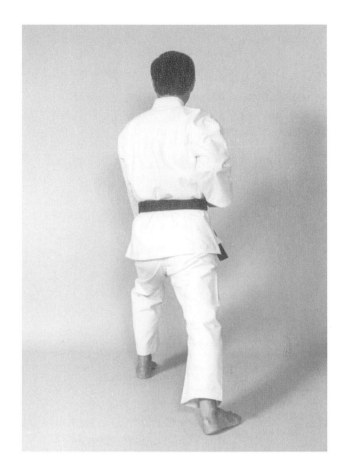

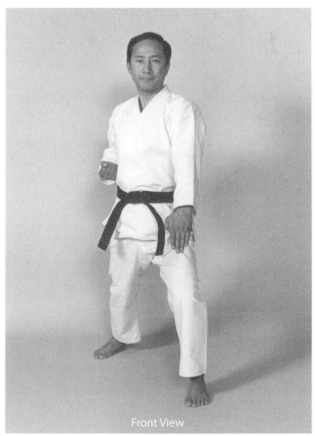

Front View

Thirtieth Position:
Tiger-Mouth Thrust and Yell

a. Slide your right foot forward.

b. Assume Right Front Stance.

c. Simultaneously execute a Right Tiger-Mouth Thrust to the throat and yell.

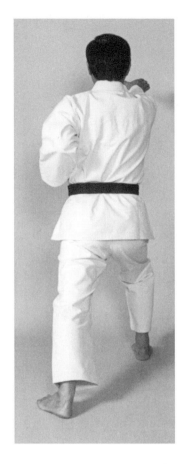

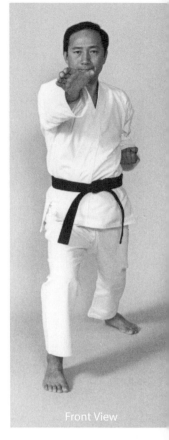

Front View

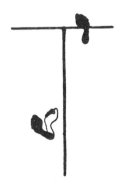

Stop

Pivoting to the left on the ball of your right foot, turn your body 180° to the left toward B. At the same time slide your left foot backward into Barrel-Pushing Ready Stance, facing B at Point A.

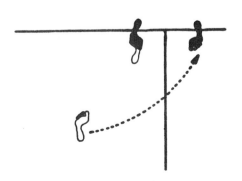

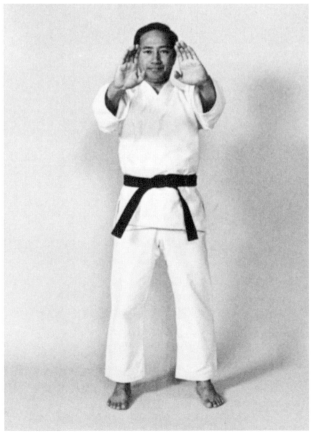

KEUMGANG (DIAMOND)

The diamond is the hardest substance known to man. It also can represent perfection and clarity: the flawless diamond is of great value. It also is a symbol of beauty, and because of this meaning, the Korean people have named the most beautiful mountain range in the Korean peninsula *Keumgang*. The theme of a diamond's strength carries into Buddhism, where that which can break off every agony of mind with the combination of wisdom and virtue is call Keumgang.

The form Keumgang moves to outline the Chinese character for mountain (山). Your movements in this form must be based on a spiritual strength that is as beautiful in its perfection as the Diamond Mountains and is as hard and adamant as the diamond, strong enough to cut off all distractions.

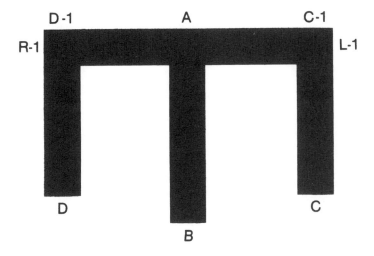

Keumgang

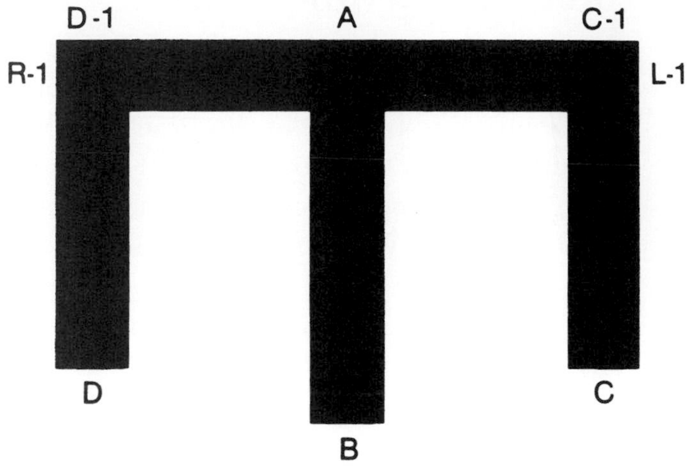

D-1   A   C-1

R-1   L-1

D   C

B

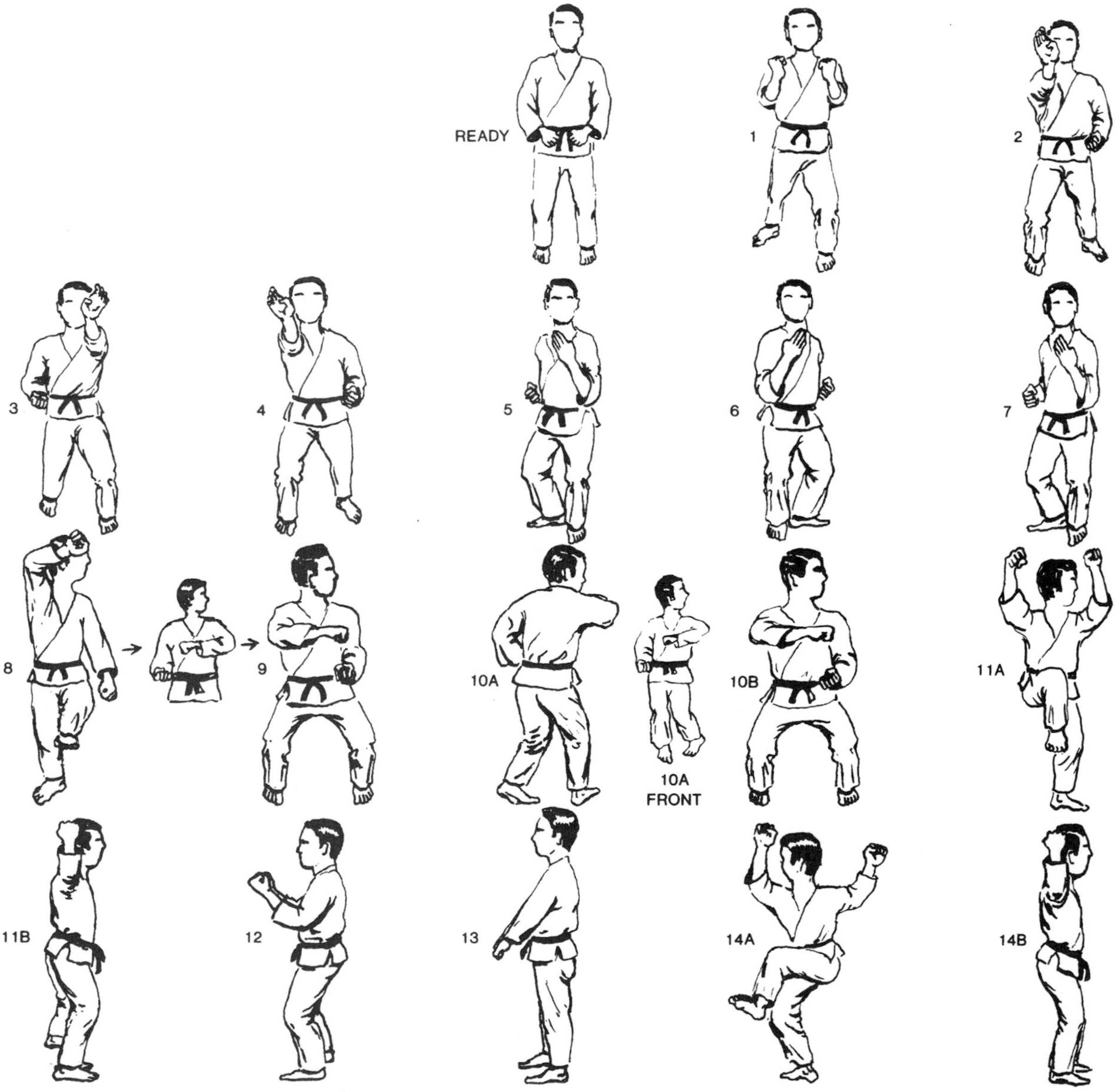

READY   1   2

3   4   5   6   7

8   9   10A   10A FRONT   10B   11A

11B   12   13   14A   14B

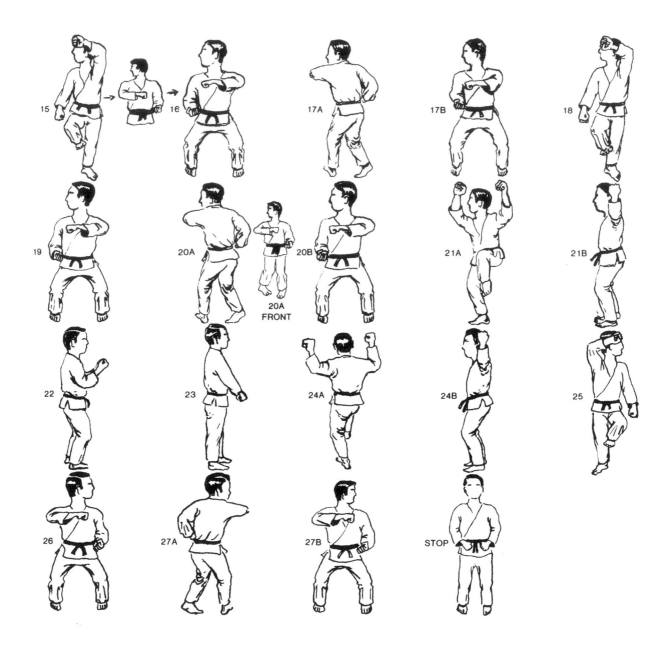

Ready.

Maintain Ready Stance, facing **B** at point **A**, eyes focused straight ahead.

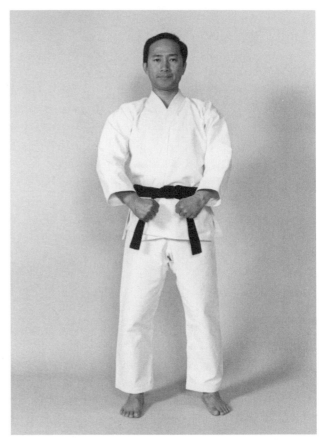

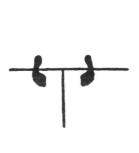

First Position:
   Spread Middle Block (Palms In)

   a. Slide your left foot forward toward **B**.

   b. Assume Left Front Stance.

   c. Simultaneously execute a Spread Middle Block, palms in.

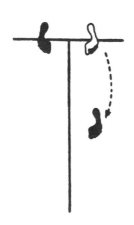

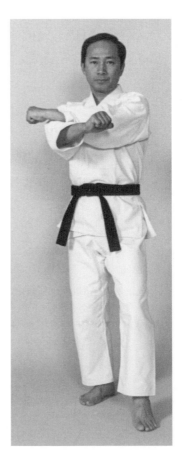

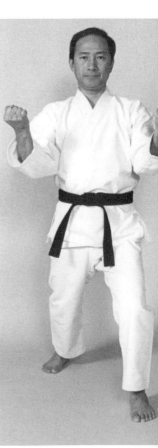

Second Position:

Palm Heel Strike to the Chin *(Batangson-Teok-Chiki)*

a. Slide your right foot forward.

b. Assume Right Front Stance.

c. Simultaneously execute a Right Palm Heel Strike to the chin.

Note: The above motion should be performed slowly with tension

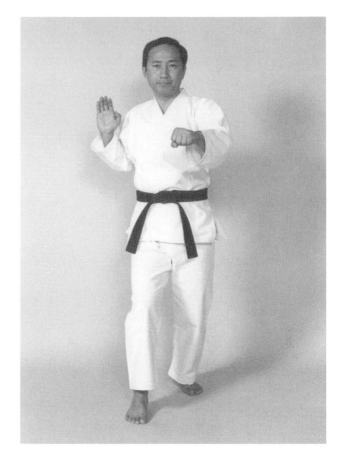

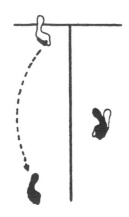

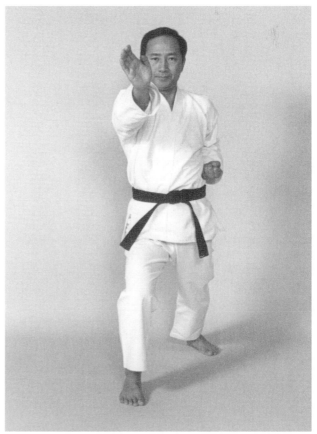

Third Position:
Palm Heel Strike to the Chin

a. Slide your left foot forward.

b. Assume Left Front Stance.

c. Simultaneously execute a Left Palm Heel Strike to the chin.

Note: The above motion should be performed slowly with tension

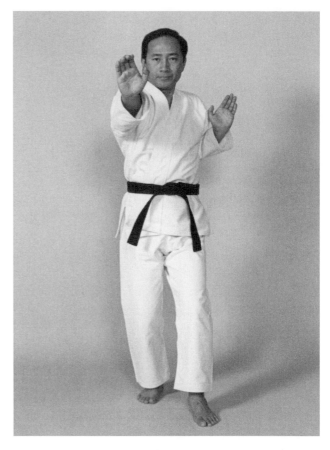

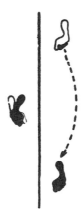

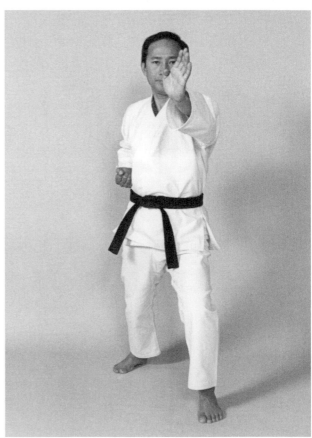

Fourth Position:
Palm Heel Strike to the Chin

a. Slide your right foot forward.

b. Assume Right Front Stance.

c. Simultaneously execute a Right Palm Heel Strike to the chin.

Note: The above motion should be performed slowly with tension.

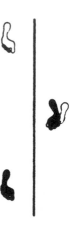

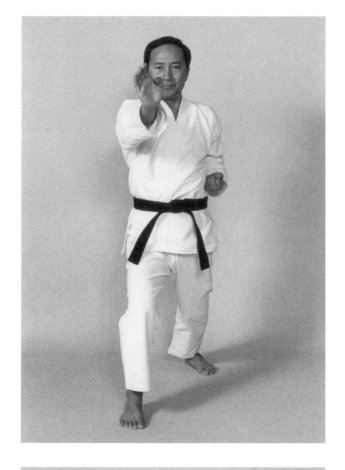

Fifth Position:
Single Knife-Hand Inside Middle Block

a. Pivoting slightly to the right on the ball of you foot, slide your right foot backward (toward **A**).

b. Assume Left Back Stance.

c. Simultaneously execute a Left Single Knife-Hand Inside Middle Block.

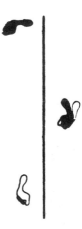

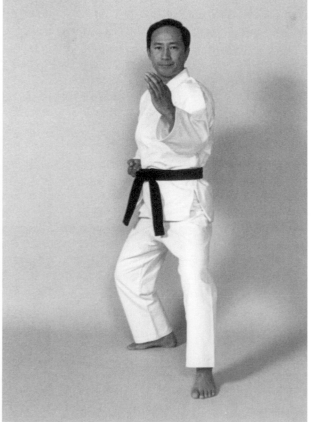

Sixth Position:
Single Knife-Hand Inside Middle Block

a. Pivoting 90° to the left on the ball of your right foot, slide your left foot backward.

b. Assume Right Back Stance.

c. Simultaneously execute a Right Single Knife-Hand Inside Middle Block.

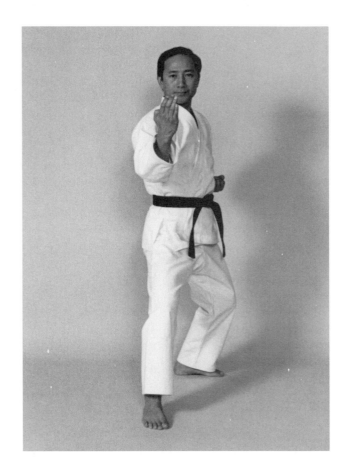

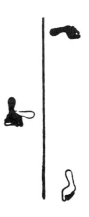

Seventh Position:
Single Knife-Hand Inside Middle Block

a. Pivoting 90° to the right on the ball of your left foot, slide your right foot backward.

b. Assume Left Back Stance.

c. Simultaneously execute a Left Single Knife-Hand Inside Middle Block.

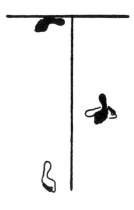

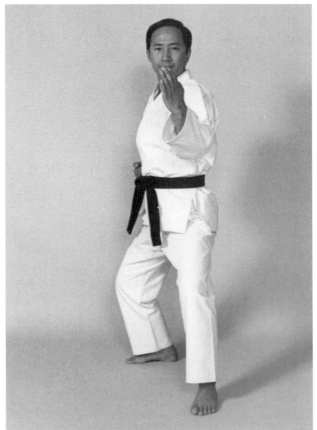

Eighth Position:

Diamond Block (Keumgang-Makki)

a. Pivoting 90° to the left on the ball of your right foot, bring your left foot next to your right knee. Body faces **B**, and head turns toward **L-1**.

b. Assume Right Crane Stance (Oreun-Haktari-Seogi).

c. Simultaneously execute a Diamond Block in Slow Motion with tension. (This is a simultaneous Right-Hand High Block and a Left-Hand Low Block to the side toward **L-1**).

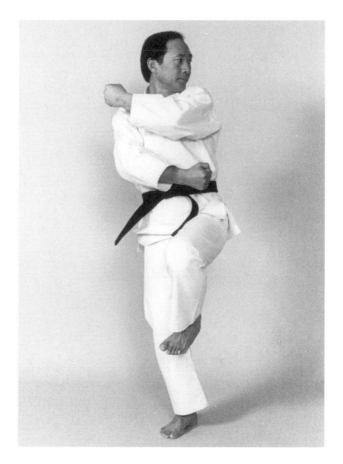

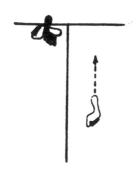

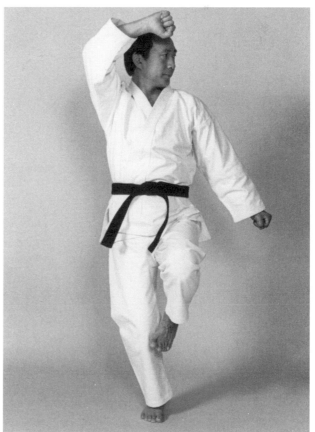

Ninth Position:
Hook Punch (Keun-Dolcheogi)

a. Bring both fists to the right, right fist at waist, palm up, and left fist at chest level, palm down. Then step out to the left with your left foot toward **L-1**.

b. Assume Horseback Stance.

c. Simultaneously execute a Right Hook Punch, palm down, to the midsection toward **L-1** and bring left fist to the waist, palm up.

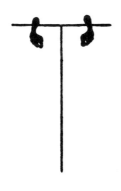

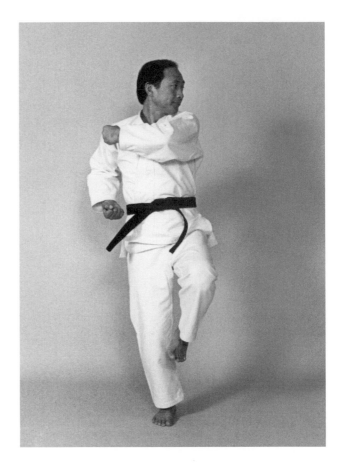

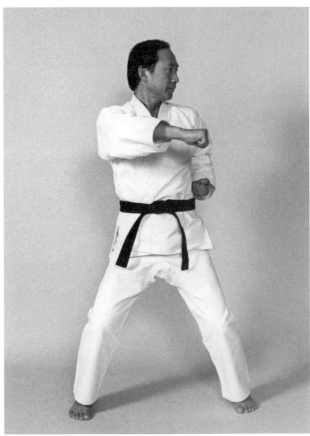

Tenth Position:
Turn with Hook Punch Preparation, Hook Punch

1. Turn with Hook Punch Preparation

a. Pivoting about 180° to the left on the ball of your left foot, slide your right foot toward **L-1** next to your left foot, about one foot length apart. At the same time bring both fists to the right, left fist at waist, palm up, and right fist at chest level, palm down.

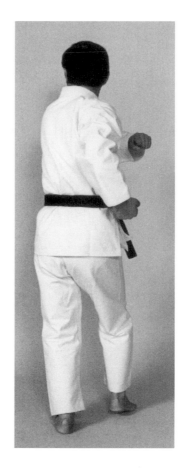
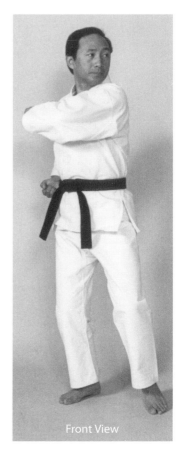

Front View

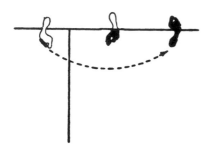

2. Hook Punch

a. Pivoting about 180° to the left on the ball of your right foot, slide your left foot backward toward **L-1** (head facing **L-1**).

b. Assume Horseback Stance.

c. Simultaneously execute a Right Hook Punch to the midsection toward **L-1**.

Note: Tenth Position, 1 and 2, should be performed rapidly as a continuous motion. The body turns a total of 360°.

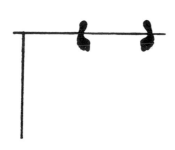

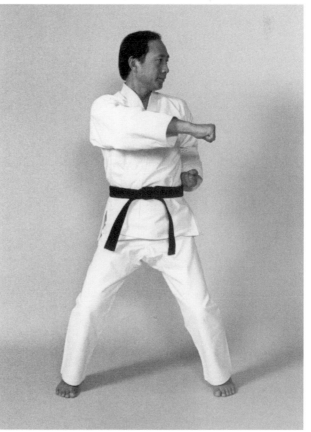

Eleventh Position:
Preparation for Mountain Block, Mountain Block (Santeul-Makki) and Yell

1. Preparation for Mountain Block
a. Pivoting slightly to the left on the ball of your left foot, raise your right knee to waist level with a tensed instep. At the same time raise both fists to head level, right fist palm out a left fist palm in.

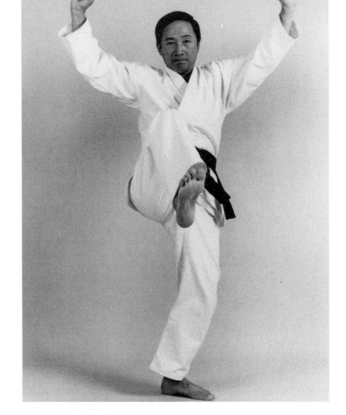

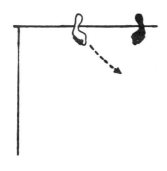

2. Mountain Block
a. Continuing to pivot to the left on the ball of your left foot, step towards **C** with your right foot (toes, body, and head facing **L**) to complete a 90° turn.

b. Assume Horseback Stance.

c. Simultaneously execute a Mountain Block and yell. (This block is completed by twisting both wrists simultaneously so that palms face in at head level on either side. The blocking surface is the outer edge of forearms.)

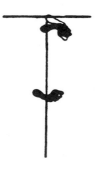

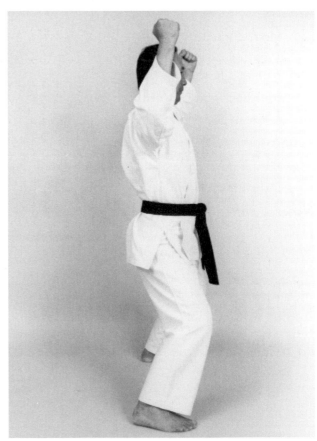

Twelfth Position:
Spread Middle Block
(Palms In)

a. Pivoting 180° to the right on the ball of your right foot, slide your left foot to the right, toward **C**, toes, body, and head facing **R**.

b. Assume Horseback Stance.

c. Simultaneously execute a Spread Middle Block, palms in. (This block is executed by crossing both forearms in front of face, palms down, and then sweeping both arms outward simultaneously, palms in.)

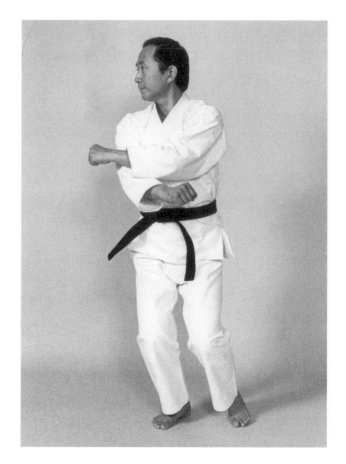

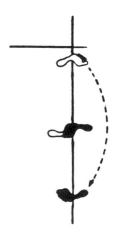

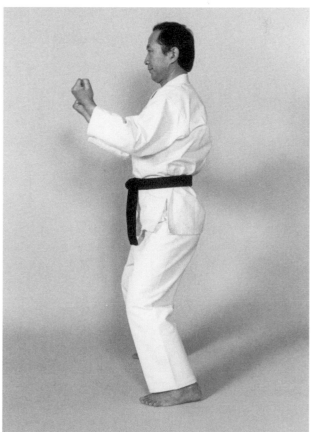

Thirteenth Position:
Spread Low Block (Palms In)

a. Keeping your right foot in place, slide your left foot slightly to the right.

b. Assume Ready Stance.

c. Simultaneously execute a Spread Low Block, palms in. (This block is executed by crossing both forearms in front of chest, palms in, and then sweeping both arms down and out simultaneously, palms in.)

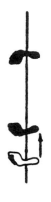

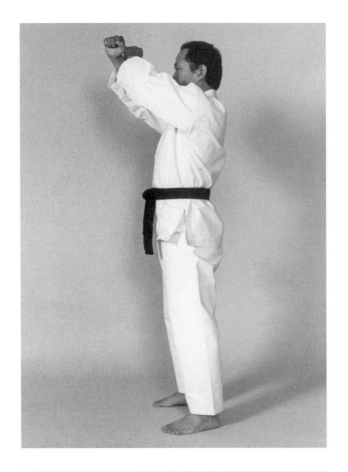

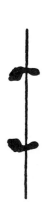

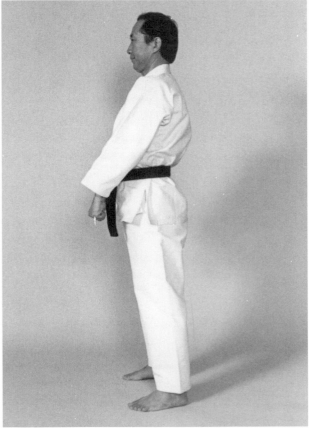

Fourteenth Position:
Preparation for Mountain Block and Yell

1. Preparation for Mountain Block

a. Pivoting slightly to the right on the ball of your right foot raise your left knee to waist level with a tensed instep. At the same time raise both fists to head level, left fist palm out right fist palm in.

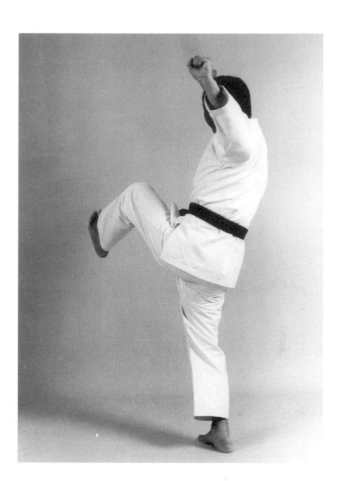

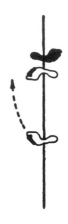

2. Mountain Block

a. Continuing to pivot to the right on the ball of your right foot, step toward **C-1** with your left foot (toes, body, and head facing **L-1**) to complete a 90° turn.

b. Assume Horseback Stance.

c. Simultaneously execute a Mountain Block and yell.

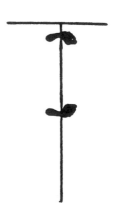

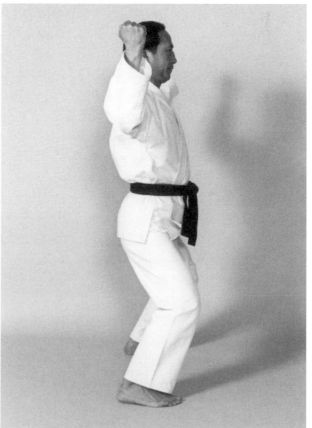

Fifteenth Position:
Diamond Block

a. Pivoting 90° to the right on the ball of your left foot, bring your right foot next to your left knee. Body faces **C**, and head turns toward **A**.

b. Assume Left Crane Stance.

c. Simultaneously execute a Diamond Block in slow motion with tension (This is a simultaneous Left-Hand High Block and a Right-Hand Low Block to the side toward **A**.)

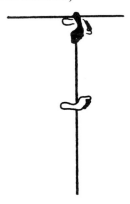

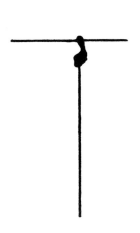

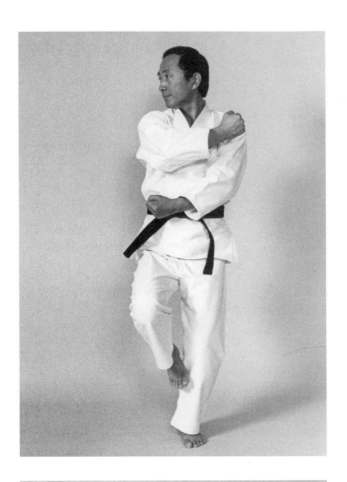

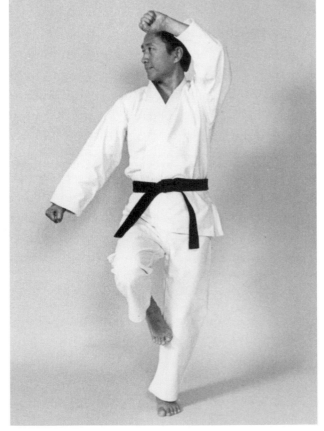

Sixteenth Position:
Hook Punch

a. Bring both fists to the left, left fist at waist, palm up, and right fist at chest level, palm down. Then step out to the right with your right foot toward **A**.

b. Assume Horseback Stance.

c. Simultaneously execute a Left Hook Punch to the midsection toward **A**.

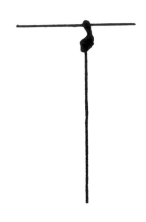

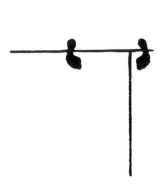

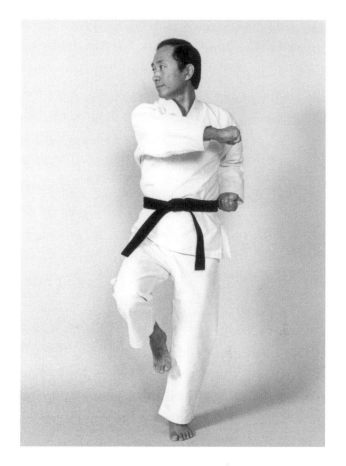

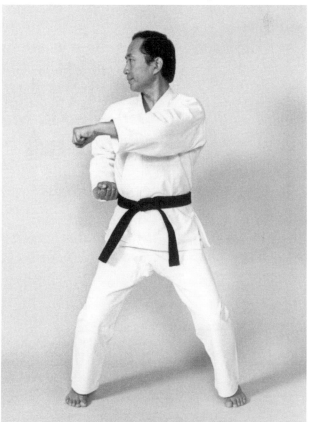

Seventeenth Position:
Turn with Hook Punch Preparation, Hook Punch

1. Turn with Hook Punch Preparation

a. Pivoting about 180° to the right on the ball of your right foot, slide your left foot toward **A** next to your right foot, about one foot length apart. At the same time, bring both fists to the left, left fist at waist, palm up, and right fist at chest level, palm down.

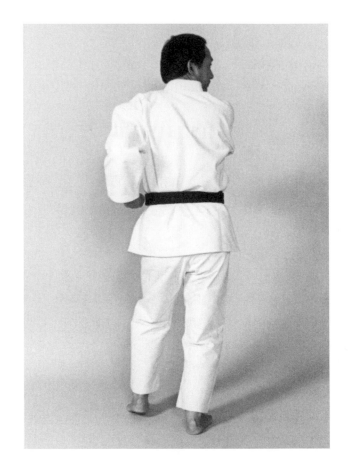

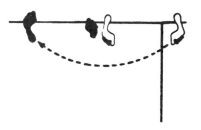

2. Hook Punch

a. Pivoting about 180° to the right on the ball of your left foot, slide your right foot backward toward **A** (Head faces **R-1**).

b. Assume Horseback Stance.

c. Simultaneously execute a Left Hook Punch to the midsection toward **R-1**.

Note: Seventeenth Position, 1 and 2 should be performed rapidly as a continuous motion. The body turns a total of 360°.

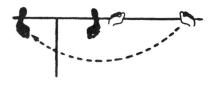

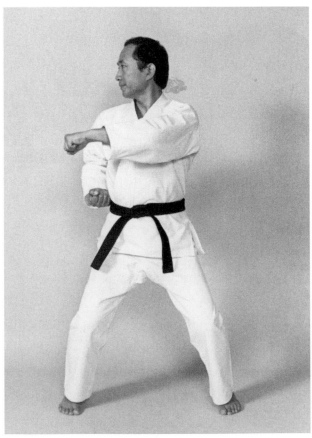

Eighteenth Position:
Diamond Block

a. Keeping your left foot in place, bring your right foot next to your left knee.

b. Assume Left Crane Stance.

c. Simultaneously execute a Diamond Block in slow motion with tension.

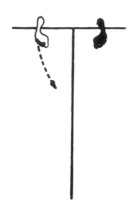

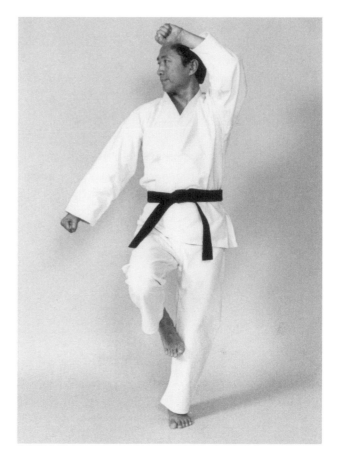

Nineteenth Position:
Hook Punch

a. Bring both fists to the left, left fist at waist, palm up, and right fist at chest level, palm down. Then step out to the right with our right foot toward **R-1**.

b. Assume Horseback Stance.

c. Simultaneously execute a Left Hook Punch to the midsection toward **R-1**.

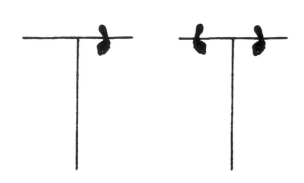

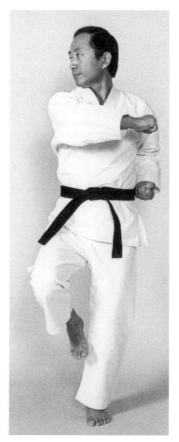

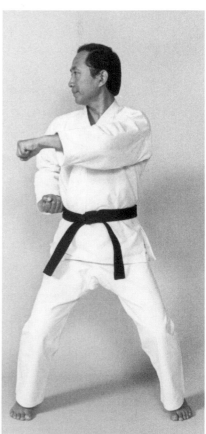

Twentieth Position:
 Turn with Hook Punch Preparation, Hook Punch

1. Turn with Hook Punch Preparation

a. Pivoting about 180° to the right on the ball of your right foot, slide your left foot toward **A** next to your right foot, about one-foot length apart. At the same time, bring both fists to the left, left fist at waist, palm up, and right fist at chest level, palm down.

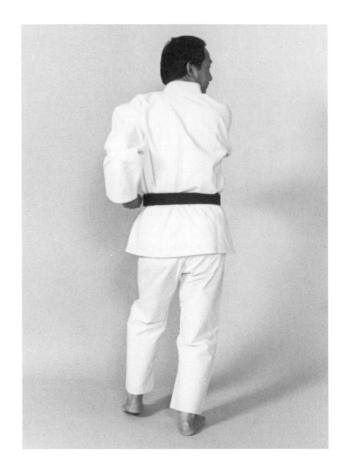

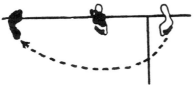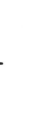

2. Hook Punch

a. Pivoting about 180° to the right on the ball of your left foot, slide your right foot backward toward **R-1** (head faces **R-1**).

b. Assume Horseback Stance.

c. Simultaneously execute a Left Hook Punch to the midsection toward **R-1**.

Note: Twentieth Position, 1 and 2, should be performed rapidly as a continuous motion. The body turns a total of 360°.

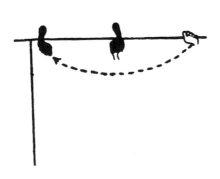

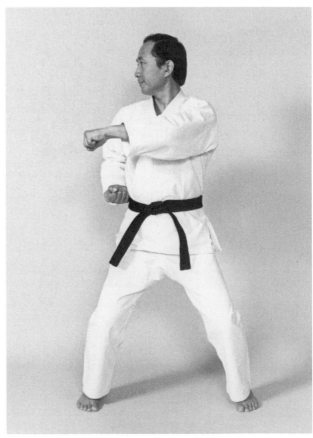

Twenty-First Position:
 Preparation for Mountain Block, Mountain Block, and Yell

1. **Preparation for Mountain Block**
a. Pivoting slightly to the right on the ball of your right foot, raise your left knee to waist level with a tensed instep. At the same time raise both fists to head level, left fist palm out and right fist palm in.

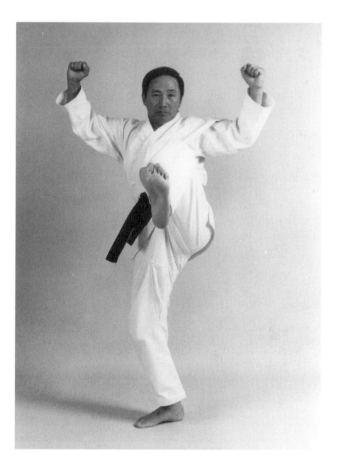

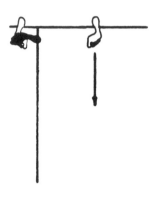

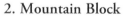

2. **Mountain Block**
a. Continuing to pivot to the right on the ball of your right foot, step toward **D** with your left foot (toes, body, and head face **R**) to complete a 90° turn.

b. Assume Horseback Stance.

c. Simultaneously execute a Mountain Block and yell.

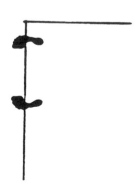

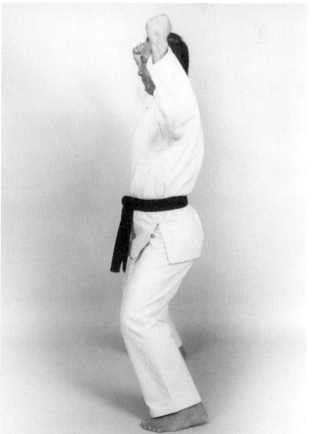

Twenty-Second Position:
  Spread Middle Block (Palms In)

a. Pivoting 180° to the left on the ball of your left foot, slide your right root to the left toward **D** (toes, body, and head face **L**).

b. Assume Horseback Stance.

c. Simultaneously execute a Spread Middle Block, palms in. This block should be performed rapidly.

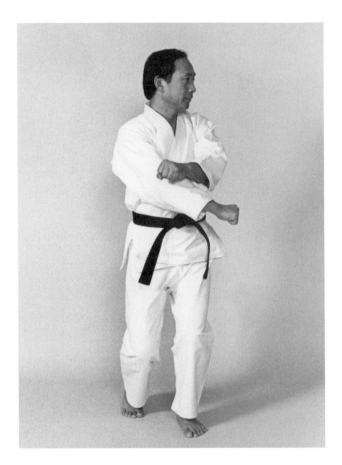

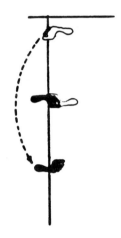

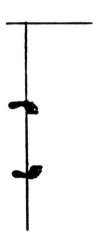

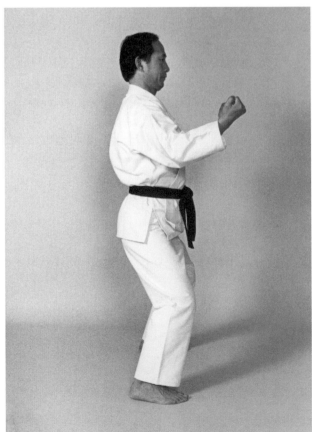

Twenty-Third Position:
Spread Low Block (Palms In)

a. Keeping your left foot in place, slide your right foot slightly to the left.

b. Assume Horseback Stance.

c. Simultaneously execute a Spread Low Block, palms in.

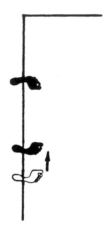

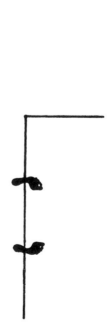

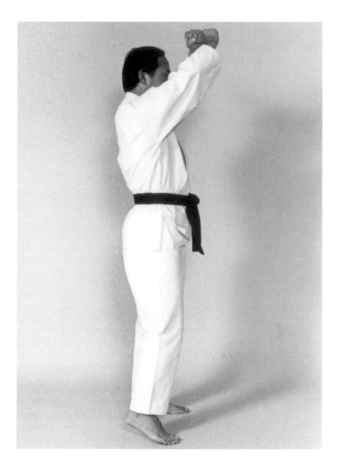

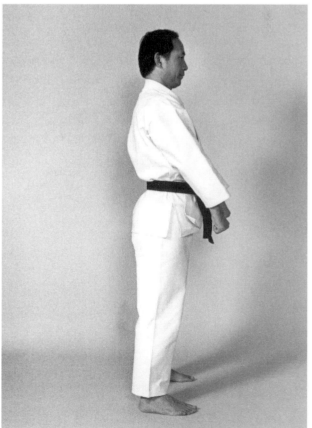

Twenty-Fourth Position:
  Preparation for Mountain Block, Mountain Block, and Yell

1. Preparation for Mountain Block

a. Pivoting slightly to the left on the ball of your left foot, raise your right knee to waist level with a tensed instep. At the same time, raise both fists to head level, right fist palm out and left fist palm in.

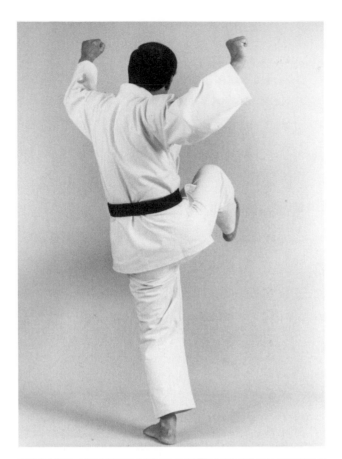

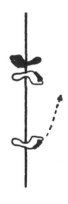

2. Mountain Block

a. Continuing to pivot to the left on the ball of your left foot, step toward **D-1** with your right foot (toes, body, and head face **R-1**) to complete a 90° turn.

b. Assume Horseback Stance.

c. Simultaneously execute a Mountain Block and yell.

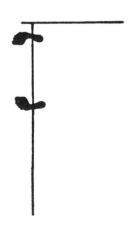

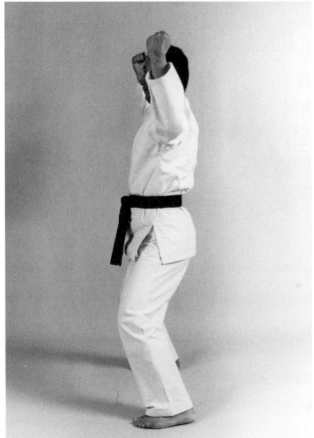

Twenty-Fifth Position:
Diamond Block

a. Pivoting 90° to the right on the ball of your right foot, bring your left foot next to your right knee. Body faces **D**, and head turns toward **A**.

b. Assume Left Crane Stance.

c. Simultaneously execute a Diamond Block in slow motion with tension.

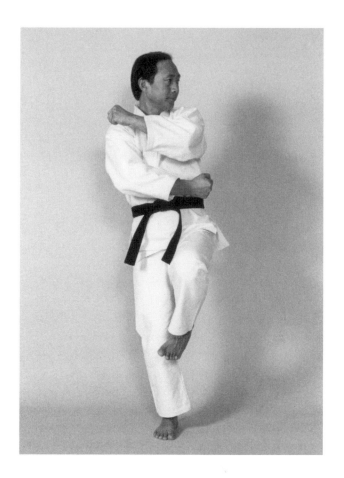

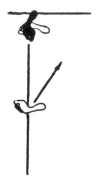

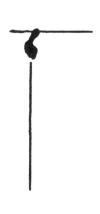

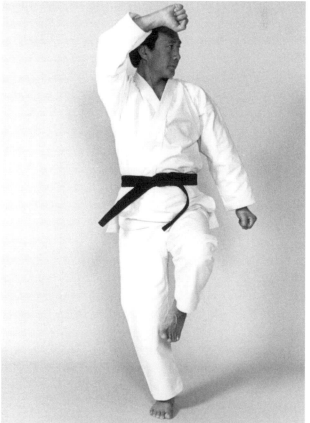

Twenty-Sixth Position:
Hook Punch

a. Bring both fists to the right, right fist at waist, palm up, and left fist at chest level, palm down. Then step out to the left with your left foot toward **A**.

b. Assume Horseback Stance.

c. Simultaneously execute a Right Hook Punch to the midsection toward **A**.

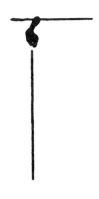

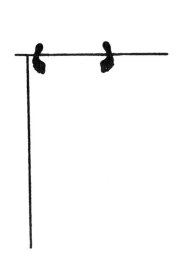

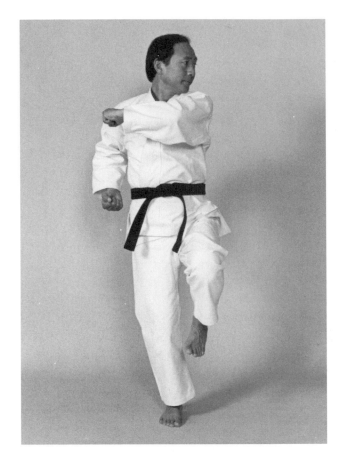

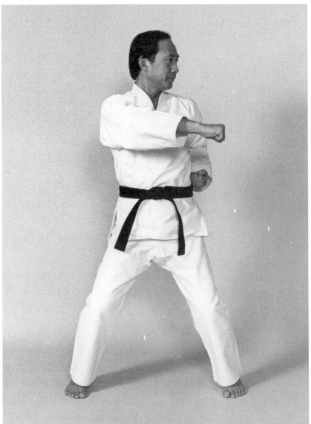

Twenty-Seventh Position:
Turn with Hook Punch Preparation, Hook Punch

1. **Turn with Hook Punch Preparation**
a. Pivoting about 180° to the left on the ball of your left foot, slide your right foot toward **A** next to your left foot, about one foot length apart. At the same time bring both fists to the right, right fist at waist, palm up, and left at chest level, palm down.

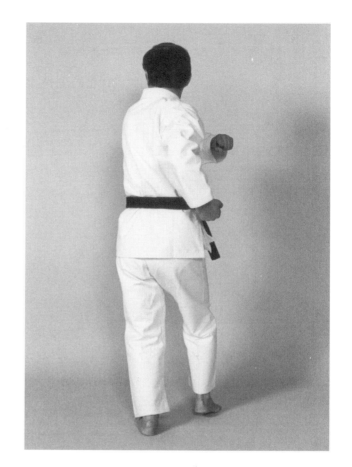

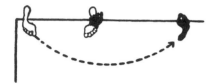

2. **Hook Punch**
a. Pivoting about 180° to the left on the ball of your right foot, slide your left foot backward toward **A** (head faces **L-1**).
b. Assume Horseback Stance.
c. Simultaneously execute a Right Hook Punch to the midsection toward **A**.

Note: Twenty-Seventh Position, 1 and 2, should be performed rapidly as a continuous motion. The body turns a total of 360°.

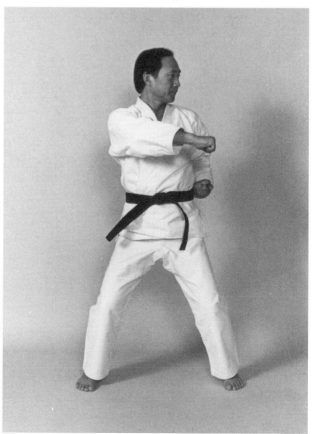

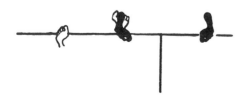

Stop

Keeping your right foot in place, slide your left foot slightly to the right. Maintain Ready Stance, face **B** at point **A**, eyes focused straight ahead.

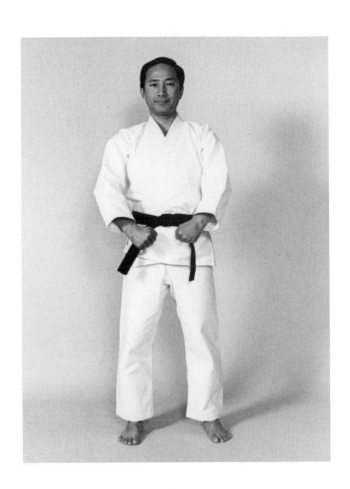

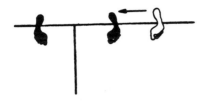

TAEBAEK (MOUNTAIN)

The mythological story about the founding of Korea says that about 4,300 years ago, the legendary Dangoon began the nation in *Taebaek*, which is currently Mount Baekdoo. This is the loftiest mountain in Korea and is thus held sacred, as the mountain reaches toward the sun, the word Taebaek has also grown to mean light, and Mount Baekdoo is regarded as the symbol of Korea.

In the form Taebaek you must demonstrate the rigor and determined will of the Korean people, displaying the respect due a sacred object. It must be performed also with the precision and agility of light.

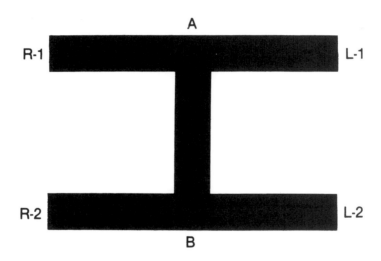

Taebaek

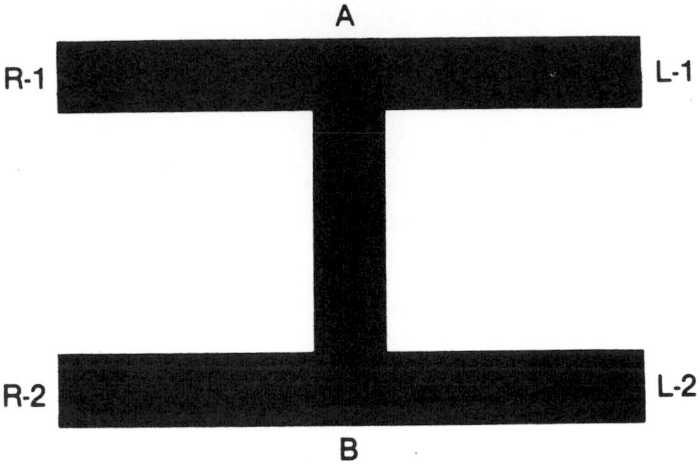

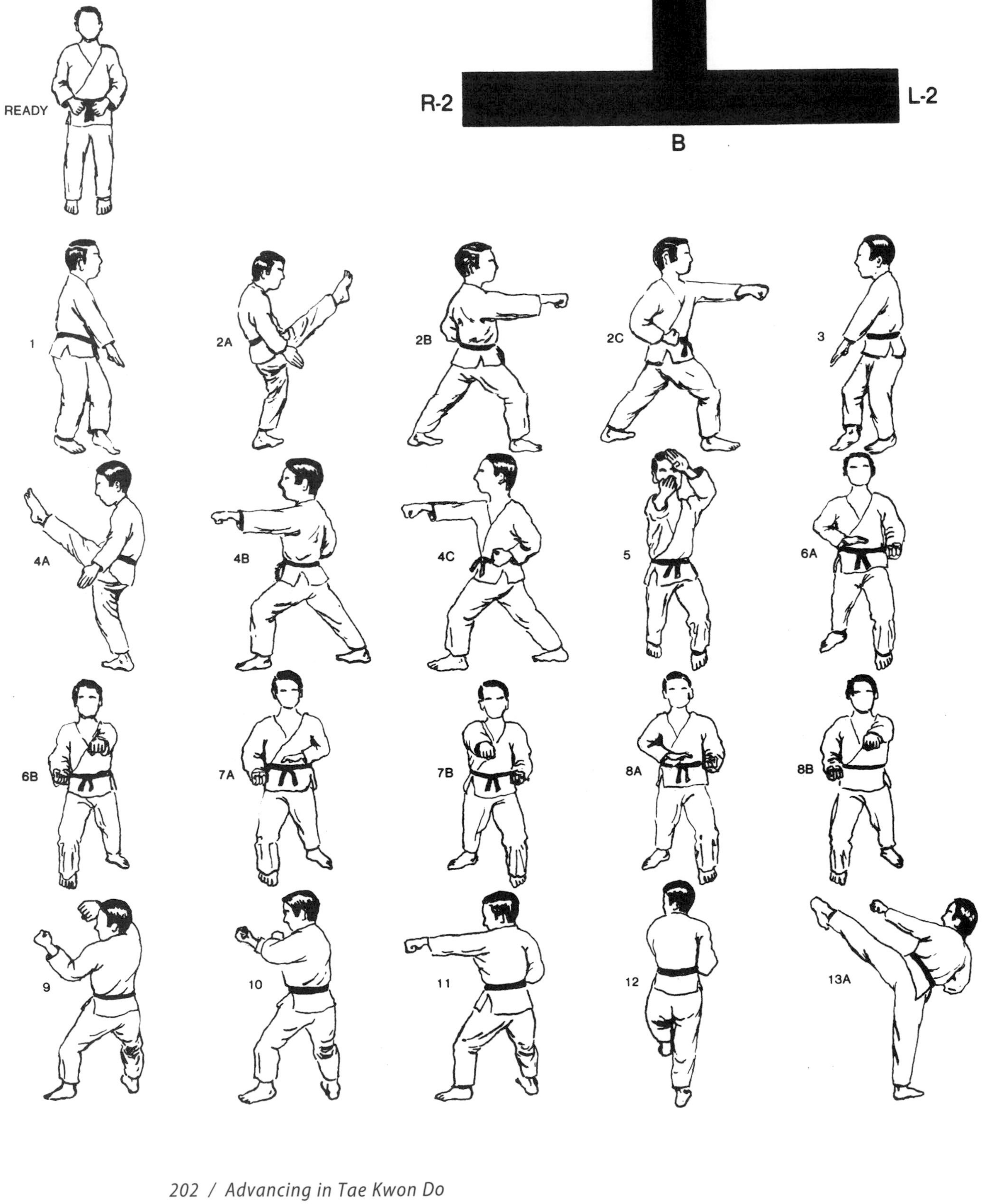

READY

1 2A 2B 2C 3

4A 4B 4C 5 6A

6B 7A 7B 8A 8B

9 10 11 12 13A

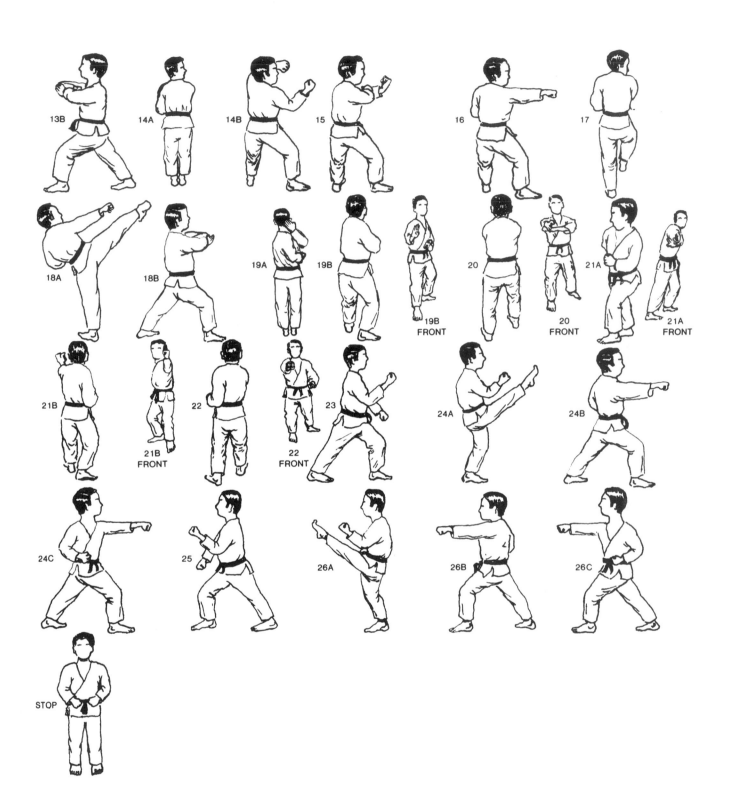

Ready

Maintain Ready Stance, facing **B** at point **A**, eyes focused straight ahead.

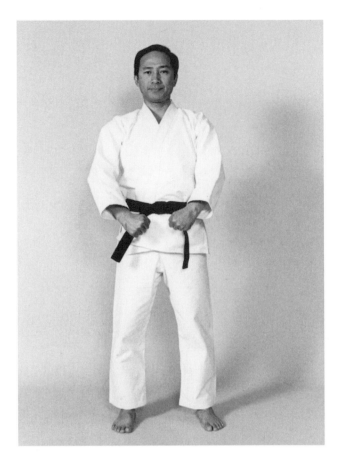

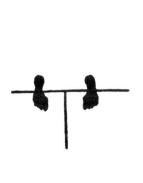

First Position:
Spread Knife-Hand Low Block

a. Slide your left foot 90° to the left (toward **L-1**).

b. Assume Left Cat Stance.

c. Simultaneously execute a Spread Knife-Hand Low Block.

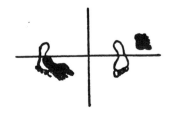

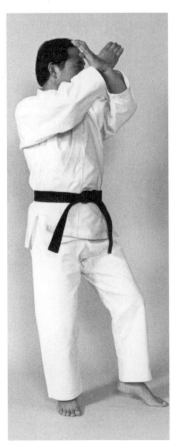

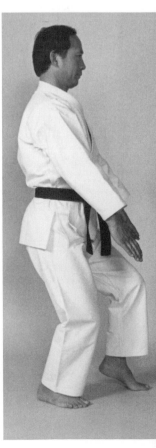

Second Position:
Front Kick, Middle Punch, Reverse Middle Punch

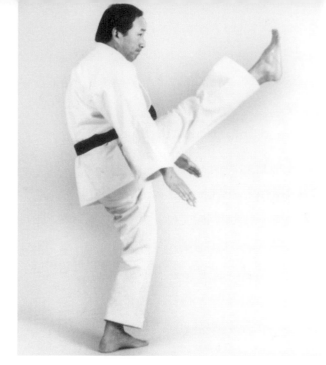

1. Front Kick

a. Execute a Front Kick with your right foot to the face.

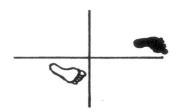

2. Middle Punch

a. Step forward with your right foot.

b. Assume Right Front Stance

c. Simultaneously execute a Right-Hand Middle Punch

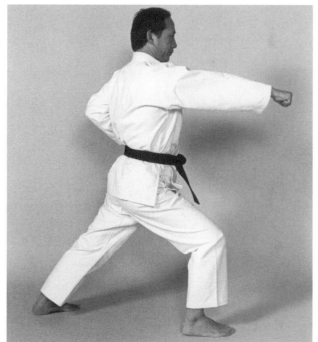

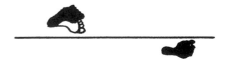

3. Reverse Middle Punch

a. Maintain the same stance.

b. Execute a Left-Hand Reverse Middle Punch

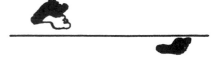

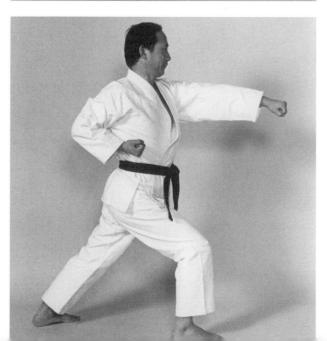

Third Position:
Spread Knife-Hand Low Block

   a. Pivoting to the right on the ball of your left foot, slide your right foot out and back in a wide arc, turning 180° to the right (toward **R-1**).

   b. Assume Right Cat Stance

   c. Simultaneously execute a Spread Knife-Hand Low Block.

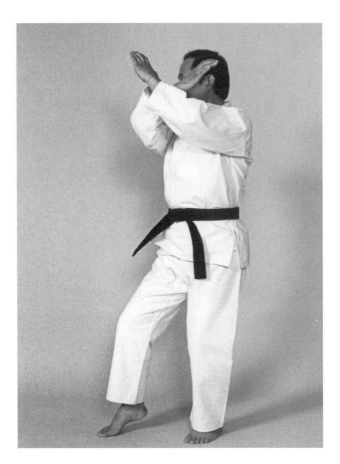

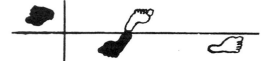

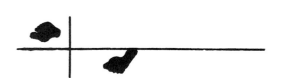

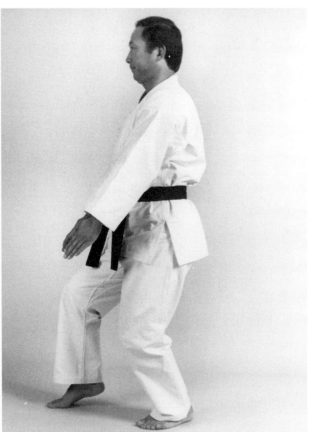

Fourth Position:
Front Kick, Middle Punch, Reverse Middle Punch

1. Front Kick

a. Execute a Front Kick with your left foot to the face.

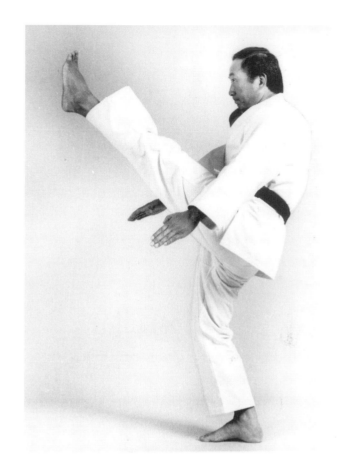

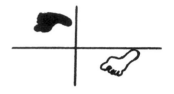

2. Middle Punch

a. Step forward with your left foot.

b. Assume Left Front Stance.

c. Simultaneously execute a Left-Hand Middle Punch.

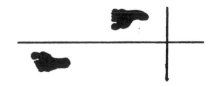

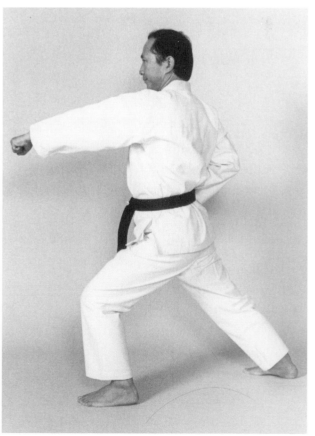

3. Reverse Middle Punch

a. Maintain the same stance.

b. Execute a Right-Hand Reverse Middle Punch.

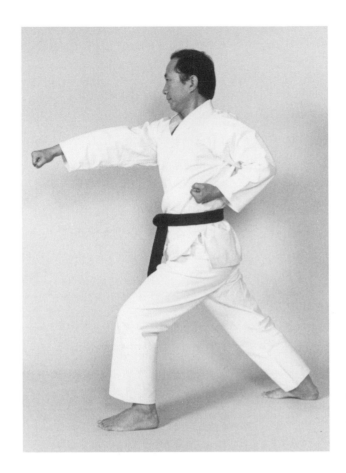

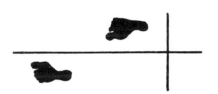

Fifth Position:
Left Knife-Hand High Block and Right Knife-Hand Strike (Jebipoom-Sonnal-Mok-Chiki)

a. Pivoting to the left on the ball of your right foot, slide your left foot out, turning 90° to the left (toward **B**).

b. Assume Left Front Stance.

c. Simultaneously execute a Knife-Hand High Block with your left hand and a Knife-Hand Strike to the neck of imaginary opponent, near **B**, with your right hand. (The blocking surface is the outer edge of left knife-hand, palm out, above forehead. The knife-hand strike to the neck is made from outside to inside with the right hand palm up.)

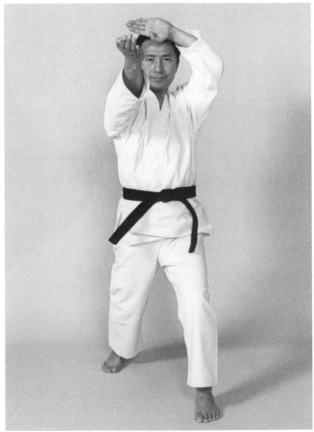

Sixth Position:
Palm Heel Block and Grab, Pull and Reverse Middle Punch

1. Palm Heel Block and Grab

a. Maintain the same stance.

b. Execute a Right Palm Heel Block in slow motion with tension and grab.

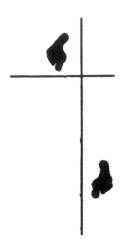

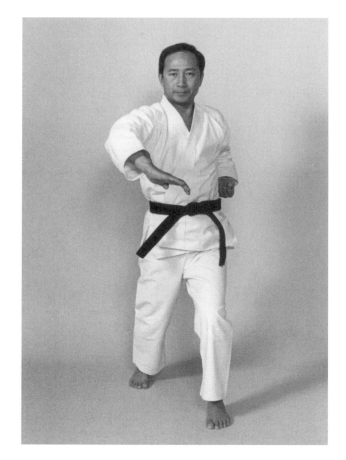

2. Reverse Middle Punch

a. Slide your right foot forward.

b. Assume Right Front Stance.

c. Simultaneously pull your right hand to the waist and at the same time execute a Left-Hand Reverse Middle Punch.

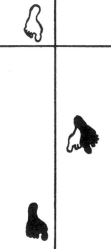

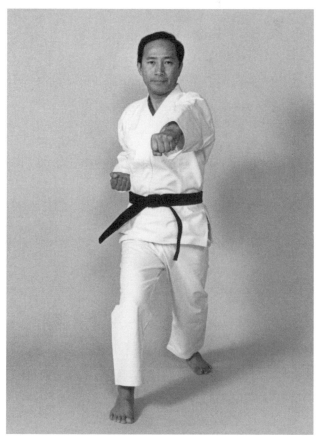

Seventh Position:
Palm Heel Block and Grab, Pull and Reverse Middle Punch

1. Palm Heel Block and Grab

a. Maintain the same stance.

b. Execute a Left Palm Heel Block in slow motion with tension and grab.

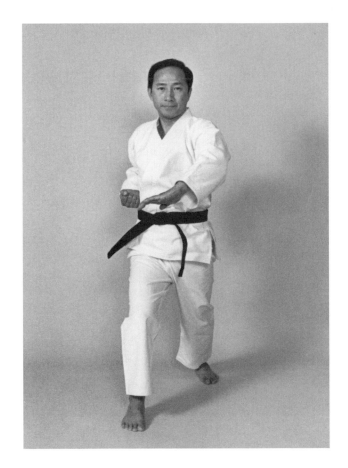

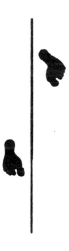

2. Reverse Middle Punch

a. Slide your left foot forward.

b. Assume Left Front Stance.

c. Simultaneously pull your left hand to the waist and at the same time execute a Right-Hand Reverse Middle Punch.

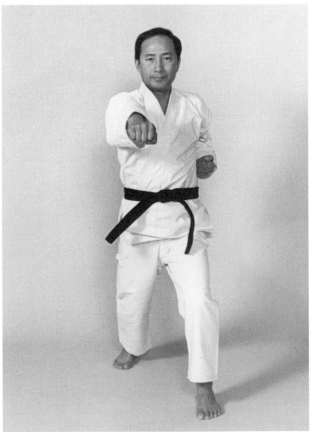

Eighth Position:
Palm Heel Block and Grab, Pull and Reverse Middle Punch

1. Palm Heel Block and Grab.

a. Maintain the same stance.

b. Execute a Right Palm Heel Block in slow motion with tension and grab.

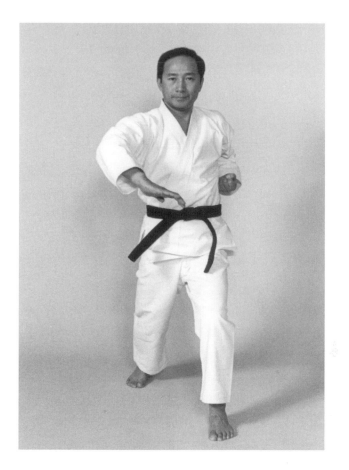

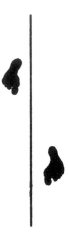

2. Reverse Middle Punch and Yell

a. Slide your right foot forward.

b. Assume Right Front Stance.

c. Simultaneously pull your right hand to the waist and at the same time execute a Left-Hand Reverse Middle Punch and yell.

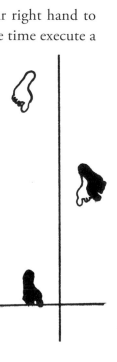

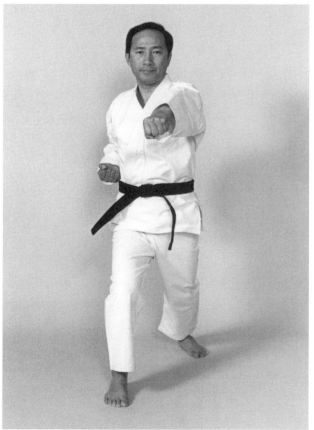

Ninth Position:
Diamond Middle Block (Geumgang-Momtong-Makki)

a. Pivoting to the left on the ball of your right foot, slide your left foot out and back to the left in a wide arc, turning 270° (three-quarters of a circle) to face **R-2**.

b. Assume a Left Back Stance.

c. Simultaneously execute a Diamond Middle Block. (Bring both fists back to right hip. Right fist at waist, palm up, and left fist, palm in, above the right fist. Execute an outside Middle Block with left forearm and a High Block with right forearm.)

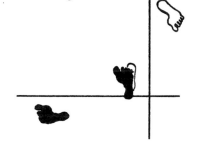

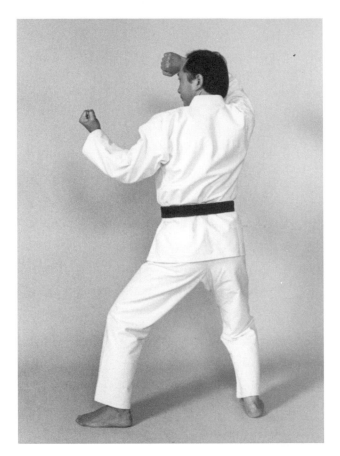

Tenth Position:
Pull and Reverse Uppercut

a. Maintain the same stance.

b. Execute a Pull and Reverse Uppercut (pulling left fist toward right shoulder, punch to the chin with your right fist, palm up).

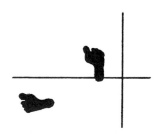

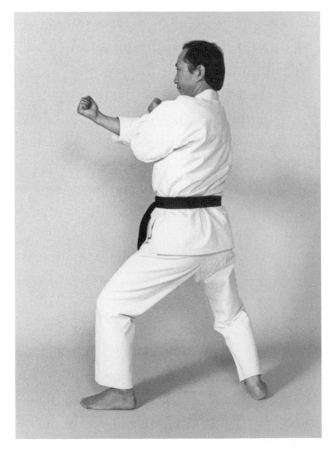

Eleventh Position:
Side Punch

a. Maintain the same stance.

b. Execute a Left Side Punch and at the same time bring your right fist to waist level, palm up.

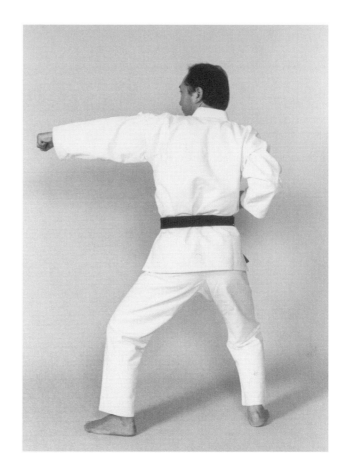

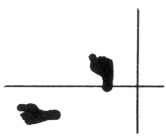

Twelfth Position:
Crane Stance (for Side Kicking)

a. Without moving your right foot, lift your left foot to the left side of your right knee.

b. Assume Right Crane Stance.

c. Simultaneously pull your left fist to the right side of your waist, palm in, over your right fist, palm up.

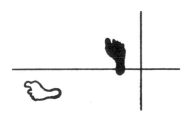

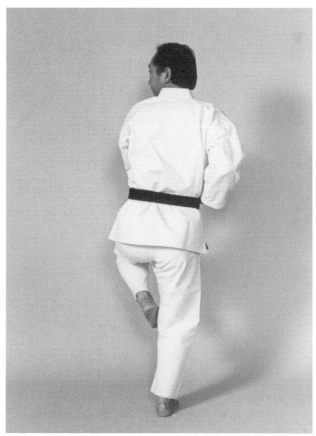

Thirteenth Position:
 Side Kick, Elbows Target Strike (Palkoop-Pyojeok-Chiki)

1. Side Kick
a. Execute a Left Side Kick and at the same time execute a High Side Punch with the left fist.

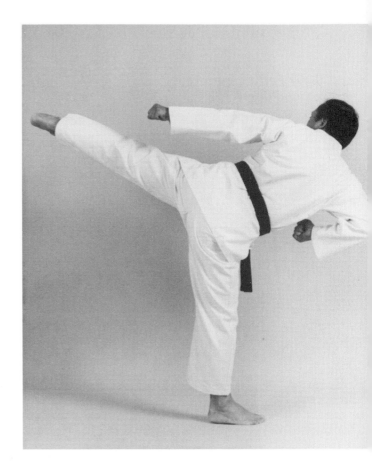

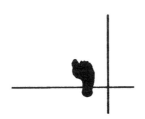

2. Elbow Target Strike
a. Immediately bring your left foot down one step forward toward **R-2**.

b. Assume Left Front Stance

c. Simultaneously execute an Elbow Strike with right elbow, striking left palm at shoulder level.

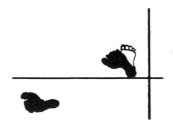

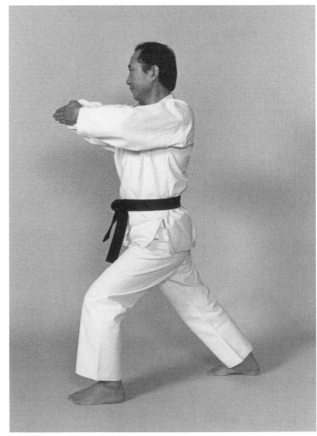

Fourteenth Position:
Close Step, Diamond Middle Block

Note: The above-mentioned movements should be performed in continuous motion.

1. Close-Step

a. Bring your left foot back next to your right foot into an informal stance at **B**, facing **A**. At the same time bring both fists back to the left side of your waist, left fist at waist, palm up, and right fist, palm in, above the left fist. Head turns toward **L-2**.

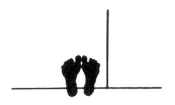

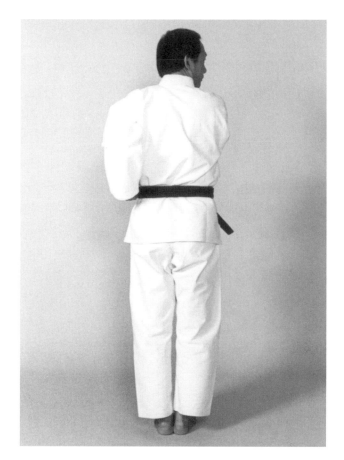

2. Diamond Middle Block

a. Immediately move your right foot to the right (toward **L-2**).

b. Assume Right Back Stance.

c. Simultaneously execute a Diamond Middle Block (Outside Middle Block with the right forearm and a High Block with left forearm).

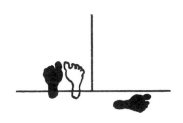

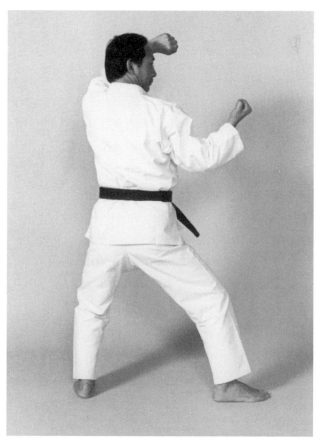

Fifteenth Position:
Pull and Reverse Uppercut

a. Maintain the same stance.

b. Execute a Pull and Reverse Uppercut. (Pulling right fist toward left shoulder, punch to the chin with your left first palm up.)

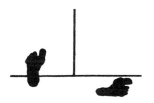

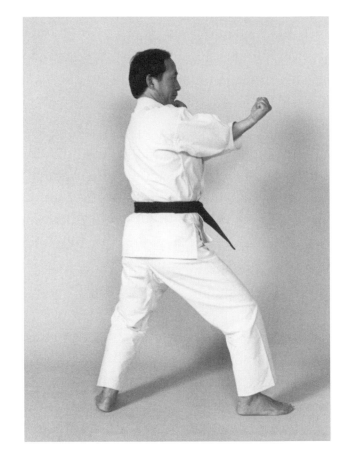

Sixteenth Position:
Side Punch

a. Maintain the same stance.

b. Execute a Right Side Punch and at the same time bring your left fist to waist level, palm up.

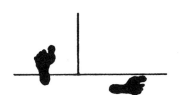

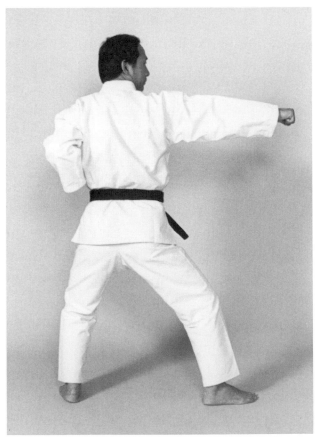

Seventeenth Position:
Crane Stance (for Side Kicking) (Haktari-Seogi)

a. Without moving your left foot, lift your right foot to the right side of your left knee.

b. Assume Left Crane Stance.

c. Simultaneously pull your right fist to the left side of your waist, palm in, over your left fist, palm up.

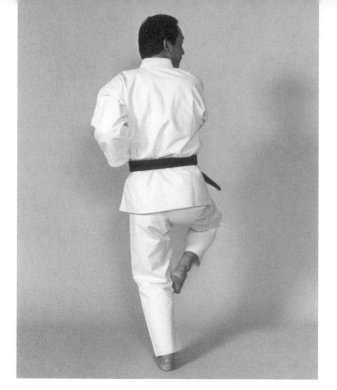

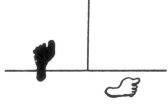

Eighteenth Position:
Side Kick, Elbow Target Strike

1. Side Kick

a. Execute a Right Side Kick and at the same time execute a High Side Punch with the right fist.

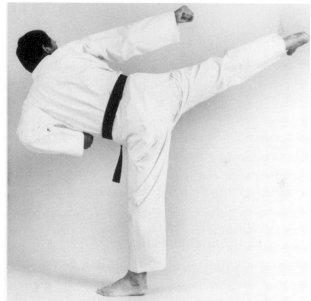

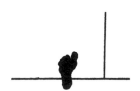

2. Elbow Target Strike

a. Immediately bring your right foot down one step forward toward L-2.

b. Assume Right Front Stance.

c. Simultaneously execute an Elbow Attack with your left elbow, striking right palm at shoulder level.

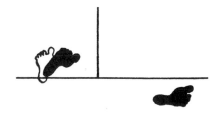

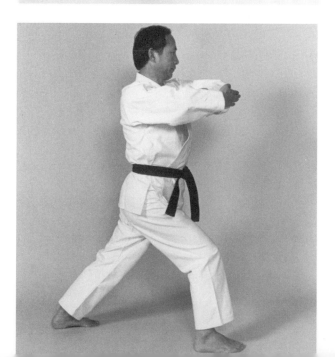

Nineteenth Position:
Close Step, Knife-Hand Middle Block

Note: These movements should be performed in continuous motion.

1. Close Step

a. Bring your right foot back next to the left foot into an informal stance at **B**, facing **A**. At the same time, bring both Knife Hands to the right to prepare for a left Knife-Hand Middle Block. Head turns toward **A**.

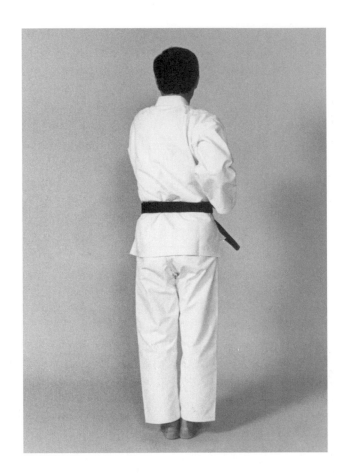

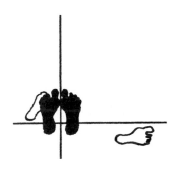

2. Knife-Hand Middle Block

a. Immediately slide your left foot forward toward **A**.

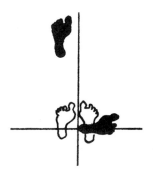

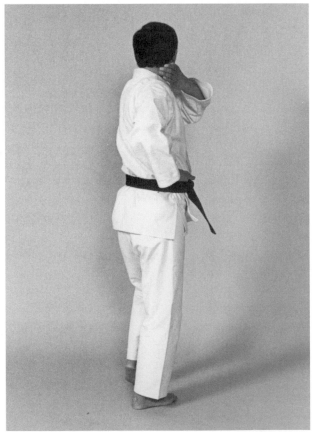

b. Assume Left Back Stance.

c. Simultaneously execute a Left Knife-Hand Middle Block.

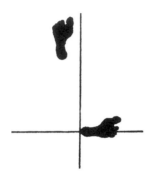

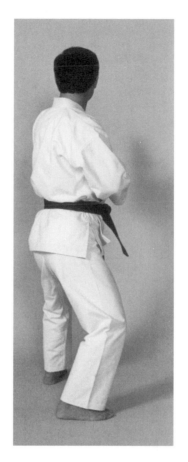

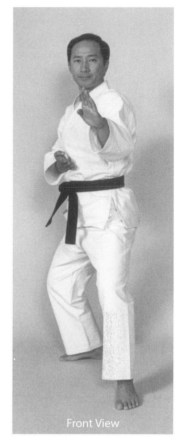

Front View

Twentieth Position:
Spear-Hand Thrust (Pyeonsonkeut-Seweo-Jiluki)

a. Slide your right foot forward.

b. Assume Right Front Stance.

c. Simultaneously execute a Right Spear-Hand Thrust

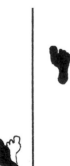

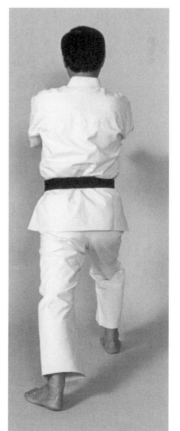

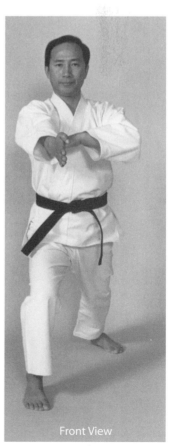

Front View

Twenty-First Position:
 Twist Spear Hand and Turn, Back-Fist Strike
 (Deung-Joomeok Chiki)

Note: If the opponent, at **B**, should grab your Spear Hand or wrist, this motion will break his hold. The above-mentioned movements should be performed in continuous motion.

1. Twist Spear Hand and Turn

a. Twist your right Spear Hand palm down and out. At the same time twist your body to the right, pivoting on the balls of your feet.

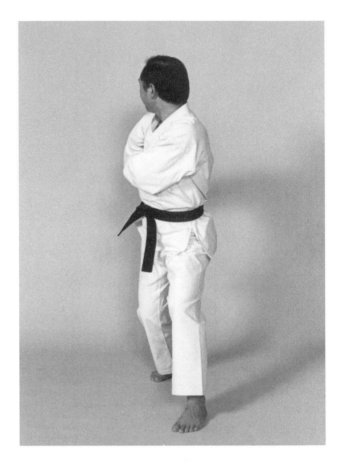

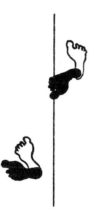

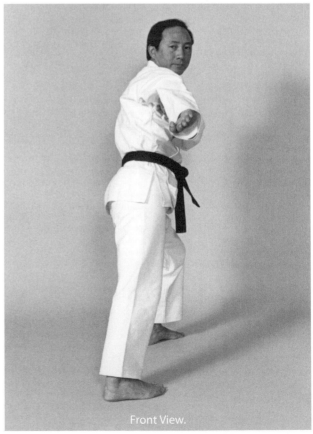

Front View.

2. Back-Fist Strike

a. Pivoting to the right on the ball of your right foot, slide your left foot out and back in a wide arc (toward **A**), one step forward.

b. Assume Left Back Stance.

c. Execute a Left Back-Fist Strike to the face.

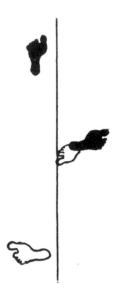

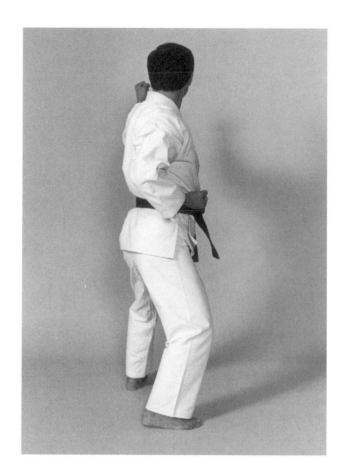

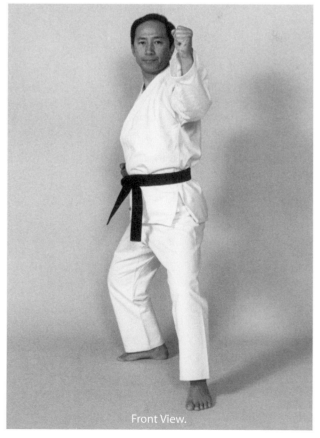

Front View.

Twenty-Second Position: Middle Punch and Yell

a. Slide your right foot forward.

b. Assume Right Front Stance.

c. Execute a Right-Hand Middle Punch and yell.

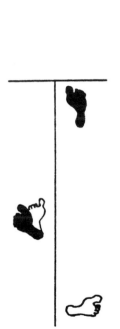

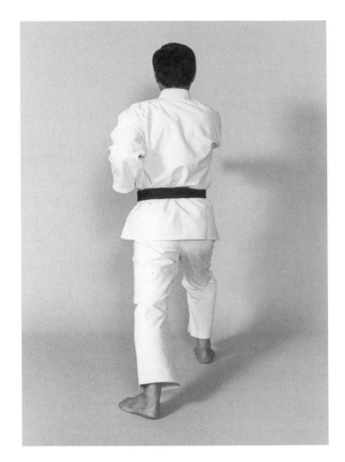

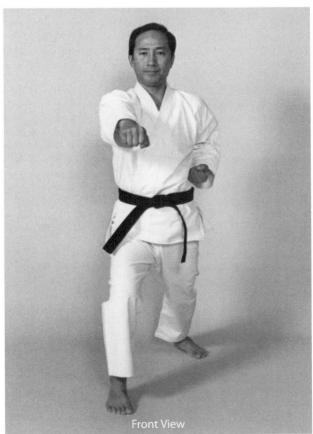

Front View

Twenty-Third Position:
Scissor Block (Gawi-Makki)

a. Pivoting to the left on the ball of your right foot, slide your left foot out and back to left in a wide arc, turning 270° (facing **L-1**).

b. Assume Left Front Stance.

c. Simultaneously execute a Right–Left Scissor Block. (This is a simultaneous Outside Middle Block with the right hand and a Low Block with the left hand.)

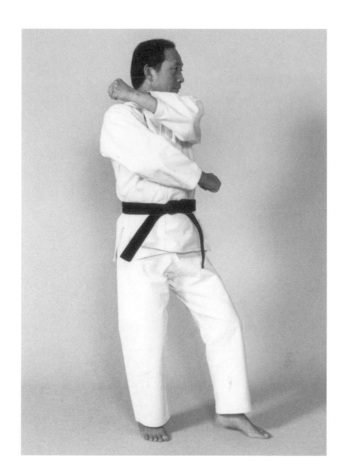

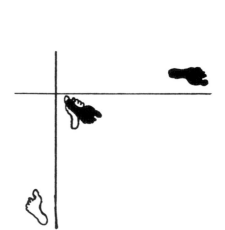

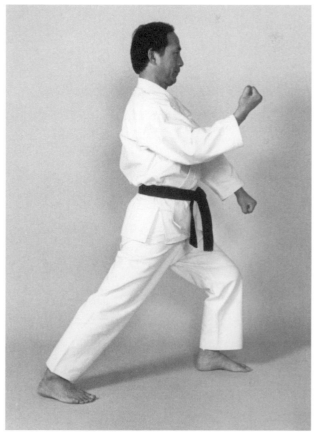

Twenty-Fourth Position:
Front Kick, Middle Punch, Reverse Middle Punch

1. Front Kick

a. Execute a Front Kick with your right foot to the face.

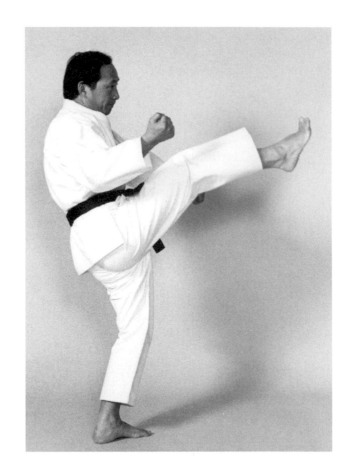

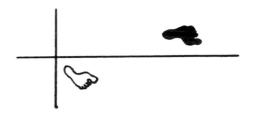

2. Middle Punch

a. Step forward with your right foot.

b. Assume Right Front Stance.

c. Simultaneously execute a Right-Hand Middle Punch.

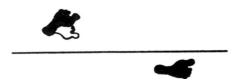

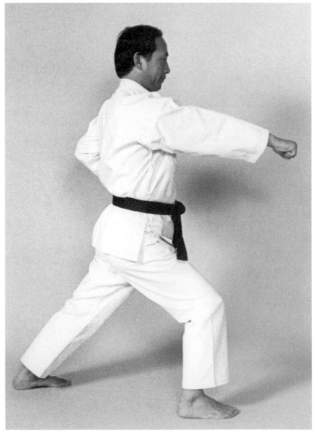

3. Reverse Middle Punch

a. Maintain the same stance.

b. Execute a Left-Hand Reverse Middle Punch.

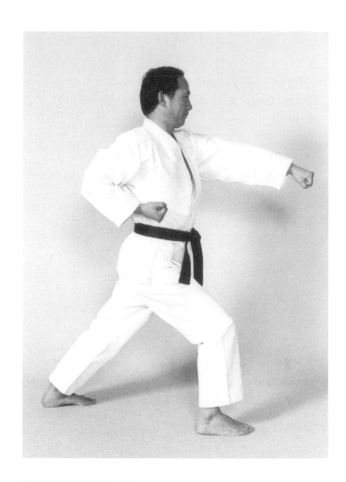

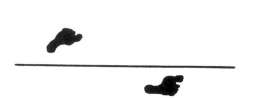

Twenty-Fifth Position:
Scissor Block

a. Pivoting to the right on the ball of your left foot, slide your right foot out and back in a wide arc, turning 180° to the right (toward **R-1**).

b. Assume Right Front Stance.

c. Simultaneously execute a Left-Right Scissor Block (Outside Middle Block with your left hand and Low Block with your right hand).

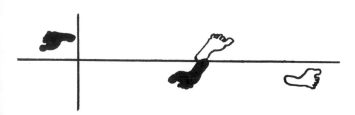

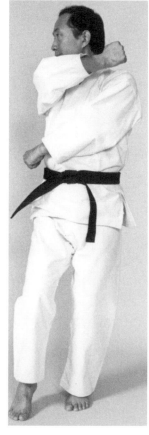

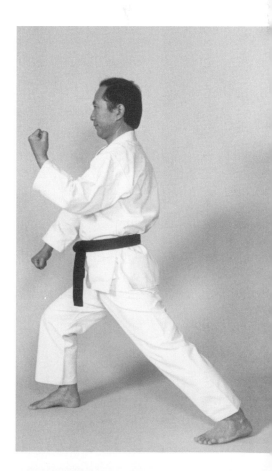

Twenty-Sixth Position:
  Front Kick, Middle Punch, Reverse Middle Punch

1. Front Kick
a. Execute a Front Kick with your left foot to the face.

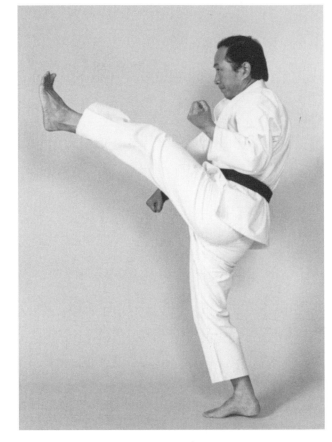

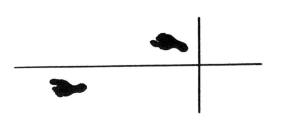

2. Middle Punch
a. Step forward with your left foot.

b. Assume Left Front Stance.

c. Simultaneously execute a Left-Hand Middle Punch.

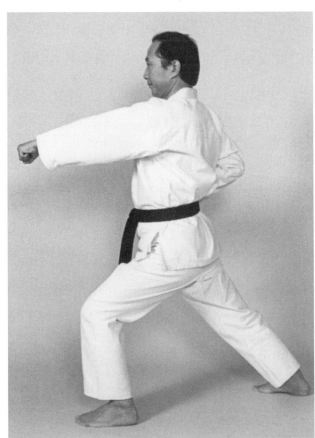

3. Reverse Middle Punch

a. Maintain the same stance.

b. Execute a Right-Hand Reverse Middle Punch.

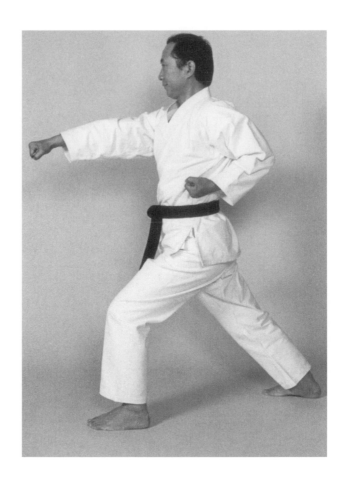

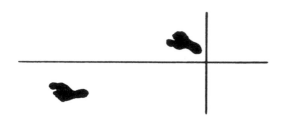

Stop

Pivoting to the left on the ball of your right foot, slide your left foot out and back, turning 90° to the left, facing **B** at point **A**. Assume Ready Stance.

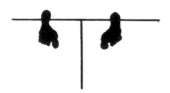

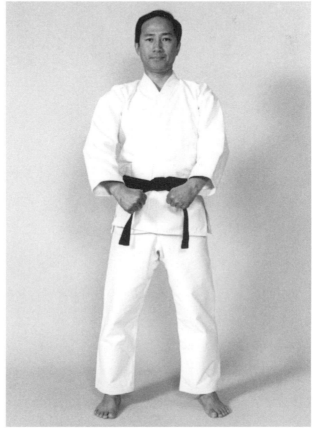

PYONGWON (PLAIN)

The plain—that broad, unbroken expanse—is the lot of ordinary human beings. It is where the day-to-day life of man unfolds. It is the fertile country which blesses man with abundant food. But the plain also can bestow a sense of majesty. A great open plain stretching out to the horizon elevates man with its majestic spirit, giving him a feeling of strength. The plain is his home; he understands it and can feel part of all that he sees. It is an impression different from that one receives when viewing the endless sea or tall mountains; both are beautiful and impressive but less friendly to the advances of man.

The form *Pyongwon* is the application of the providence of the plain—its abundance and grace as well as its vastness—which welcomes man as a part of itself rather than challenging him to conquer it. In this form you must demonstrate the majestic but friendly spirit of the vast plain.

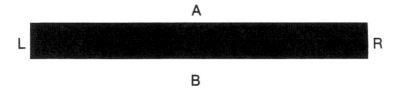

Pyongwon

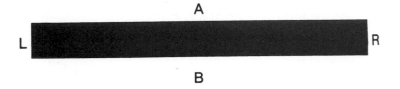

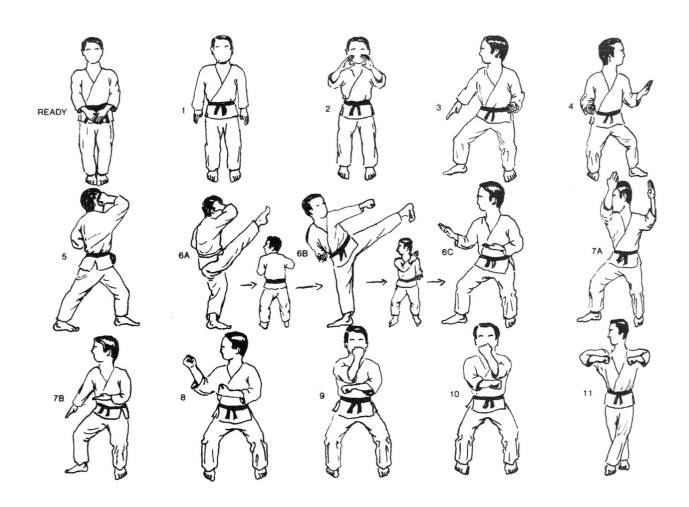

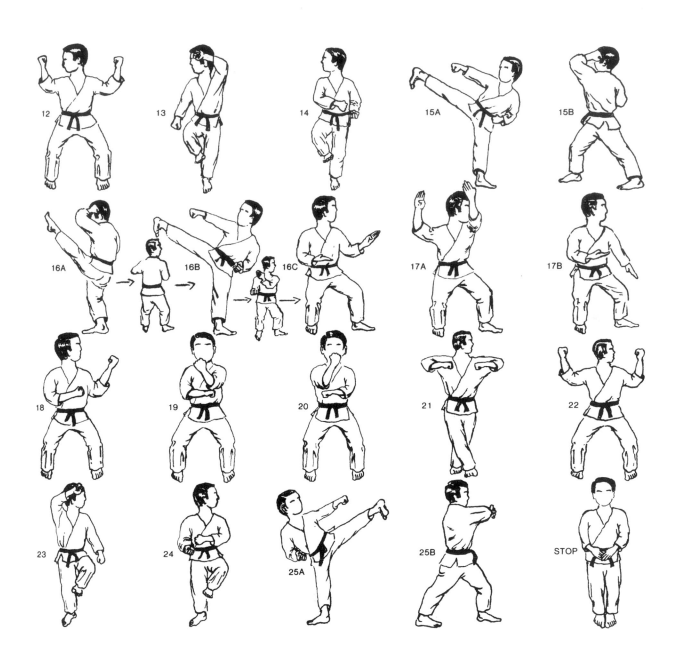

Ready (Cross-Hand Ready): (Gyopson-Choonbi)
Maintain an Informal Stance, facing **B** at point **A**, eyes focused straight ahead, with both open hands positioned in front of abdomen, palms in, and left hand crossing over right hand.

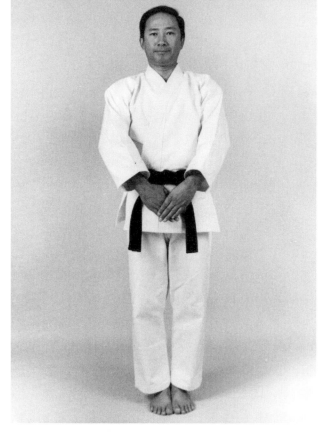

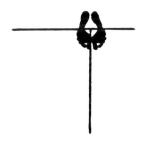

First Position:
  Spread Knife-Hand Low Block
  a. Slide your right foot slightly to the right.

  b. Assume Normal Stance (feet apart in parallel position).

  c. Simultaneously raise both hands to chest level, wrists crossing each other, palms in, and execute a spread Knife-Hand Low Block, palms in, near upper thighs. (This block is performed in slow motion with arms tensed. Exhale slowly and forcefully while executing block.)

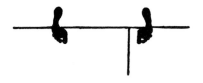

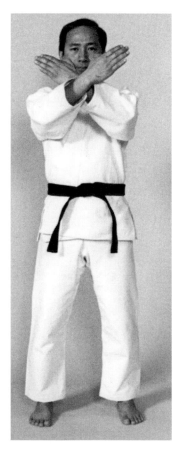

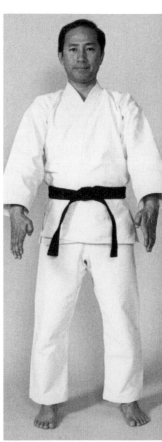

Second Position:
Barrel Pushing
a. Maintain the same stance.

b. Raise both hands up slowly, with tension, to neck level and execute a Barrel Pushing motion. (Inhale while raising hands and exhale while pushing.)

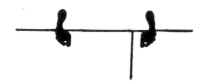

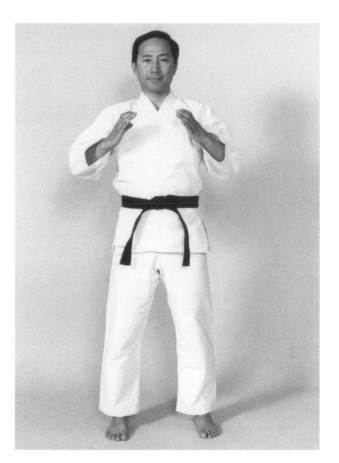

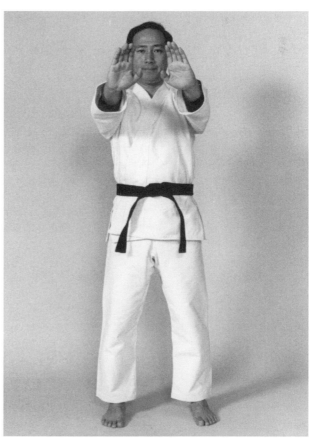

Third Position:
Single Knife-Hand Low Block

a. Keeping your left foot in place, slide your right foot 90° to the right (toward **R**).

b. Assume Right Back Stance.

c. Simultaneously execute a Single Right Knife-Hand Low Block, left fist at waist level, palm up.

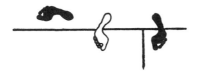

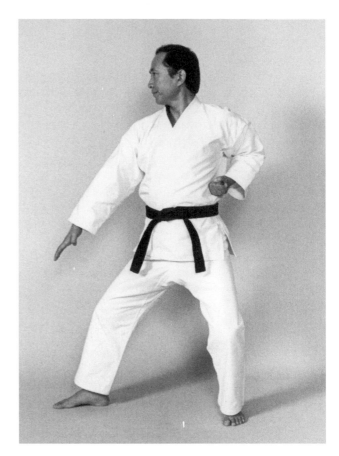

Fourth Position:
Single Knife-Hand Middle Block

a. Maintain both feet in the same location. Pivot 90° to the left on the heel of your right foot and slide your left foot 90° to the left (toward **L**). Face turns toward **L**.

b. Assume Left Back Stance.

c. Simultaneously execute a Single Left Knife-Hand Middle Block.

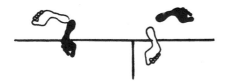

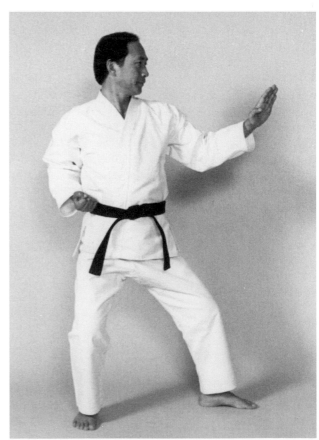

Fifth Position:
Elbow Strike

a. Slide your left foot slightly forward.

b. Assume Left Front Stance.

c. Simultaneously execute a Right Elbow Strike to the chin.

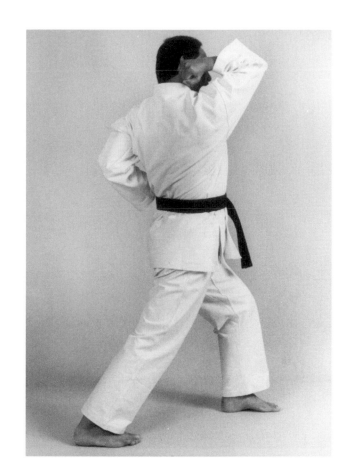

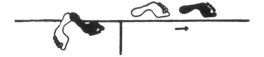

Sixth Position:
Front Kick, Turning Side Kick, Knife-Hand Middle Block

1. Front Kick

a. Execute a Front Kick with your right foot.

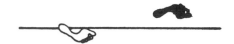

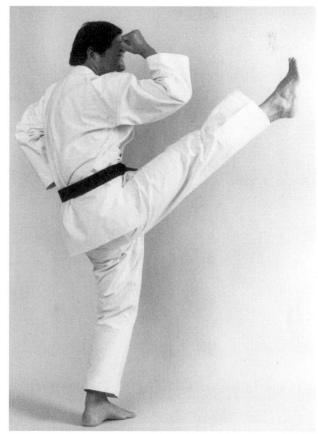

2. Turning Side Kick

a. Step forward with your right foot.

b. Immediately execute a Turning Side Kick with your left foot toward **L** and at the same time execute a Left Side Punch.

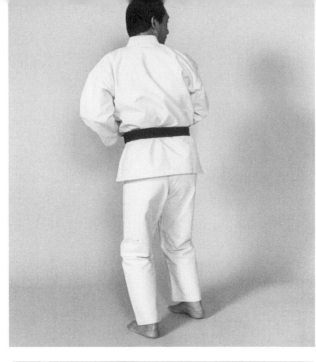

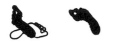

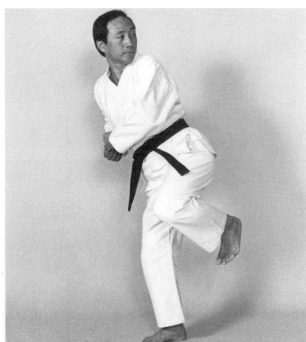

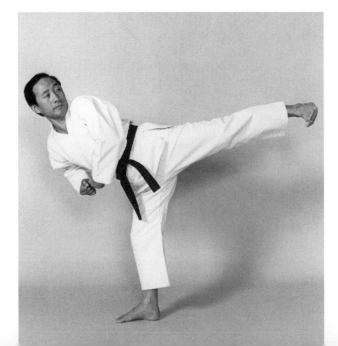

3. Knife-Hand Middle Block

a. Bringing your left foot down, slide your right foot 90° to the right (toward **R**). Face turns toward **R**.

b. Assume Right Back Stance.

c. Simultaneously execute a Right Knife-Hand Middle Block.

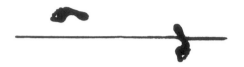

Seventh Position:
Circling Motion, Knife-Hand Low Block

1. Circling Motion

a. Maintain the same stance.

b. Bring both hands back near left shoulder area and make a large circle above the head.

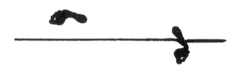

2. Knife-Hand Low Block

a. Continuing the Circling Motion, execute a Right Knife-Hand Low Block.

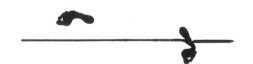

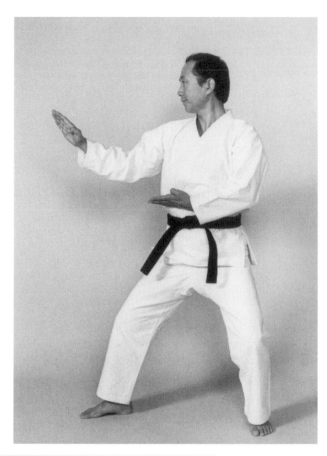

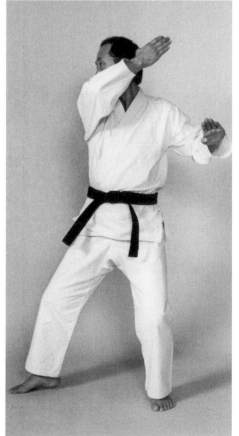

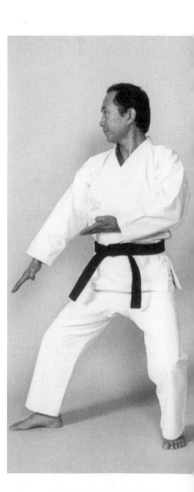

Eighth Position:
Double-Hand High Block (Geodeureo-Eolgool-Makki)

a. Keeping your left foot in place, slightly move your right foot toward **R** and at the same time turn it 90° (toward **B**). Head continues to face **R**.

b. Assume Horseback Stance.

c. Simultaneously execute a Double-Hand High Block.

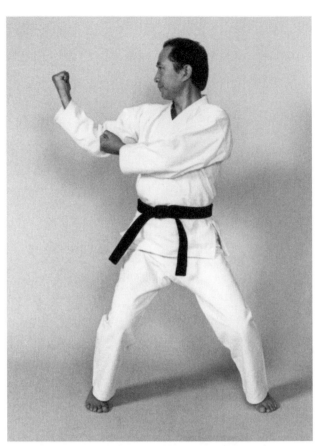

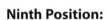

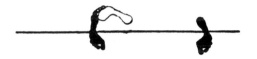

Ninth Position:
Uppercut Punch (Dangyo-Teok-Chiki) and Yell

a. Keeping your left foot in place, lift your right foot and stamp down.

b. Assume Horseback Stance.

c. As you lift your right foot, bring your right fist back, palm out, at head level, and face turns toward **B**. As you stamp your right foot down, simultaneously execute a Right Uppercut Punch to the chin (place left fist, palm down, under right elbow) and yell.

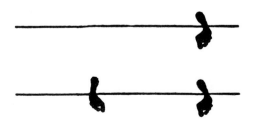

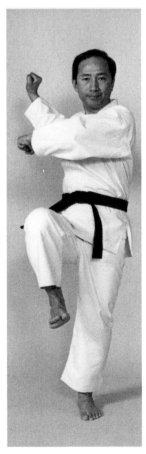

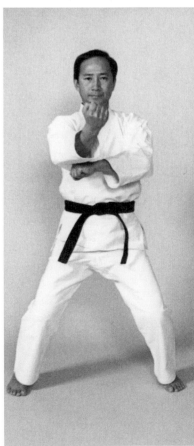

Tenth Position:
Uppercut Punch

a. Maintain the same stance.

b. Bring your left fist back, palm out, at head level and execute a Left Uppercut to the chin (place right fist, palm down, under left elbow).

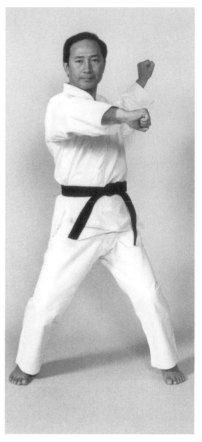
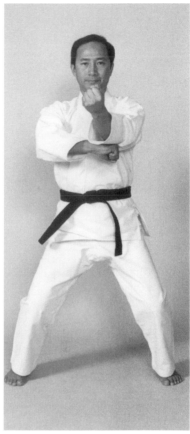

Eleventh Position:
Yoke Strike *(Meonge-Chiki)*

a. Keeping your right foot in place, cross over it with your left foot. Face turns toward **R**.

b. Assume Left Cross Stance.

c. Simultaneously execute a Yoke Strike (simultaneous outward Elbow Strike).

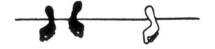

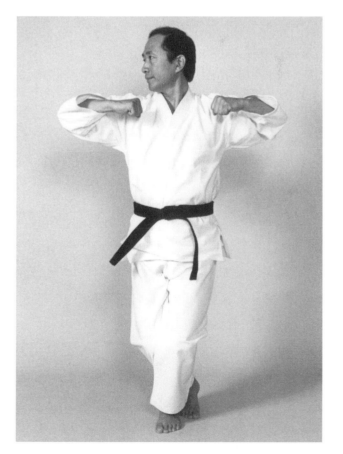

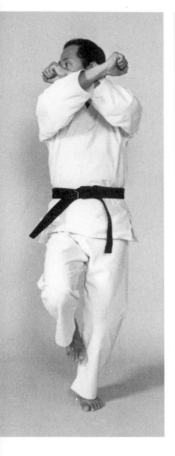
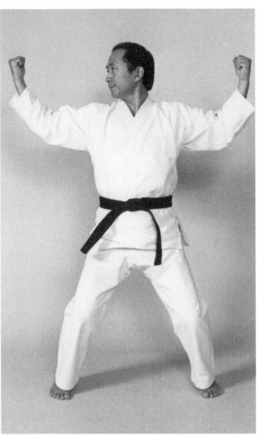

Twelfth Position:
Spread Mountain Block *(Hechyo-Santeul-Makki)*

a. Keeping your left foot in place, move your right foot to the right (toward **R**).

b. Assume Horseback Stance.

c. Simultaneously execute a Mountain Block. (Cross both fists in front of face and snap them out and to the side palm in at head level. Both elbows are bent at a 90° angle, arms tensed. Blocking surface is the inner edge of forearms.)

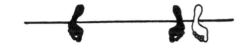

Thirteenth Position:
Diamond Block *(Keumgang-Makki)*

a. Keeping your left foot in place, raise your right foot to the side of your left knee.

b. Assume Left Crane Stance.

c. Simultaneously execute a Diamond Block. (This is a simultaneous Left-Hand High Block and a Right-Hand Low Block to the side.)

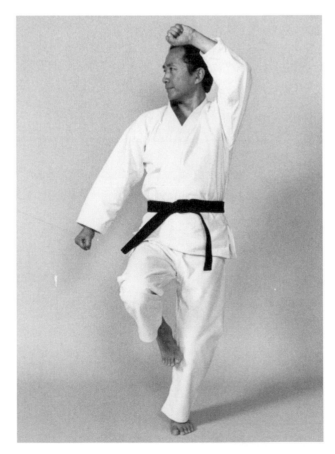

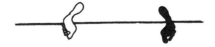

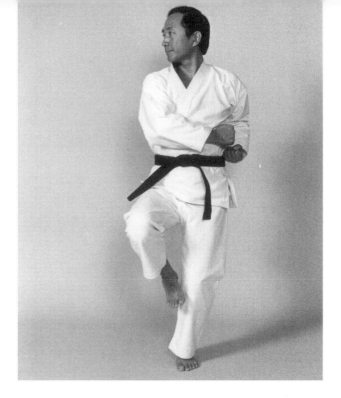

Fourteenth Position:
Crane Stance (for Side Kicking)

   a. Maintain the same stance (Left Crane Stance).

   b. Pull both fists back to your left hip, left fist at waist level, palm up, and right fist, palm in, over left fist.

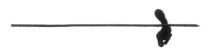

Fifteenth Position:
Side Kick, Elbow Strike

1. Side Kick

   a. Execute a Side Kick with your right foot toward **R** and at the same time execute a Right Side Punch.

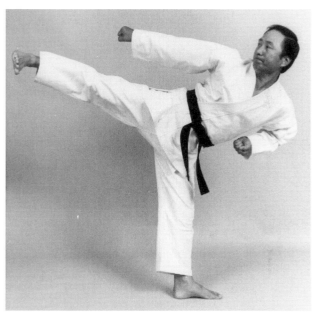

2. Elbow Strike

   a. Immediately bring your right foot one step forward toward **R**.

   b. Assume Right Front Stance.

   c. Simultaneously execute a Left Elbow Strike to the chin.

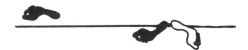

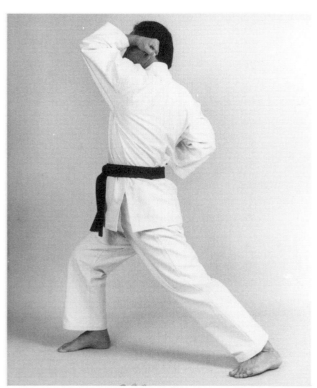

241 / The Forms (Poomsae): Pyongwon

Sixteenth Position:
Front Kick, Turning Side Kick, Knife-Hand Middle Block.

1. Front Kick

a. Execute a Front Kick toward **R** with your left foot.

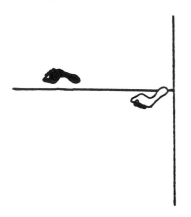

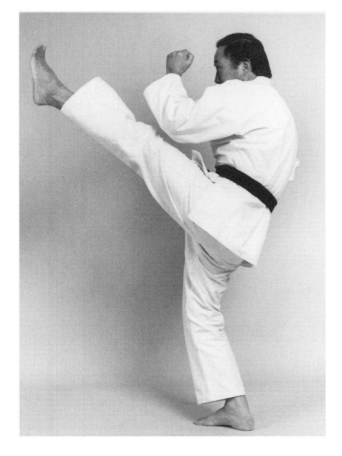

2. Turning Side Kick

a. Step forward with your left foot.

b. Immediately execute a Turning Side Kick with your right foot toward **R** and at the same time execute a Right Side Punch.

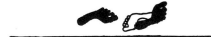

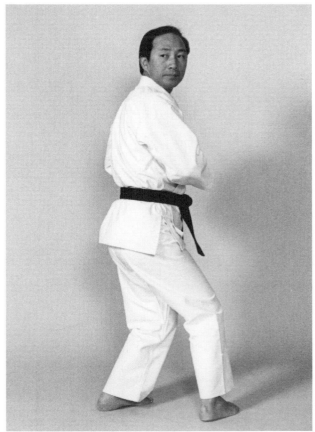

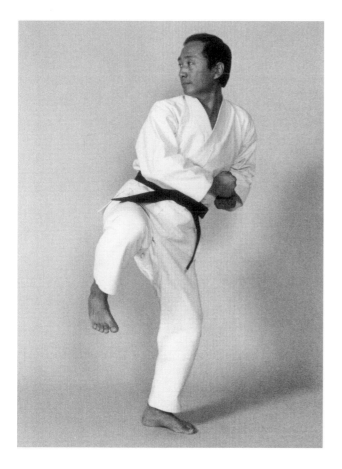

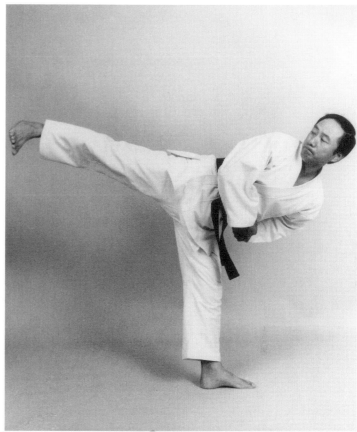

3. Knife-Hand Middle Block

a. Bringing your right foot down, slide your left foot 90° to the left (toward **L**). Face turns toward **L**.

b. Assume Left Back Stance.

c. Simultaneously execute a Left Knife-Hand Middle Block.

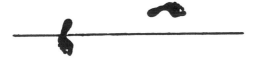

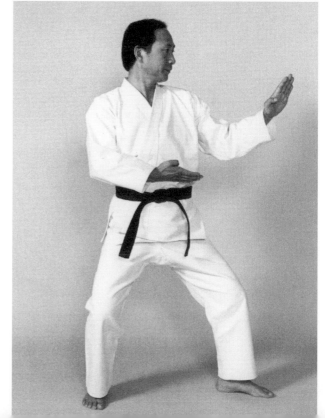

Seventeenth Position:
Circling Motion, Knife-Hand Low Block

1. Circling Motion

a. Maintain the same stance.

b. Bring both hands back near right shoulder area and make a large circle above head.

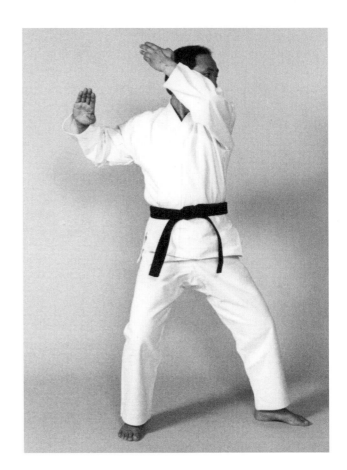

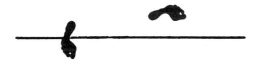

2. Knife-Hand Low Block

a. Continuing the Circling Motion, execute a Left-Hand Low Block.

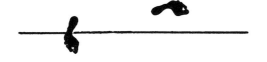

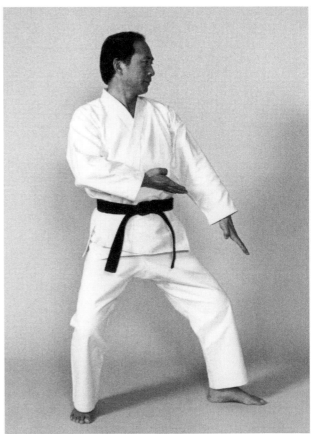

Eighteenth Position:
Double-Hand High Block

a. Keeping your right foot in place, slightly move your left foot toward L and at the same time turn in 90° (toward **B**). Head continues to face L.

b. Assume Horseback Stance.

c. Simultaneously execute Double-Hand High Block.

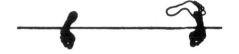

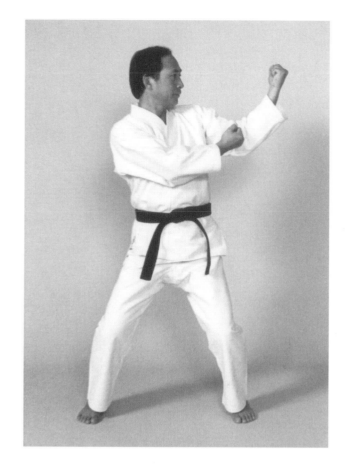

Nineteenth Position:
Uppercut Punch and Yell

a. Keeping your right foot in place, lift your left foot and stamp down.

b. Assume Horseback Stance.

c. As you lift your left foot, bring your left fist back, palm out, at head level, and face turns toward **B**. As you stamp your left foot down, simultaneously execute a Left Uppercut Punch to the chin (place right fist, palm down, under left elbow) and yell.

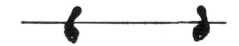

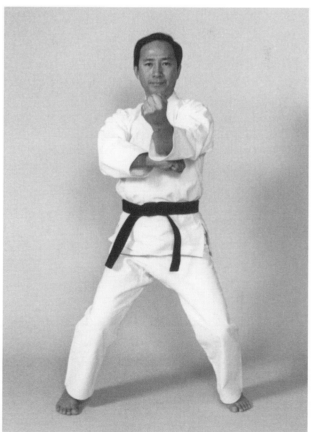

Twentieth Position:
Uppercut Punch

a. Maintain the same stance.

b. Bring your right fist back, palm out, at head level and execute a Right Uppercut Punch to the chin (place left fist, palm down, under right elbow).

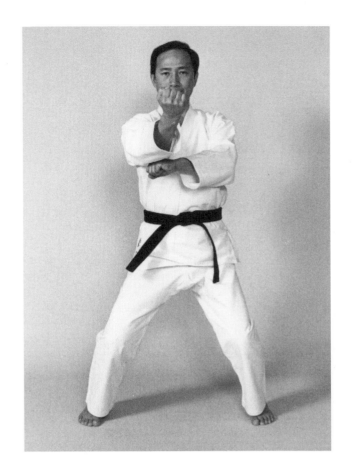

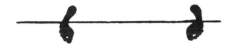

Twenty-First Position:
Yoke Strike

a. Keeping your left foot in place, cross over it with your right foot. Face turns toward L.

b. Assume Right Cross Stance.

c. Simultaneously execute a Yoke Strike (simultaneous outward Elbow Strikes).

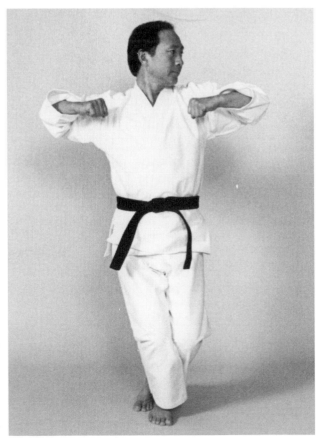

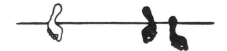

Twenty-Second Position: Spread Mountain Block

a. Keeping your right foot in place, move your left foot to the left (toward **L**).

b. Assume Horseback Stance.

c. Simultaneously execute a Mountain Block. (Cross both fists in front of face and snap them out and to the side palm in at head level. Both elbows are bent at a 90° angle, arms tensed. Blocking surface is the inner edge of forearms.)

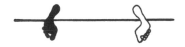

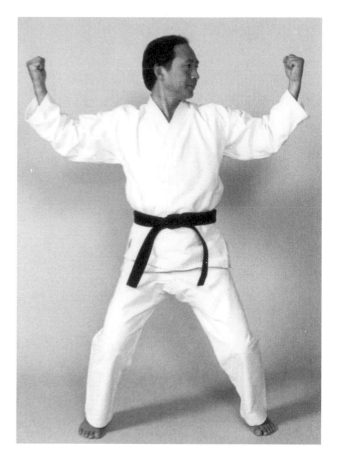

Twenty-Third Position: Diamond Block

a. Keeping your right foot in place, raise your left foot to the side of your right knee.

b. Assume Right Crane Stance.

c. Simultaneously execute a Diamond Block. (This is a simultaneous Right-Hand High Block and a Left-Hand Low Block to the side.)

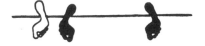

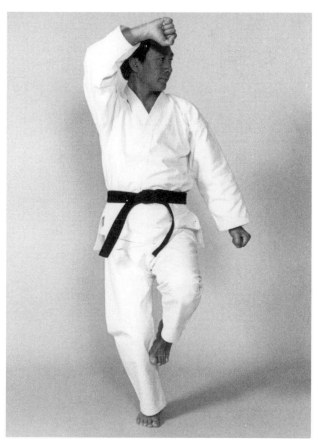

Twenty-Fourth Position:
Crane Stance (for Side Kicking)

a. Maintain the same stance (Right Crane Stance).

b. Pull both fists back to your right hip, right fist at waist level palm up and left fist palm in over right fist.

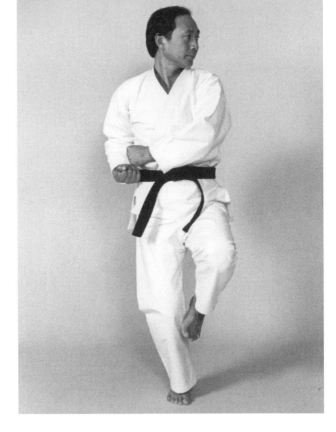

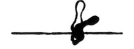

Twenty-Fifth Position:
Side Kick, Elbow Target Strike (Palkoop-Pyojeok-Chiki)

1. Side Kick

a. Execute a Side Kick with your left foot toward L and at the same time execute a Left Side Punch.

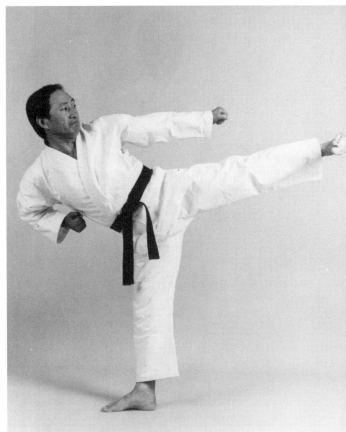

2. Elbow Target Strike

a. Immediately bring your left foot one step forward toward **L**.

b. Assume Left Front Stance.

c. Simultaneously execute a Right Elbow Strike (striking left palm at shoulder level).

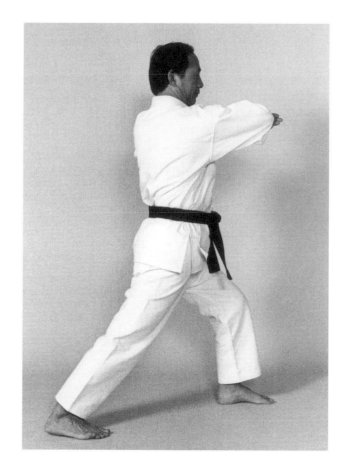

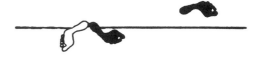

Stop

Pivoting 90° to the right on the ball of your left foot, bring your right foot next to your left foot and assume Cross-Hand Informal Stance (left hand crossing over right hand), facing **B** at point **A**.

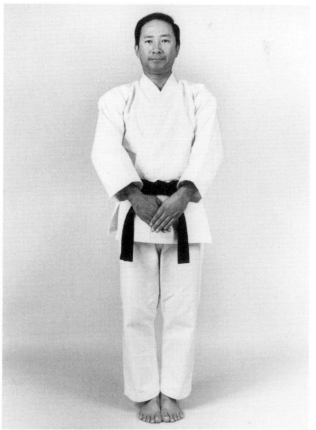

Sipjin (Decimal)

The decimal system, our standard numerical system, is based on ten. It is infinite—hundreds, thousands, millions, billions, and on—beyond the capability of any language to describe it. In this sense, the decimal system represents endless development and growth—but a very orderly and predictable growth that fosters stability. It is a very human system rather than just an arbitrary progression, for it is based on man's first computer—his ten fingers. Unlike the binary system, which was designed for a machine's artificial intelligence, the decimal system is innately man's.

The form *Sipjin* outlines the Chinese character that means ten (十). To demonstrate the key characteristics of the decimal system in the form, you must seek stability with every movement, giving change a systematic, orderly progression.

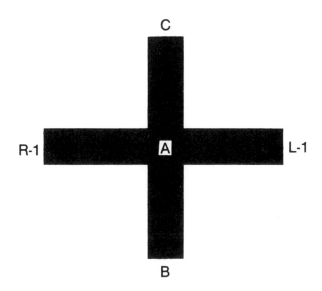

Sipjin

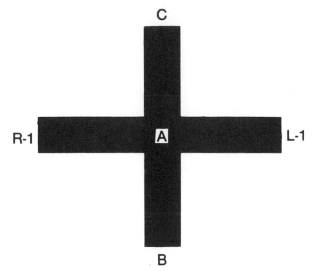

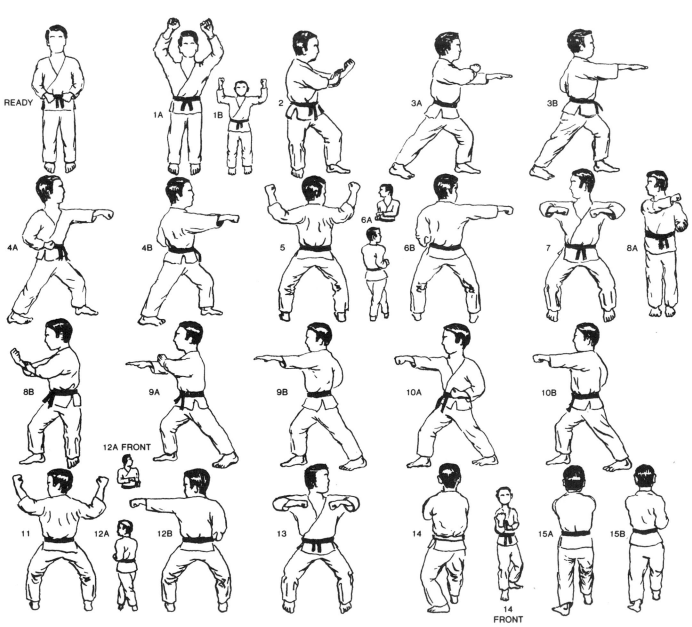

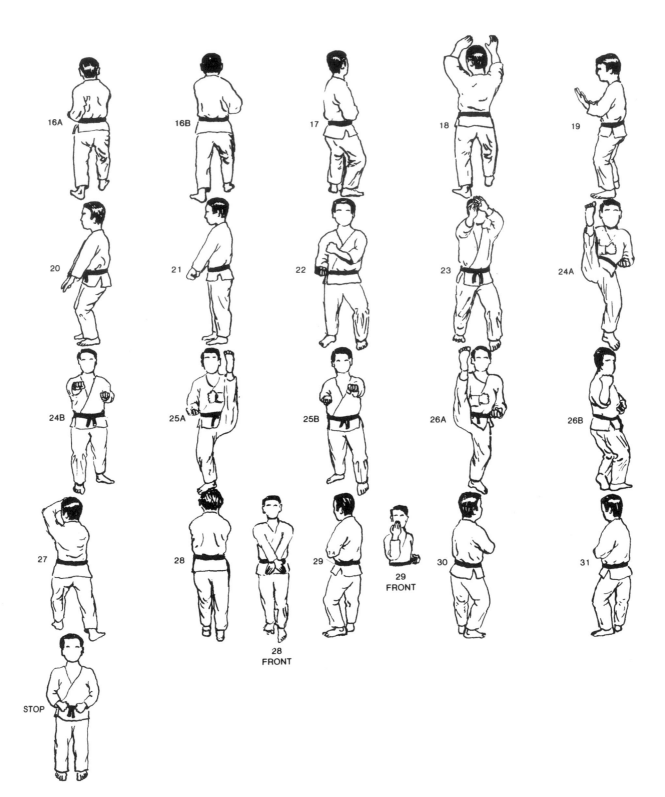

16A   16B   17   18   19

20   21   22   23   24A

24B   25A   25B   26A   26B

27   28   29   29 FRONT   30   31

28 FRONT

STOP

Ready

Maintain Ready Stance, facing **B** at point **A**, eyes focused straight ahead.

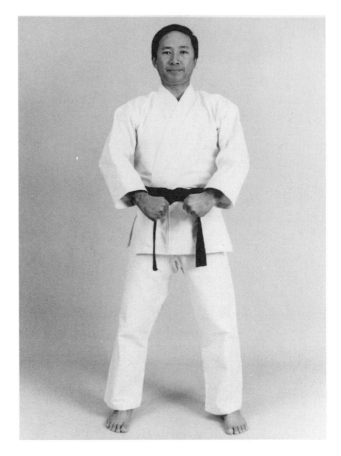

First Position:
   Bull Block *(Hwangso-Makki)*, Mountain Block *(Santeul-Makki)*

1. Bull Block

a. Maintain the same stance (Ready Stance).

b. Raise both fists slowly, arms tensed. When fists reach chest level, snap arms upward, over head, and execute a Bull Block. (Arms form the shape of a bull's horns with fists palm out. Blocking surface is the outer edge of forearm.)

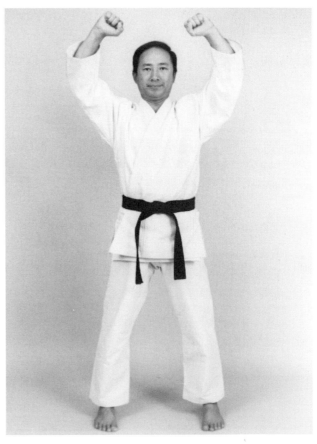

2. Mountain Block

a. Maintain the same stance.

b. Execute a Mountain Block. (Snap both fists out and to the side, palms in, at head level. Both elbows are bent at a 90° angle, arms tensed. Blocking surface is the inner edge of forearm.)

Note: The above two blocks, 1 and 2, should be performed in a continuous motion.

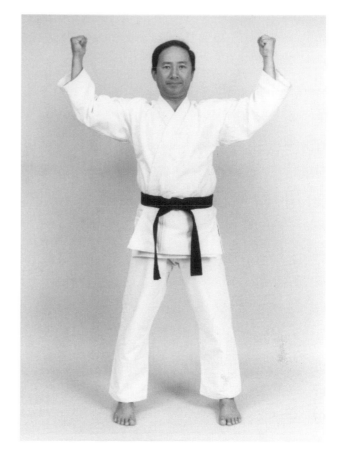

Second Position:
Hand-Supported Middle Block (*Sonbadak-Geodeuro-Momtong-Makki*)

a. Slide your left foot 90° to the left toward **L-1**.

b. Assume Left Back Stance.

c. Simultaneously execute a Hand-Supported Middle Block. (Outside Middle Block with your left hand, and simultaneously support with your right hand by placing your open hand on the inside of the left forearm.)

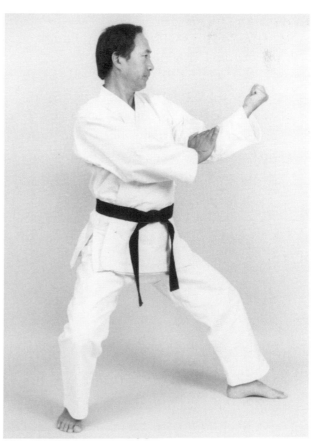

Third Position:
 Arm Twist, Spear-Hand Thrust (Palm Down)
 (Pyonson-Keut-Eopeo-Jiluki)

1. Arm Twist

a. Pivoting to the left on the ball of your right foot, slide your left foot slightly forward.

b. Assume Left Front Stance.

c. Simultaneously, opening your left fist, twist your left arm to the right and straighten forward, palm down. This motion should be performed slowly with tension.

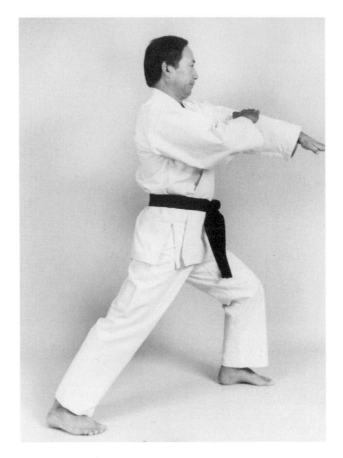

2. Spear-Hand Thrust (Palm Down)

a. Maintain the same stance.

b. Move your Right Spear Hand slowly forward with tension. Then execute a Spear-Hand Thrust with your right hand, palm down, rapidly with power.

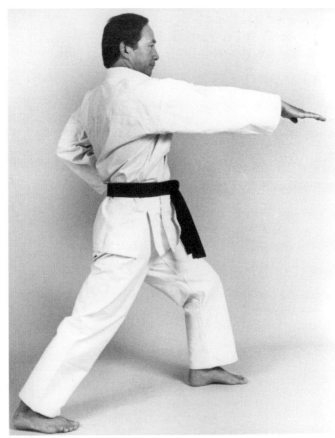

Fourth Position:
Double Middle Punch *(Momtonent-Doobeon-Jiluki)*

1. Middle Punch

a. Maintain the same stance.

b. Execute a Right-Hand Middle Punch.

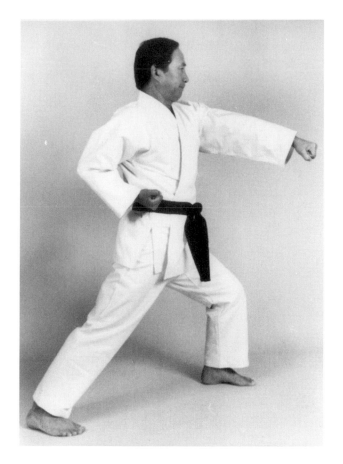

2. Reverse Middle Punch

a. Maintain the same stance.

b. Execute a Left-Hand Reverse Middle Punch.

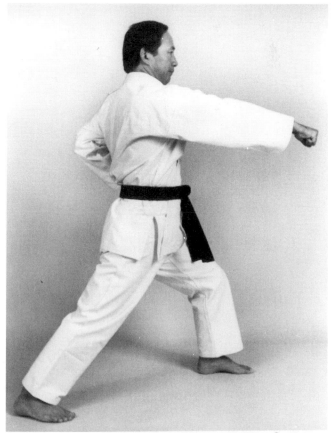

Fifth Position:
Spread Mountain Block *(Hechyo-Santeul-Makki)*

a. Pivoting 90° to the left on the ball of your left foot, step forward with your right foot toward **L-1**.

b. Assume Horseback Stance, body facing **C**. Head continues to face **L-1**.

c. Simultaneously execute a Spread Mountain Block. (Cross wrists in front of face, palms out, then sweep both forearms simultaneously outward and to the sides, snapping both wrists, palms in, at head level.)

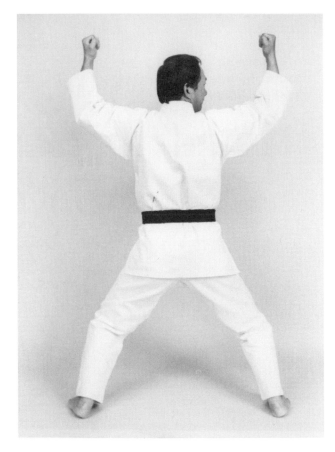

Sixth Position:
Cross Stance, Side Punch, and Yell

1. Cross Stance

a. Lift your left foot and cross over your right foot. At the same time, bring your right fist to waist level, palm up, and place left arm at chest level, left fist palm down.

b. Assume Left Cross Stance.

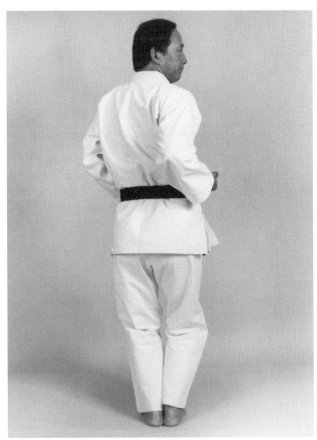

2. Side Punch

a. Keeping your left foot in place, move your right foot to the right (toward **L-1**).

b. Assume Horseback Stance.

c. Simultaneously execute a Right Side Punch and yell.

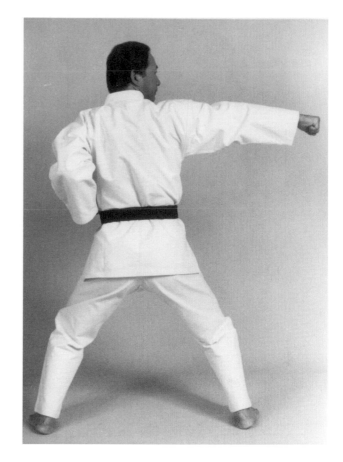

Seventh Position:
Yoke Strike *(Meong-E Chiki)*

a. Pivoting 180° to the left on the ball of your left foot, step your right foot 180° to the left (counterclockwise toward **R-1**). Body is facing **B**, and face is turned toward **R-1**.

b. Assume Horseback Stance.

c. Simultaneously execute a Yoke Strike (simultaneous outward Elbow Strikes).

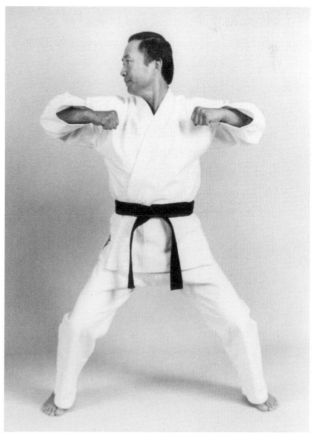

Eighth Position:
Close Step, Hand-Supported Middle Block
(Sonbadak-Geodeuro-Momton-Makki)

1. Close Step

a. Draw your left foot in next to your right foot.

b. At the same time, place your right fist near left shoulder level, palm down, and place your left fist near waist, palm down.

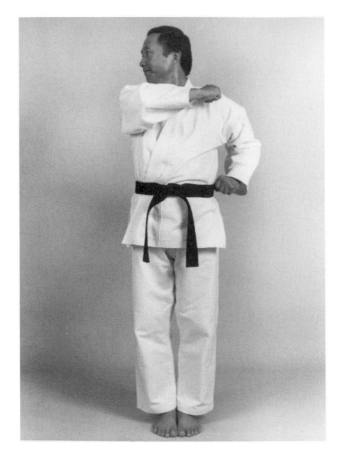

2. Hand-Supported Middle Block

a. Slide your right foot one step out to the right side toward **R-1**

b. Assume Right Back Stance.

c. Simultaneously execute a Hand-Supported Middle Block. (Outside Middle Block with your right hand and simultaneously support with your left hand by placing your open hand on the inside of the right forearm.)

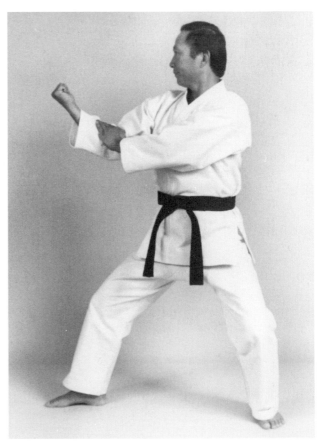

Ninth Position:
Arm Twist, Spear-Hand Thrust (Palm Down)
(Pyonsonkeut-Eopeo-Jiluki)

1. Arm Twist

a. Pivoting to the right on the ball of your left foot, slide your right foot slightly forward.

b. Assume Right Front Stance.

c. Simultaneously, opening your right fist, twist your right arm to the left and straighten forward, palm down. This motion should be performed slowly with tension.

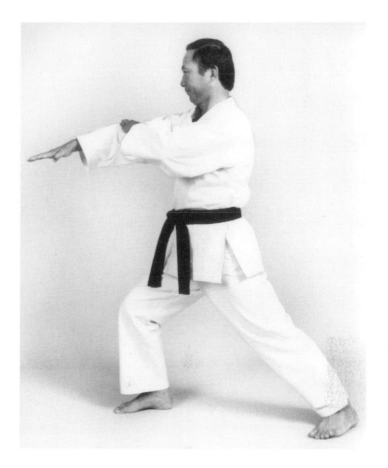

2. Spear-Hand Thrust (Palm Down)

a. Maintain the same stance.

b. Move your left Spear Hand slowly forward with tension. Then execute a Spear-Hand Thrust with your left hand, palm down, rapidly with power.

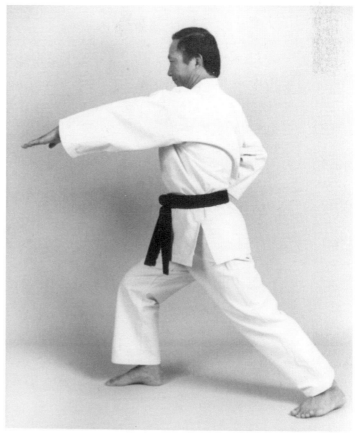

Tenth Position:
Double Middle Punch (Momtong-Doobeon-
Jiluki)

1. Middle Punch

a. Maintain the same stance.

b. Execute a Left-Hand Middle Punch.

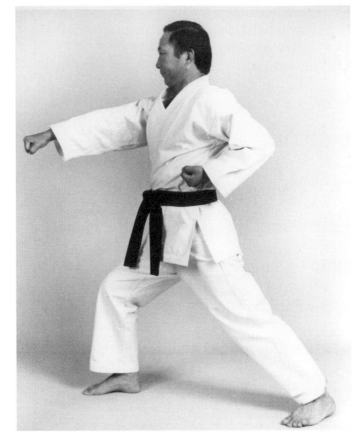

2. Reverse Middle Punch

a. Maintain the same stance.

b. Execute a Right-Hand Reverse Middle Punch.

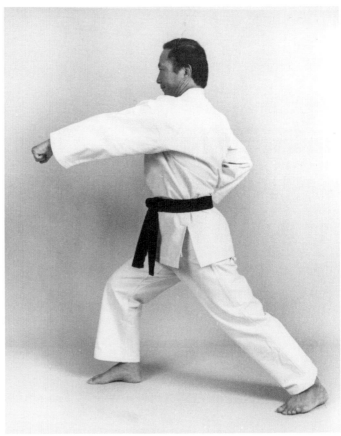

Eleventh Position:
Spread Mountain Block

a. Pivoting 90° to the right on the ball of your right foot, step forward with your left foot toward **R-1**.

b. Assume Horseback Stance, body facing **C**. Head continues to face **R-1**.

c. Simultaneously execute a Spread Mountain Block

Twelfth Position:
Cross Stance, Slide Punch, and Yell

1. Cross Stance

a. Lift your right foot and cross over your left foot. At the same time, bring your left fist to waist level, palm up, and place right arm at chest level, right fist palm down.

b. Assume Right Cross Stance.

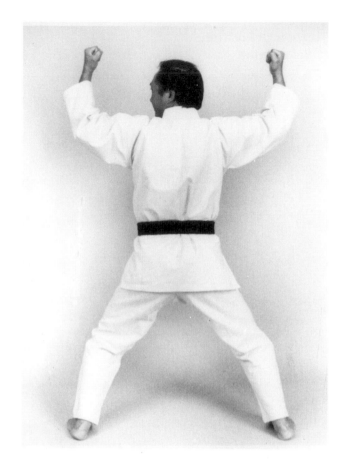

2. Side Punch

a. Keeping your right foot in place, move your left foot to the left toward **R-1**.

b. Assume Horseback Stance.

c. Simultaneously execute a Left Side Punch and yell.

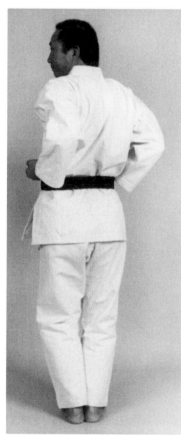

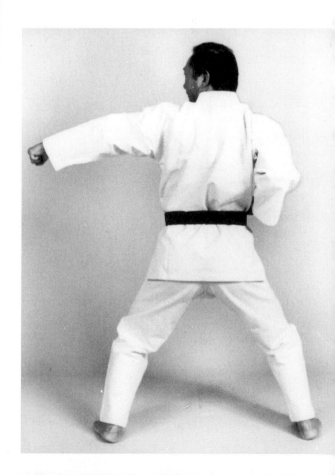

Thirteenth Position:
Yoke Strike

a. Pivoting 180° to the right on the ball of your right foot, step your left foot 180° to the right (clockwise towards **L-1**). Body is facing **B**, and face is turned toward **L-1**.

b. Assume Horseback Stance.

c. Simultaneously execute a Yoke Strike (simultaneous outward Elbow Strikes).

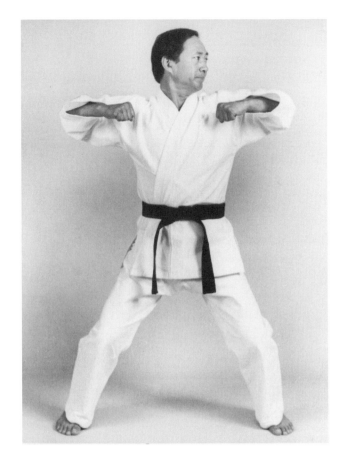

Fourteenth Position:
Hand-Supported Middle Block

a. Pivoting 90° to the right on the ball of your left foot, slide your right foot back and 180° to the right in an arc toward **C**.

b. Assume Right Back Stance.

c. Simultaneously execute a Hand-Supported Right-Hand Outside Middle Block. It is the same blocking motion as in the Eighth Position.

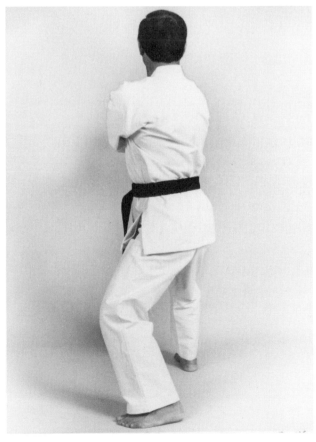

Fifteenth Position:
Arm Twist, Spear-Hand Thrust (Palm Down)

1. Arm Twist

a. Pivoting to the right on the ball of your left foot, slide your right foot slightly forward.

b. Assume Right Front Stance.

c. Simultaneously, opening your right fist, twist your right arm to the left and straighten forward, palms down. This motion should be performed slowly with tension.

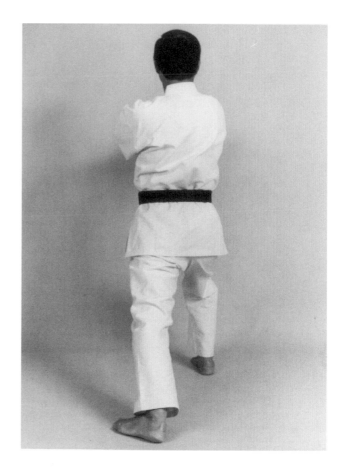

2. Spear-Hand Thrust (Palm Down)

a. Maintain the same stance.

b. Move your left Spear-Hand slowly forward with tension. Then execute a Spear-Hand Thrust with your left hand, palm down, rapidly with power.

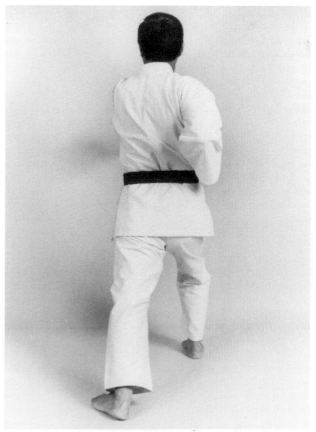

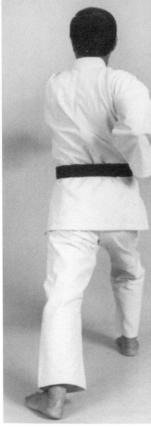
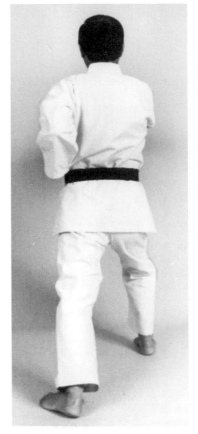

Sixteenth Position:
Double Middle Punch

1. Middle Punch

a. Maintain the same stance.

b. Execute a Right-Hand Middle Punch.

2. Reverse Middle Punch

a. Maintain the same stance.

b. Execute a Left-Hand Reverse Middle Punch.

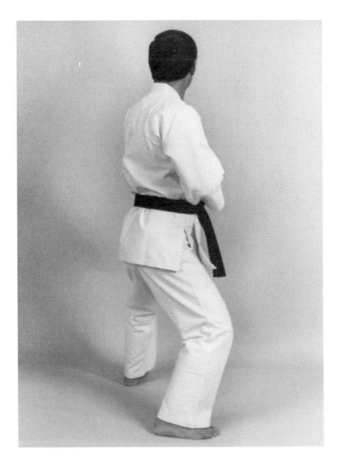

Seventeenth Position:
Knife-Hand Low Block

a. Slide your left foot forward

b. Assume Left Back Stance.

c. Simultaneously execute a Left Knife-Hand Low Block (right fist assisting, palm down).

Eighteenth Position:
Boulder Pushing (Bawi-Milki)

a. Slide your right foot forward.

b. Assume Right Front Stance.

c. Simultaneously bring both open hands outside to the right, palms out, slightly above waist level. Then push both open palms forward, elbows slightly bent, wrists tensed, as if pushing a huge boulder (execute in slow motion).

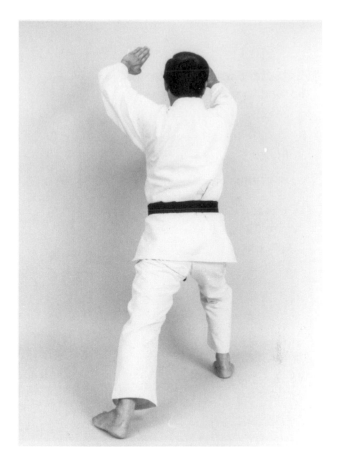

Nineteenth Position:
Spread Knife-Hand Middle Block (Palms In) (Sonnal-Deung-Hechyo-Makki)

a. Pivoting to the left on the ball of your left foot, slide your right foot in an arc to the left, body and head facing **R**.

b. Assume Horseback Stance.

c. Simultaneously execute a Spread Knife-Hand Middle Block, palms in. Cross wrists in front of chest, open palm out. Then sweep both forearms simultaneously outward, snapping both wrists, palm in, at shoulder level. The blocking surfaces are the inner forearms.

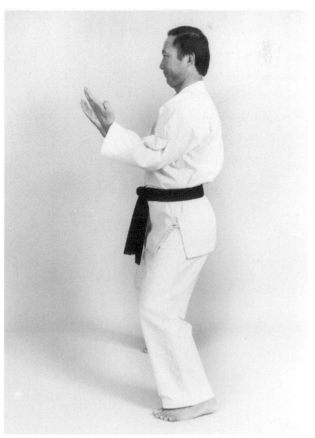

Twentieth Position:
Spread Knife-Hand Block

a. Maintain the same stance.

b. Simultaneously execute a Spread Knife-Hand Low Block in slow motion with tension.

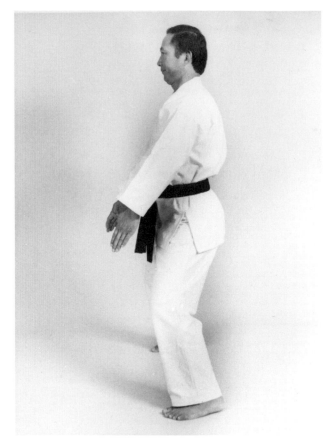

Twenty-First Position:
Clenched Fists

a. Maintaining your feet in the same position, straighten knees slowly.

b. Simultaneously clench your fists.

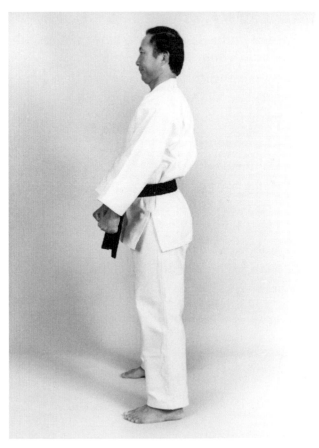

Twenty-Second Position:
Pull-Left Block (Keureo-Olliki)

a. Pivoting to the left on the ball of your right foot, slide your left foot in an arc to the left (toward **B**).

b. Assume Left Front Stance.

c. Simultaneously pull your left forearm, palm down, from your middle left side and raise upward to the right side of upper chest, palm in. (This is a blocking motion in which the inner forearm is used to pull the attacker's kicking leg and to lift it to make the opponent lose his balance.)

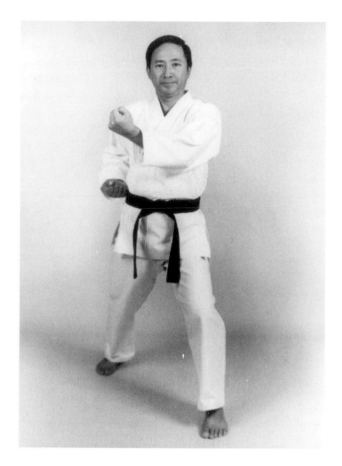

Twenty-Third Position:
Boulder Pushing

a. Maintain the same stance.

b. Execute a Boulder Pushing in slow motion (see Eighteenth Position).

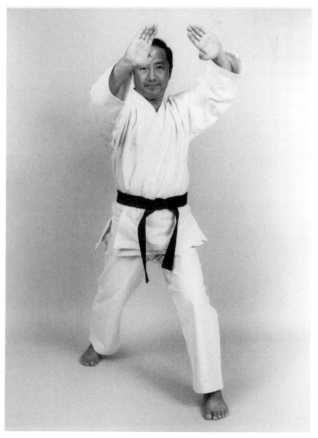

Twenty-Fourth Position:
 Front Kick, Two-Fisted Punch *(Chettari-Jiluki)*

1. Front Kick

a. Pull both fists back to the left side of the waist, left fist palm up and right fist palm in over left fist.

b. Simultaneously execute a Right Front Kick.

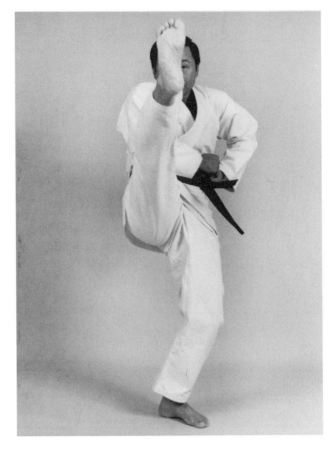

2. Two-Fisted Punch

a. Step forward with your right foot.

b. Assume Right Front Stance.

c. Simultaneously execute a Two-Fisted Punch. (This is a Middle Punch with your right fist and a Middle Punch with your left fist, in which the left arm is only extended halfway. Both punches are executed simultaneously.)

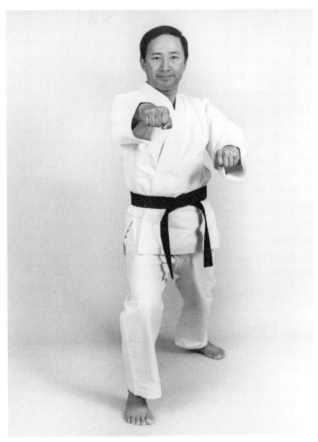

Twenty-Fifth Position:
Front Kick, Two-Fisted Punch

1. Front Kick

a. Pull both fists back to the right side of the waist, right fist palm up and left fist palm in over right fist.

b. Simultaneously execute a Left Front Kick.

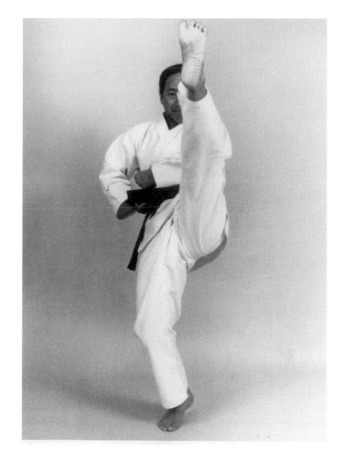

2. Two-Fisted Punch

a. Step forward with your left foot.

b. Assume Left Front Stance.

c. Simultaneously execute a Two-Fisted Punch. (This is a Middle Punch with your right fist and a Middle Punch with your left fist, in which the right arm is only extended halfway. Both punches are executed simultaneously.)

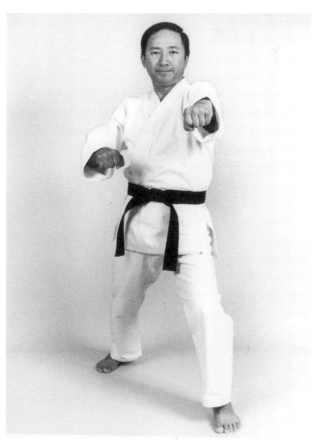

Twenty-Sixth Position:
Front Kick, Back Fist Strike (Left Had Assisting) *(Deung-Joomeok-Geodeuro-Olgool-Chikl)*

1. Front Kick

a. Pull both fists back to the left side of the waist, left fist palm up and right fist palm in over left fist.

b. Simultaneously execute a Right Front Kick.

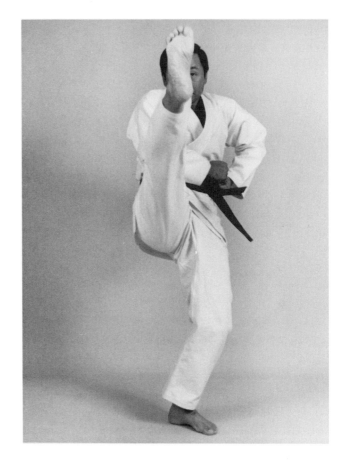

2. Back-Fist Strike (Left Hand Assisting)

a. Immediately lunge a long step forward, bringing weight down on your right foot with a stamp and drawing ball of your left foot close into position behind the right heel, standing with knees slightly bent.

b. Assume Right Cross Stance.

c. Simultaneously execute a Right Back Fist Strike, Left Hand Assisting, palm up.

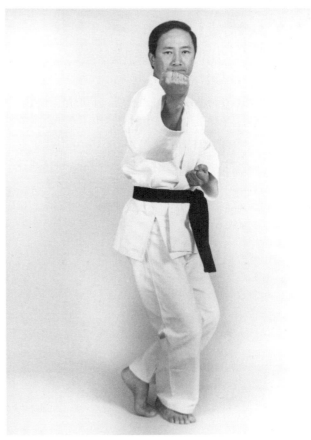

Twenty-Seventh Position:
Boulder Pushing

a. Pivoting to the left 180° on the ball of your right foot, slide your left foot backward and take one step toward **A** with your left foot as you turn toward **A**.

b. Assume Left Front Stance.

c. Simultaneously execute a Boulder Pushing in slow motion with tension toward **A**.

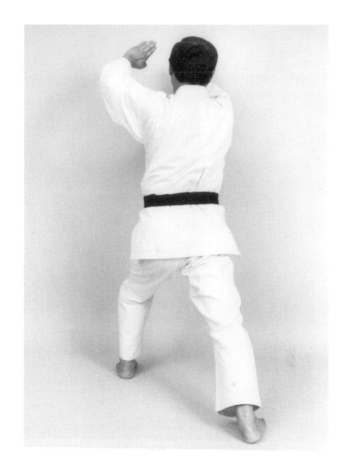

Twenty-Eighth Position:
Knife-Hand X Block *(Sohnnal-Otkolo-Makki)*

a. Keeping the same position with your right foot, slide your left foot backwards slightly.

b. Assume Left Cat Stance.

c. Simultaneously execute a Knife-Hand Low X Block.

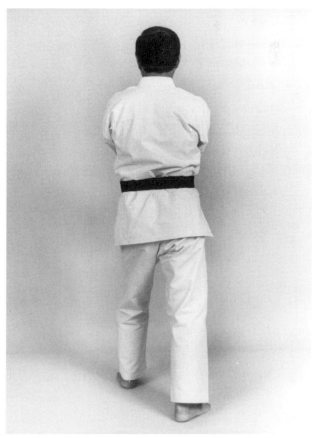

Twenty-Ninth Position:
Ridge-Hand Middle Block

a. Slide your right foot forward.

b. Assume Right Back Stance.

c. Simultaneously execute a Right Ridge-Hand Middle Block.

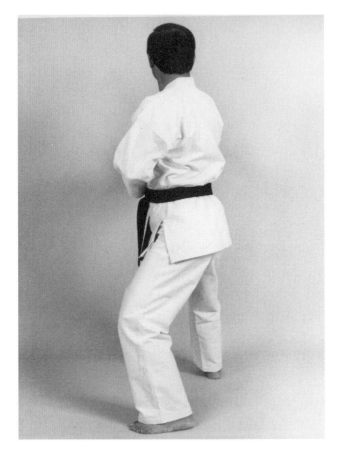

Thirtieth Position:
Two-Fisted Punch (Chettari-Jiluki)

a. Slide your left foot forward

b. Assume Left Back Stance.

c. Simultaneously execute a Two-Fisted Punch. (Your left arm is completely extended, and your right arm is only extended halfway.)

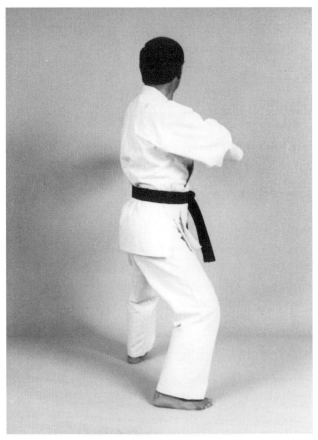

Thirty-First Position:
Two-Fisted Punch

a. Slide your right foot forward.

b. Assume Right Back Stance.

c. Simultaneously execute a Two-Fisted Punch. (Your right arm is completely extended and your left arm is only extended halfway.)

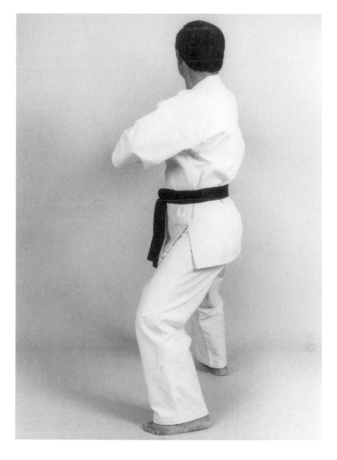

Stop

Pivoting to the left on the ball of your right foot, turn your body 180° to the left toward **B**. At the same time, slide your left foot backward into Ready Stance, facing **B** at point **A**.

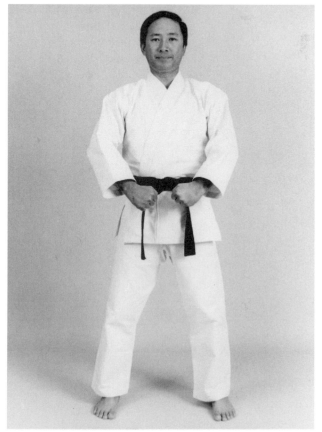

JITAE (EARTH)

According to Oriental beliefs, all life comes from and returns to the earth. The earth is endlessly bountiful, yielding the fruit that sustains mankind. It is also completely accepting, as all living things eventually become earth again. The earth hides its greatest power deep within its hot core, only occasionally allowing it to well up in volcanoes or to shake the buildings of civilization, reminding man how weak he is in comparison with the supreme strength of the earth.

In the form *Jitae* you must demonstrate the properties of the earth, showing the vigor of life as it stems from the power welling up from strong muscles and from a deep powerful core.

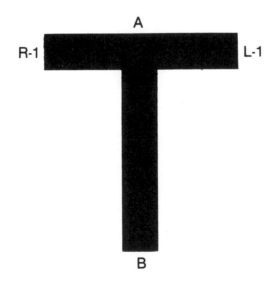

Jitae

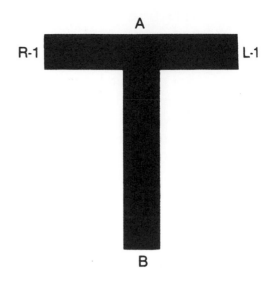

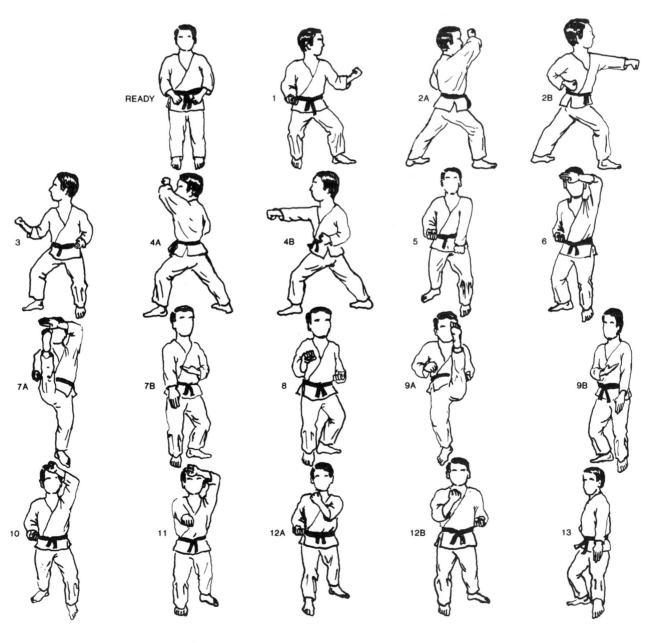

READY   1   2A   2B   3   4A   4B   5   6   7A   7B   8   9A   9B   10   11   12A   12B   13

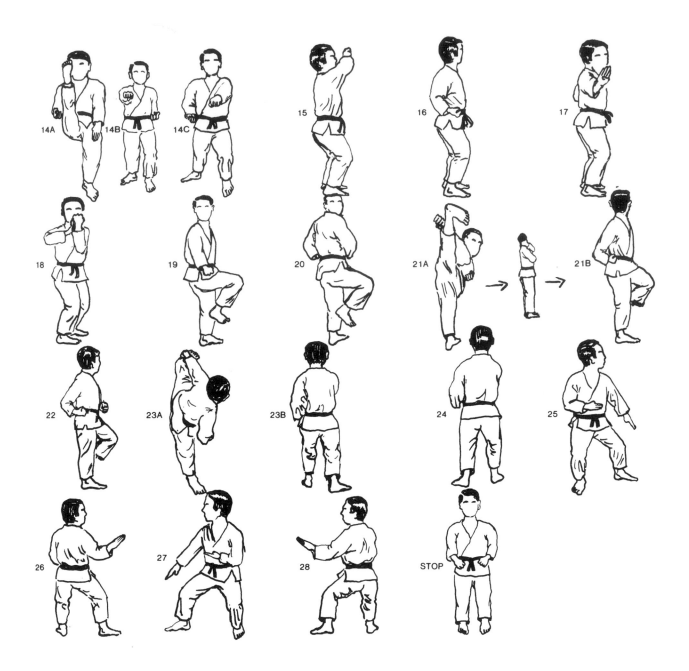

Ready

Maintain Ready Stance, facing B at point A, eyes focused straight ahead.

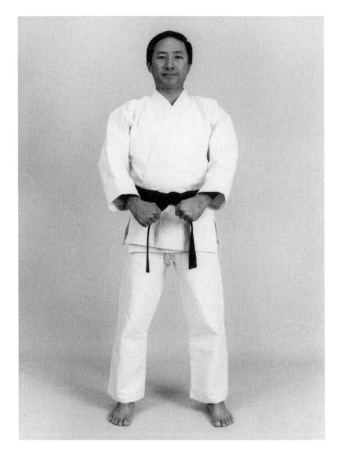

First Position:
Outside Middle Block

a. Slide your left foot 90° to the left (toward **L-1**).

b. Assume Left Back Stance.

c. Simultaneously execute an Outside Middle Block with your left hand.

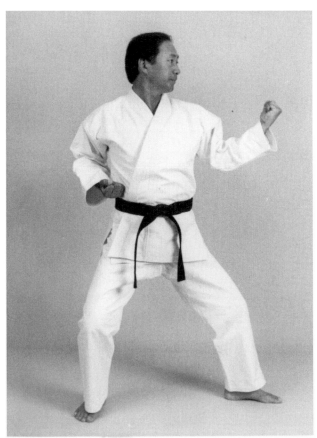

Second Position:
High Block, Reverse Middle Punch

1. High Block

a. Slide your right foot forward with tension.

b. Assume Right Front Stance.

c. Simultaneously execute a Right-Hand High Block in a slow motion with full tension. While executing the block, exhale slowly and fully.

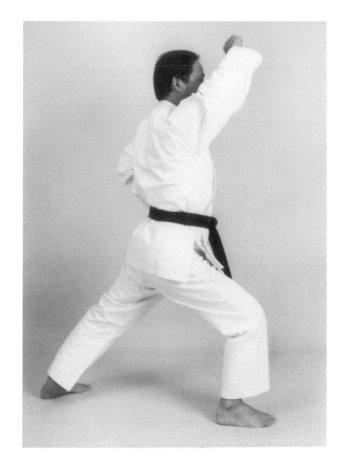

2. Reverse Middle Punch

a. Maintain the same stance.

b. Execute a Left-Hand Reverse Middle Punch with full tension.

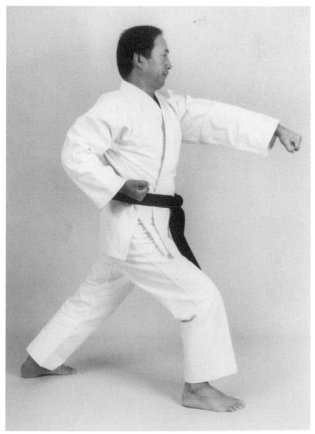

Third Position:
Outside Middle Block

a. Pivoting to the right on the ball of your left foot, slide your right foot out and back in a wide arc, turning 180° to the right (toward **R-1**).

b. Assume Right Back Stance.

c. Simultaneously execute an Outside Middle Block with your right hand.

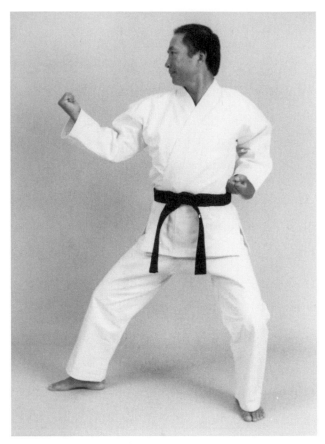

Fourth Position:
High Block, Reverse
Middle Punch

1. High Block

a. Slide your left foot forward.

b. Assume Left Front Stance.

c. Simultaneously execute a Left-Hand High Block in slow motion with full tension.

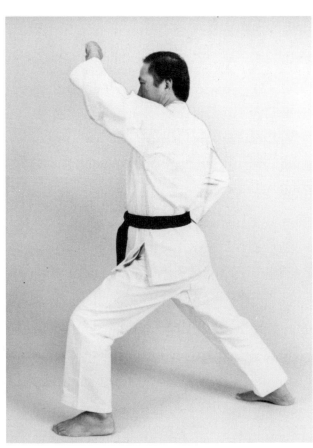

2. Reverse Middle Punch

a. Maintain the same stance.

b. Execute a Left-Hand Reverse Middle Punch with full tension.

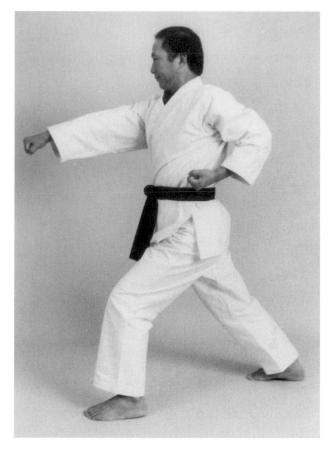

Fifth Position:
Low Block

Note: The two positions, Fifth and Sixth, should be performed in rapid sequence.

a. Pivoting to the left on the ball of your right foot, slide your left foot out to the left, turning 90° (toward **B**).

b. Assume Left Front Stance.

c. Simultaneously execute a Left-Hand Low Block.

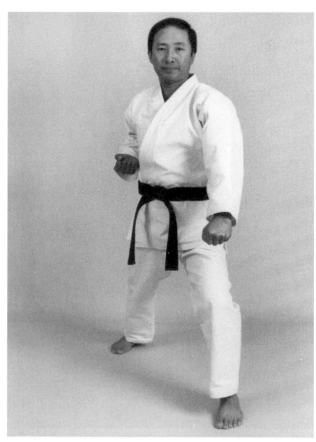

Sixth Position:
Single Knife-Hand High Block

Note: The two positions, Fifth and Sixth, should be performed in rapid sequence.

a. Pivoting your right foot to the right in place, slide your left foot slightly backward.

b. Simultaneously execute a Left Single Knife-Hand High Block

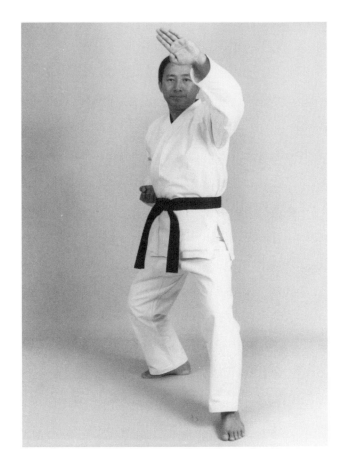

Seventh Position:
Front Kick, Knife-Hand Low Block

1. Front Kick
a. Execute a Front Kick with your right foot.

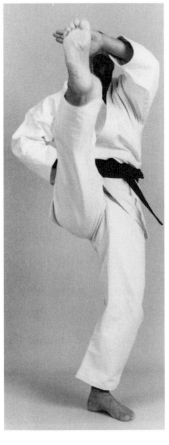
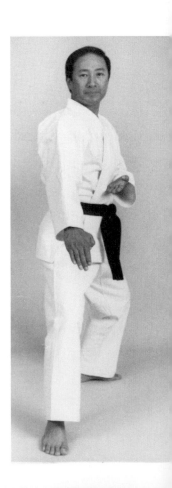

2. Knife Low Block
a. Step forward with your right foot.

b. Assume Right Back Stance.

c. Simultaneously execute a Right Knife-Hand Low Block.

Eighth Position:
  Outside Middle Block (Palm Out) *(Bakat-Palmok-Bakat-Makki)*

a. Maintain the same stance.

b. Execute an Outside Middle Block, palm out, with your right hand in slow motion with tension (the block should be performed with proper breathing motion).

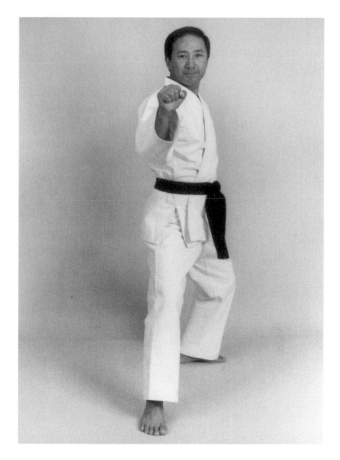

Ninth Position:
  Front Kick, Knife-Hand Low Block

1. Front Kick
a. Execute a Front Kick with your left foot.

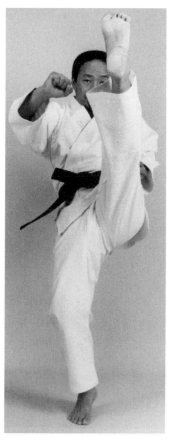

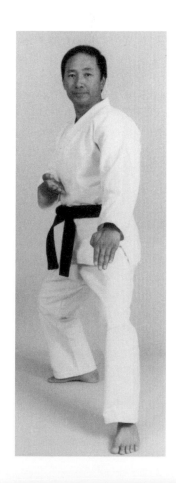

2. Knife-Hand Low Block
a. Step forward with your left foot.

b. Assume Left Back Stance.

c. Simultaneously execute a Left Knife-Hand Low Block.

Tenth Position:
High Block

a. Pivoting your right foot to the left in place, slide your left foot slightly forward.

b. Assume Left Front Stance.

c. Simultaneously execute a Left-Hand High Block (in slow motion with tension).

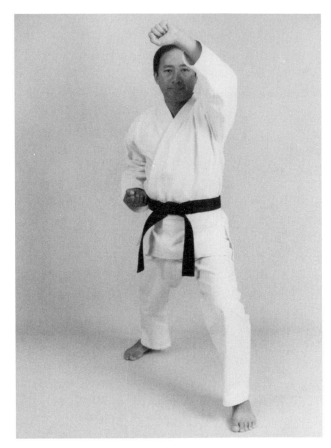

Eleventh Position:
Diamond Punch (Keumgang-Jiluki)

a. Slide your right foot forward.

b. Assume Right Front Stance.

c. Simultaneously execute a Diamond Punch (High Block with your left hand and Middle Punch with your right hand).

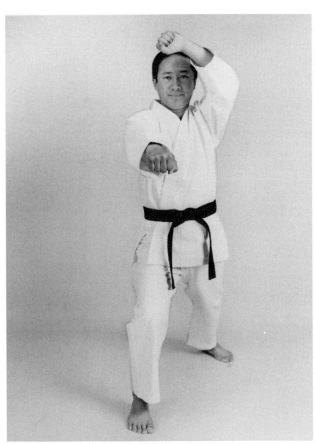

Twelfth Position:
Inside Middle Block, Inside Middle Block

Note: The blocks, 1 and 2, should be performed in rapid sequence.

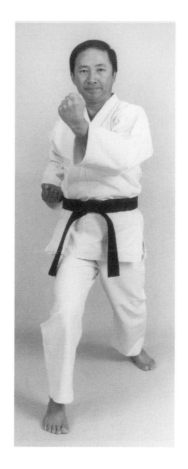
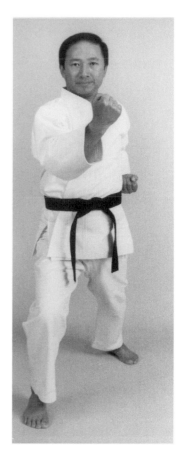

1. Inside Middle Block

a. Maintain the same stance.

b. Execute an Inside Middle Block with your left hand.

2. Inside Middle Block

a. Maintain the same stance.

b. Execute an Inside Middle Block with your right hand.

Thirteenth Position:
Single Knife-Hand Low Block

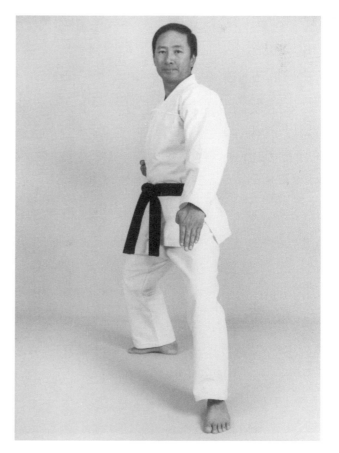

a. Slide your right foot backward toward **A**.

b. Assume Left Back Stance.

c. Simultaneously execute a Single Left Knife-Hand Low Block.

Fourteenth Position:
Front Kick, Double-Hand Middle Punch

1. Front Kick

a. Execute a Front Kick with your right foot.

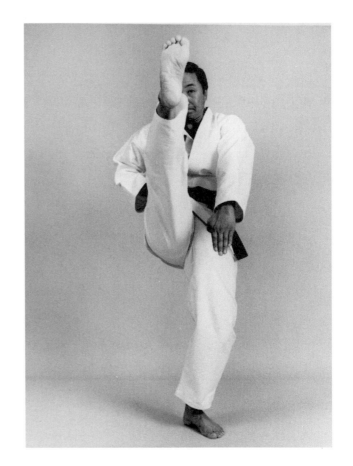

2. Reverse Middle Punch

a. Step backward with your right foot toward **A**. Body continues facing **B**.

b. Assume Left Front Stance.

c. Simultaneously execute a Reverse Middle Punch with your right hand.

3. Middle Punch

a. Consecutively execute a Middle Punch with your left hand.

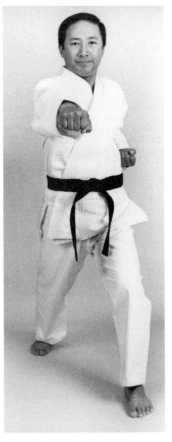

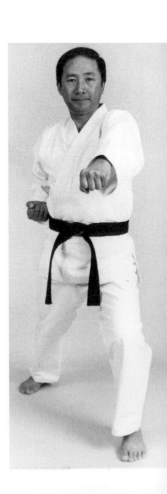

Fifteenth Position:
Bull Block *(Hwangso-Makki)*

a. Pivoting your right foot to the left, slide your left foot backward toward **A**.

b. Assume Horseback Stance, body facing **L**.

c. Simultaneously execute a Bull Block (toward **L**).

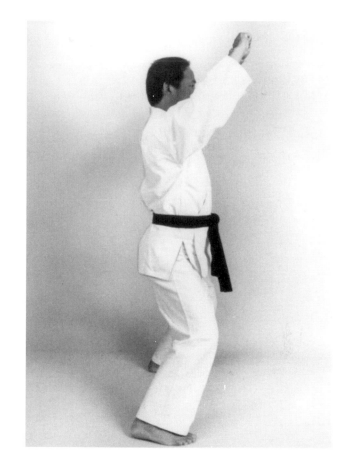

Sixteenth Position:
Low Block to the Side

a. Maintaining the same stance, turn your face toward **A**.

b. Simultaneously execute a Low Block to the left side (toward **A**) with your left hand.

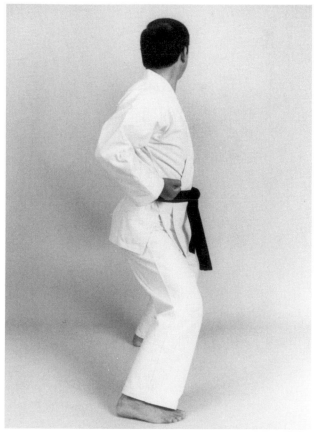

Seventeenth Position:
Single Knife-Hand Outside Middle Block

a. Maintaining the same stance, turn your face toward **B**.

b. Simultaneously execute a single Right Knife-Hand Outside Middle Block.

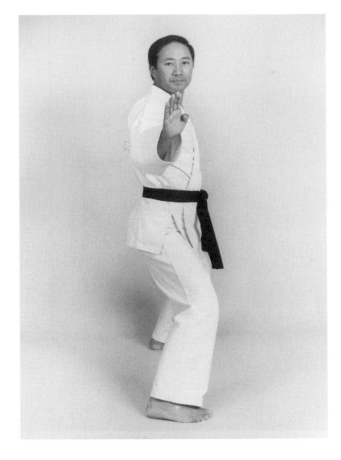

Eighteenth Position:
Hammer-Fist Target Punch (*Mejoomeok-Pyojeok-Emiki*) and Yell

a. Maintain the same stance.

b. Execute a Left-Hand Hammer-Fist Target Punch toward **B**, left Hammer Fist hitting right open hand, and yell.

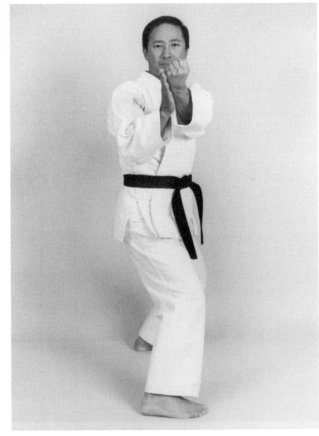

Nineteenth Position:
Low Block to the Side

Note: The next six positions, Nineteenth through Twenty-Fourth, should be performed in rapid sequence.

a. Maintaining your left foot in place, raise your right foot to your left knee.

b. Assume Left Crane Stance.

c. Simultaneously execute a Low Block to the right side toward **B** with your right hand.

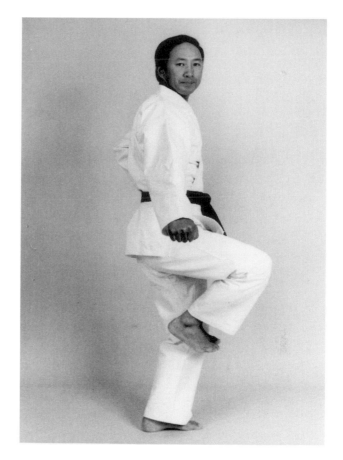

Twentieth Position:
Left Crane Stance with Hand Positions for Side Kick *(Oen-Jageun-Dolcheogi)*

a. Maintain the same stance.

b. Bring both fists to your left side, left fist palm up at waist level and right fist palm in over left fist.

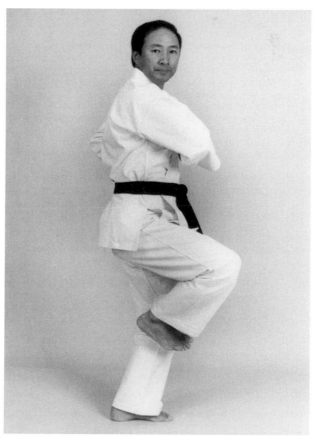

Twenty-First Position:
Side Kick, Low Block to the Side

1. Side Kick

a. Execute a Side Kick with your right foot toward **B**.

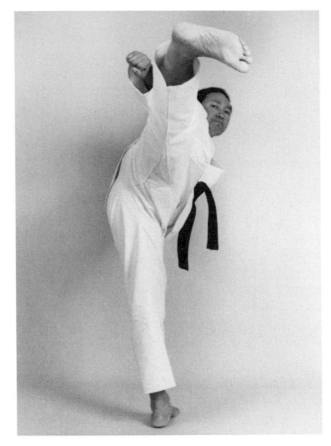

2. Low Block to the Side

a. With a jumping motion, bring your right foot down placing it next to your left foot and at the same time raise your left foot to your right knee.

b. Assume Right Crane Stance. Face turns toward **A**, body facing **L**.

c. Simultaneously execute a Low Block to the left side toward **A** with your left hand.

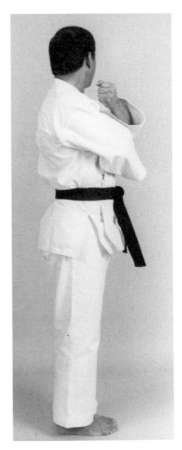
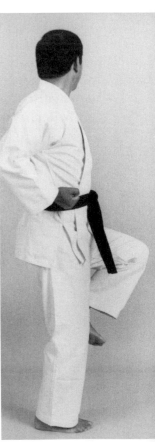

Twenty-Second Position:
Right Crane Stance with Hand Positions for Side Kick *(Oreun-Jageun-Dolcheogi)*

a. Maintain the same stance.

b. Bring both fists to your right side, right fist palm up to waist level and left fist palm in over right fist.

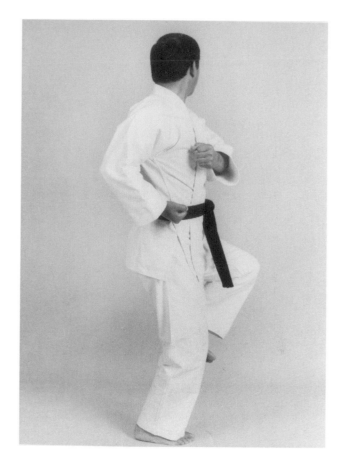

Twenty-Third Position:
Side Kick, Reverse Middle Punch

1. Side Kick

a. Execute a Side Kick with your left foot toward **A**.

2. Reverse Middle Punch

a. Step forward with your right foot toward **A**.

b. Assume Left Front Stance.

c. Simultaneously execute a Reverse Middle Punch with your right hand.

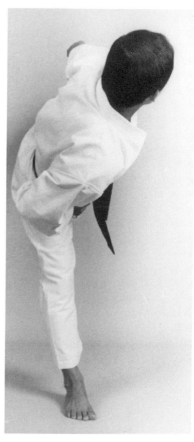

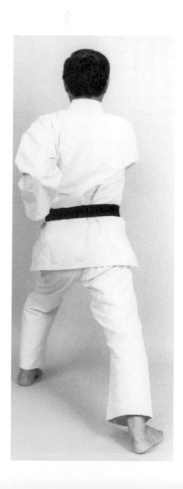

Twenty-Fourth Position:
Middle Punch and Yell

Note: The six positions, Nineteenth through Twenty-Fourth, should be performed in rapid sequence.

a. Slide your right foot forward.

b. Assume Right Front Stance.

c. Simultaneously execute a Right-Hand Middle Punch and yell.

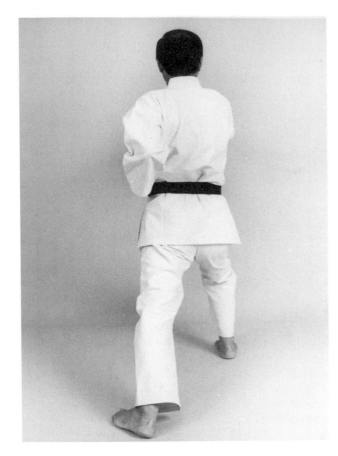

Twenty-Fifth Position:
Knife-Hand Low Block

a. Pivoting to the left on the ball of your right foot, slide your left foot out and back to the left in a wide arc, turning 270° (facing **L-1**).

b. Assume Left Back Stance.

c. Simultaneously execute a Left Knife-Hand Low Block

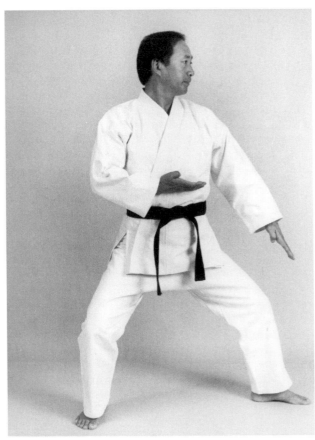

**Twenty-Sixth Position:
Knife-Hand Middle Block**

a. Slide your right foot forward.

b. Assume Right Back Stance.

c. Simultaneously execute a Right Knife-Hand Middle Block.

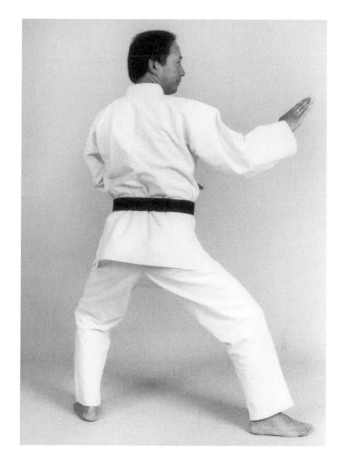

**Twenty-Seventh Position:
Knife-Hand Low Block**

a. Pivoting to the right on the ball of your left foot, slide your right foot out and back in a wide arc, turning 180° to the right (toward **R-1**).

b. Assume Right Back Stance.

c. Simultaneously execute a Right Knife-Hand Low Block.

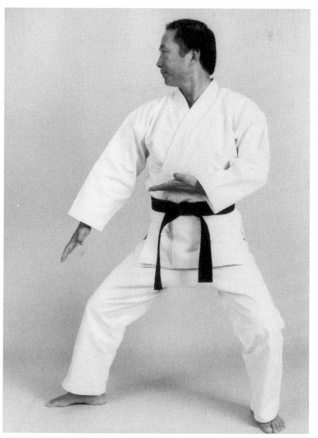

Twenty-Eighth Position:
Knife-Hand Middle Block

a. Slide your left foot forward.

b. Assume Left Back Stance.

c. Simultaneously execute a Left Knife-Hand Middle Block.

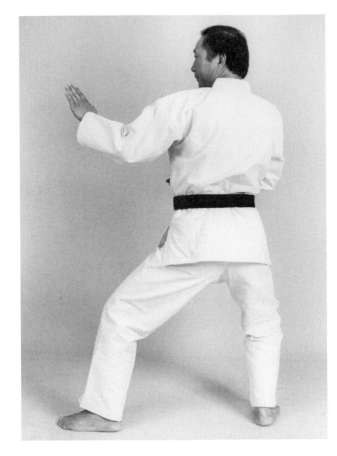

Stop

Pivoting to the left on the ball of your right foot, slide your left foot out and back, turning 90° to the left, facing **B** at point **A**. Assume Ready Stance.

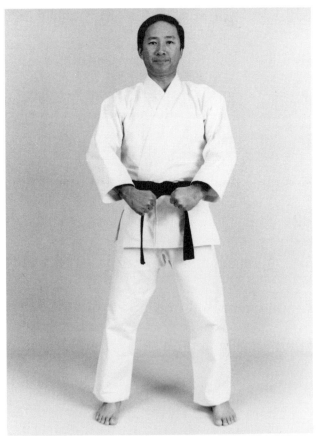

CHEONKWON (SKY)

Since ancient times, Orientals have worshiped the sky as the ruler of the Universe and of mankind. The sky is the highest, the most supreme. They have also thought that the sky controls everything in nature. And so, in the eyes of finite human beings, the infinite sky is awesome, touching the mysterious and profound world of man's imagination. Man has always envied the bird's capacity for flight, aspiring to become, even for a moment, part of the sky, and thus throughout the development of civilization he has used his yearning to reach higher and higher into the heavens.

In the motions of the form *Cheonkwon*, you must demonstrate the piety and awe that the sky commands as well as the vitality it sparks in man's imagination, driving him to strive upward. The form should show a man's feelings as he looks up from earth and is reminded of an eagle flying off into the clouds.

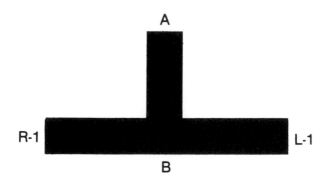

Cheonkwon

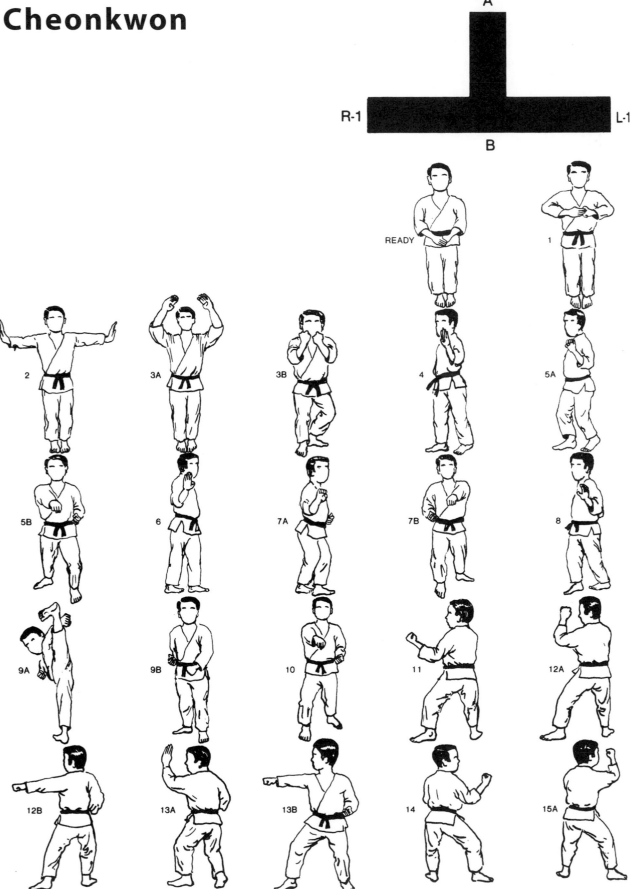

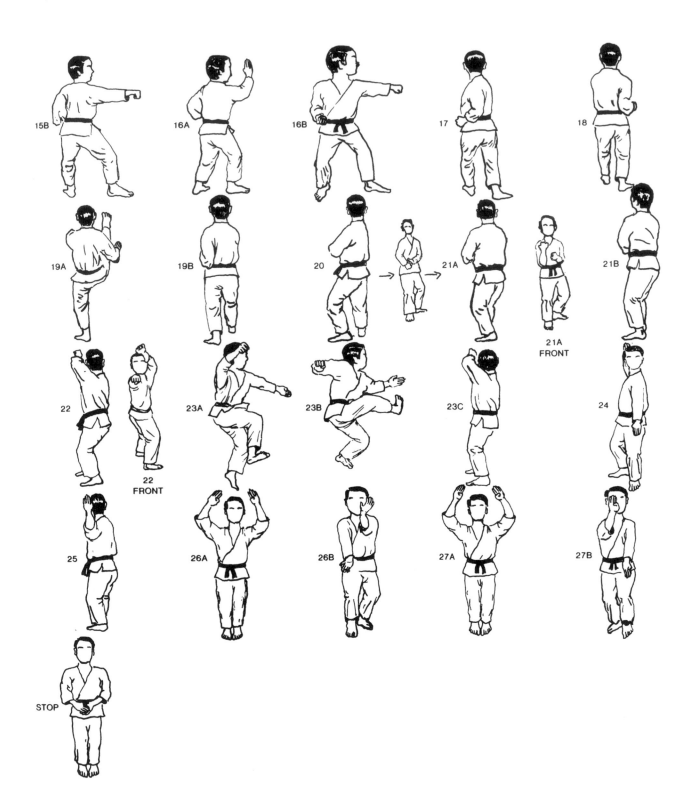

Ready (Cross-Hand Ready) *(Gyopsohn-Choonbi)*

Maintain an Informal Stance, facing **B** at point **A**, eyes focused straight ahead, with both open hands positioned in front of abdomen, palms in, right hand crossing over left hand.

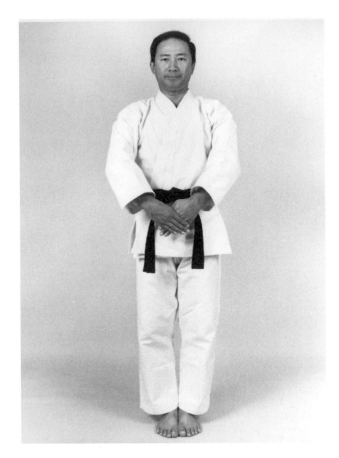

First Position: Folded Hands *(Gyop-Sohn)*

a. Maintain the same stance.

b. Bring both open hands very close to body up to chest level in slow motion, right hand on top of left hand. (Tips of fingers should be aligned with wrists of opposite hand.) Inhale while performing this motion.

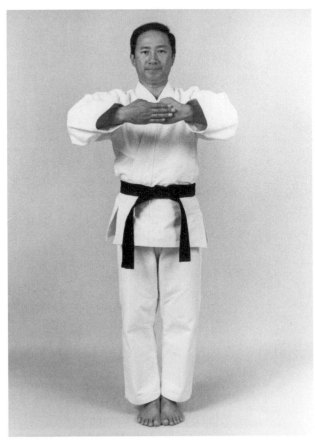

Second Position:
Open Wing (Nalgae-Pyogi)

a. Maintain the same stance.

b. Spread both hands to the sides at shoulder level in slow motion with tension, palms out, exhaling while performing this motion.

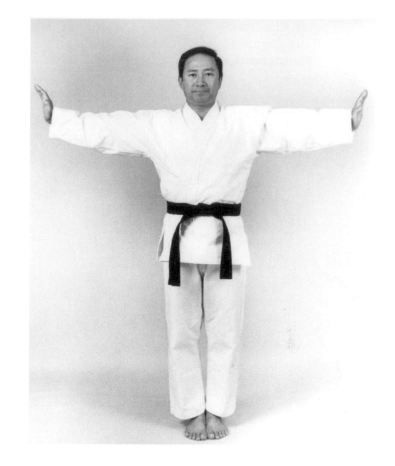

Third Position:
Knife-Hand Bull Block, Middle-Knuckle Fist Punch (Bamjoomeok-Soseum-Chiki)

1. Knife-Hand Bull Block

a. Maintain the same stance.

b. Bring both open hands down and cross in front of body, right hand over left hand, and continue to raise hands (palms out) to prepare for Knife-Hand Bull Block. The above movements should be performed as one continuous motion.

c. Execute a Knife-Hand Bull Block.

2. Middle-Knuckle Fist Punch (Both Fists)

a. Circle both hands downward in a wide arc in slow motion

b. Stamp backward with your left foot.

c. Assume Right Back Stance.

d. Simultaneously execute a Middle-Knuckle Fist Punch (with both fists).

Note: Third Position, 1 and 2 should be performed in a rapid continuous motion.

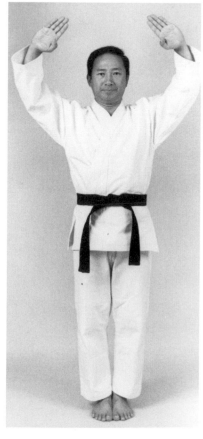

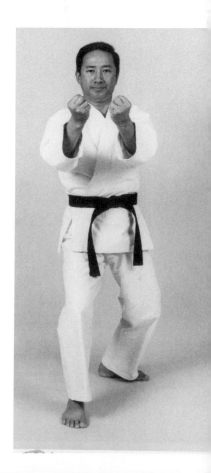

Fourth Position:
Single Knife-Hand Outside Middle Block (Hansonnal-Jebipoom-Momtong-Bakat-Makki)

a. Pivoting to the right on the ball of your right foot, slide your left foot slightly backward toward **L**. Body turns toward **R** and head continues to face **B**.

b. Assume Right High Front Stance (toward **R**).

c. Simultaneously execute a Left Single Knife-Hand Outside Middle Block (toward **B**).

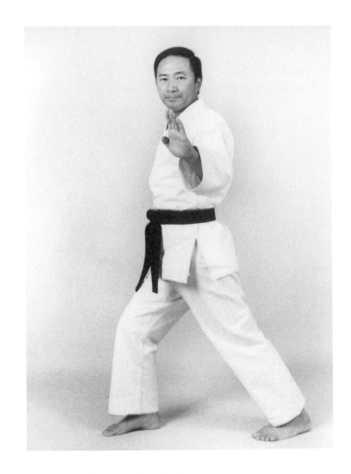

Fifth Position:
Twist and Grab, Pull and Reverse Middle Punch

1. Twist and Grab
a. While twisting your wrist, circle your left Knife Hand to the left, then grab.

2. Pull and Reverse Middle Punch
a. Pulling your left hand to the waist, slide your left foot forward toward **B** in slow motion.

b. Assume Left Front Stance.

c. Simultaneously execute a Right-Hand Reverse Middle Punch (in slow motion with tension).

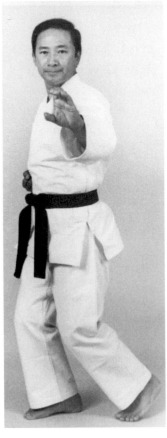

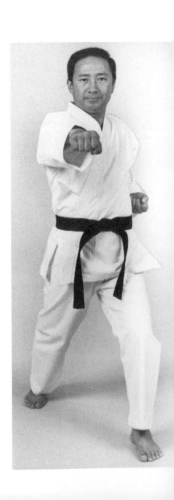

Sixth Position:
Single Knife-Hand Outside Middle Block

a. Pivoting to the left on the ball of your left foot, slide your right foot slightly backward toward **R**. Body turns toward **L**, and head continues to face **A**.

b. Assume Left High Front Stance (toward **L**).

c. Simultaneously execute a Right Single Knife-Hand Outside Middle Block (toward **B**).

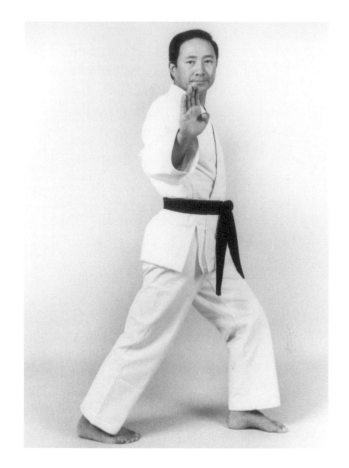

Seventh Position:
Twist and Grab, Pull and Reverse Middle Punch

1. Twist and Grab

a. While twisting your wrist, circle your Right Knife-Hand to the right, then grab.

2. Pull and Reverse Middle Punch

a. Pulling your right hand to the waist, slide your right foot forward toward **B** in slow motion.

b. Assume Right Front Stance.

c. Simultaneously execute a Left-Hand Reverse Middle Punch (in slow motion with tension).

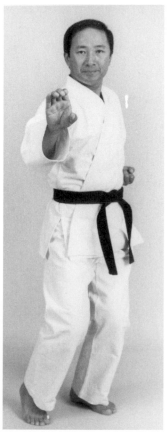
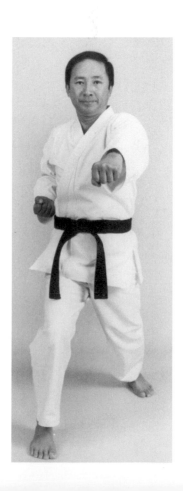

Eighth Position:
Single Knife-Hand Outside Middle Punch

a. Pivoting to the right on the ball of your right foot, slide your left foot slightly backward toward **L**. Body turns toward **R** and head continues to face **B**.

b. Assume Right High Front Stance (toward **R**).

c. Simultaneously execute a Left Single Knife-Hand Outside Middle Block (toward **B**).

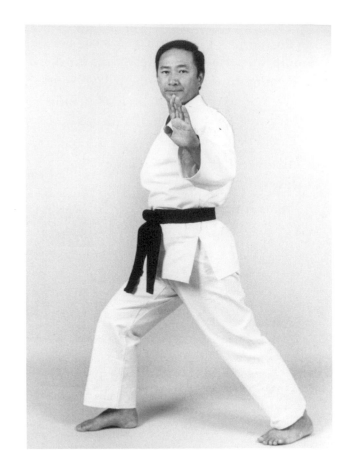

Ninth Position:
Twist and Grab, Pull and Side Kick, and Yell, Low Block

1. Twist and Grab, Pull and Side Kick, and Yell

a. While twisting your wrist, circle your left Knife Hand to the left, then grab.

b. Pulling your left hand, execute a Side Kick with your left foot and yell.

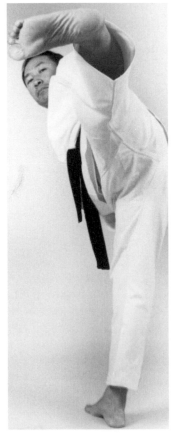

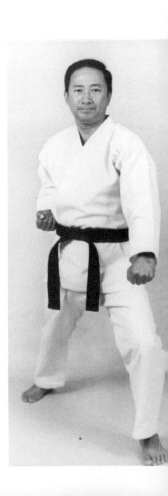

2. Low Block

a. Step forward with your left foot toward **B**.

b. Assume Left Front Stance.

c. Simultaneously execute a Left-Hand Low Block.

Tenth Position:
Middle Punch

a. Slide your right foot forward.

b. Assume Right Front Stance.

c. Simultaneously execute a Right-Hand Middle Punch.

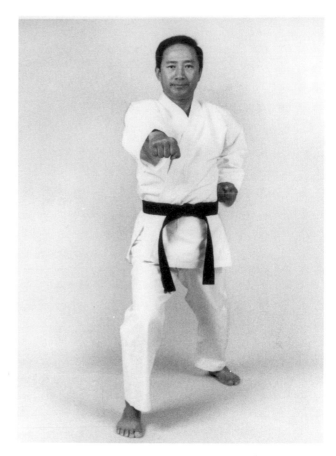

Eleventh Position:
Double-Hand Middle Block

a. Pivoting to the left on the ball of your right foot, slide your left foot out and back to the left in a wide arc, turning 270° (three-quarters of a circle) to face **R-1**.

b. Assume Left Back Stance.

c. Simultaneously execute a Double-Hand Middle Block with your left inner forearm.

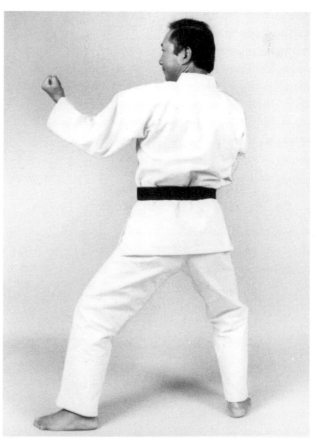

Twelfth Position:
Outside Middle Block (Palm Out), Side Punch

1. Outside High Block (Palm Out)

a. Maintain the same stance.

b. Circling your left fist inside to outside (counterclockwise), execute a Left-Hand Outside High Block, palm out. Your right hand remains in place.

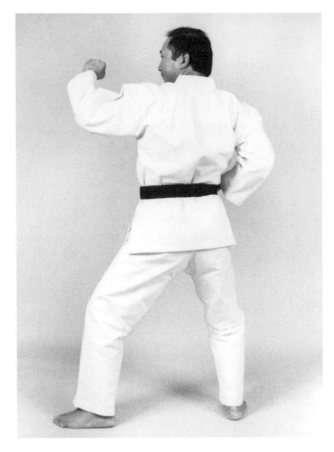

2. Side Punch

a. Maintain the same stance.

b. Execute a Left Side Punch.

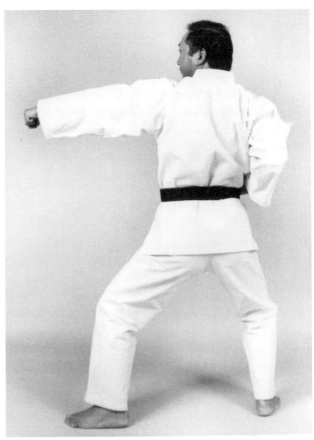

Thirteenth Position:
Single Knife-Hand Outside High Block, Grab and Pull and Side Punch

1. **Single Knife-Hand Outside High Block, Grab and Pull.**

a. Maintain the same stance, but shift your weight to your left foot in preparation to move forward.

b. Circling your Left Knife Hand inside to outside (counterclockwise), execute a Left Single Knife-Hand Outside High Block.

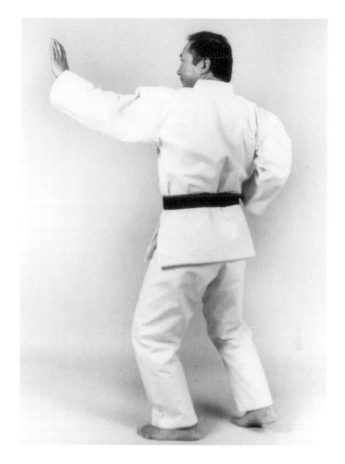

2. **Grab and Pull, Side Punch**

a. Slide your right foot forward.

b. Assume Right Back Stance.

c. Simultaneously grabbing and pulling with your left hand to the waist, execute a Right Side Punch.

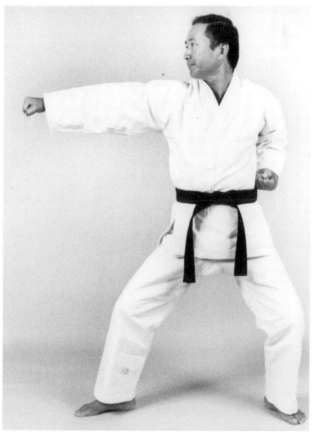

Fourteenth Position:
Double-Hand Middle Block

a. Pivoting to the right on the ball of your left foot, slide your right foot out and back in a wide arc, turning 180° to the right (toward **L-1**).

b. Assume Right Back Stance.

c. Simultaneously execute a Double-Hand Middle Block with your right inner forearm.

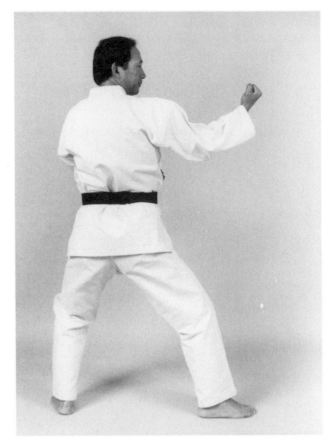

Fifteenth Position:
Outside Middle Block (Palm Out), Side Punch

1. Outside High Block (Palm Out)

a. Maintain the same stance.

b. Circling your right fist inside to outside (clockwise), execute a Right-Hand Outside High Block, palm out. Your left hand remains in place.

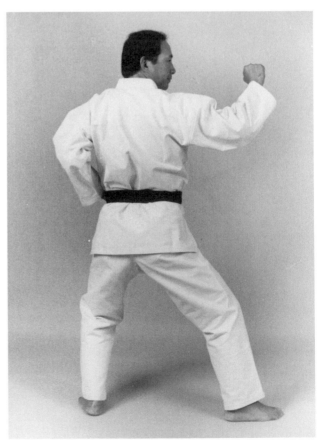

2. Side Punch
a. Maintain the same stance.

b. Execute a Right Side Punch.

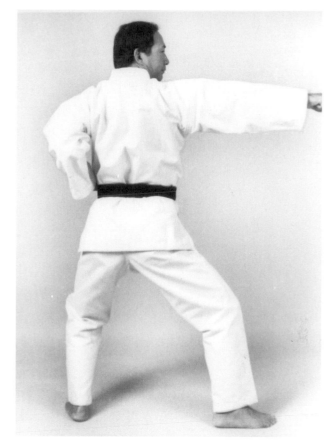

Sixteenth Position:
Single Knife-Hand Outside High Block, Grab and Pull, and Side Punch

1. Single Knife-Hand Outside High Block

a. Maintain the same stance, but shift your weight to the right foot in preparation to move forward.

b. Circling your Right Knife Hand inside to outside (clockwise), execute a Right Single Knife-Hand Outside High Block.

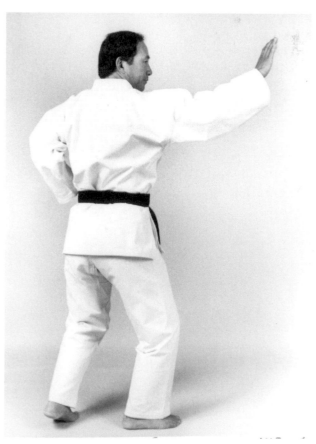

2. Grab and Pull, Side Punch

a. Slide your left foot forward

b. Assume Left Back Stance.

c. Simultaneously grabbing and pulling with your right hand to the waist, execute a Left Side Punch.

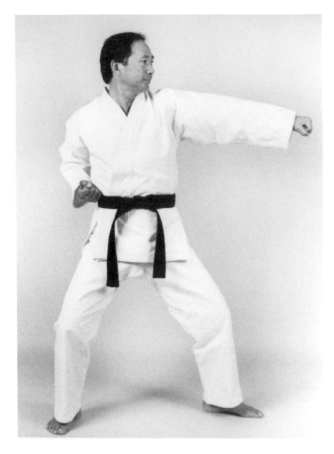

Seventeenth Position: Outside Middle Block

a. Pivoting to the left on the ball of your right foot, slide your left foot out, turning 90° to the left (toward **A**).

b. Assume Left Front Stance.

c. Simultaneously execute a Right-Hand Outside Middle Block.

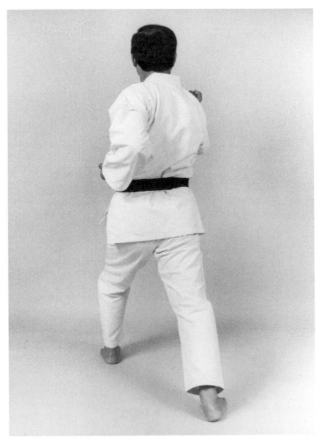

Eighteen Position:
Middle Punch

a. Maintain the same stance.

b. Execute a Left-Hand Middle Punch.

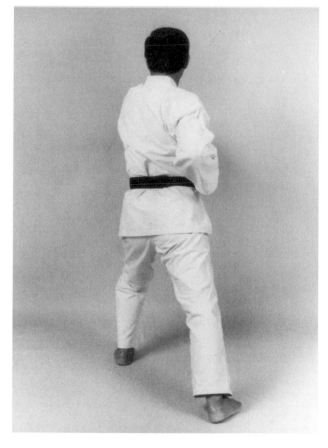

Nineteenth Position:
Front Kick, Middle Punch

1. Front Kick

a. Execute a Front Kick with your right foot.

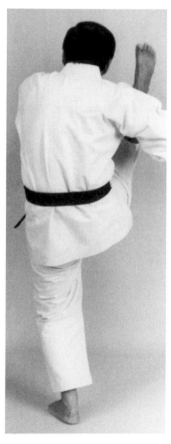

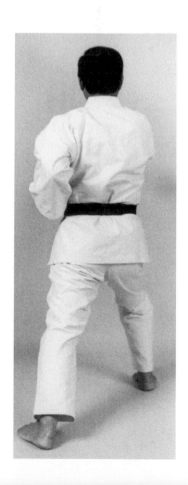

2. Middle Punch

a. Step forward with your right foot toward **A**.

b. Assume Right Front Stance.

c. Simultaneously execute a Right-Hand Middle Punch.

Twentieth Position:
Knife-Hand Low Block

a. Pivoting to the left on the ball of your left foot, slide your right foot slightly backward.

b. Assume Right Back Stance.

c. Simultaneously execute a Right Knife-Hand Low Block.

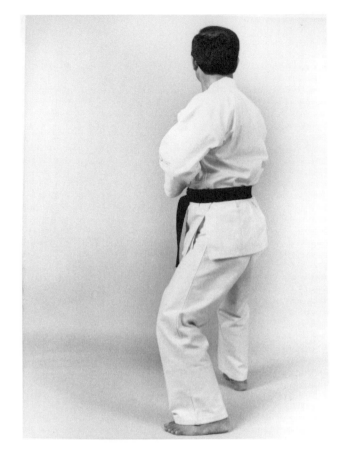

Twenty-First Position:
Open-Hand Wrist Middle Block, Knife-Hand Low Block

1. Open-Hand Wrist Middle Block

a. Hop half a step forward and at the same time hit your open left palm with the wrist of your open right hand at stomach level.

b. Assume Right Back Stance.

c. Simultaneously execute a Right Wrist Middle Block (hand open and palms in), your open left hand placed at left side of abdomen, palm down.

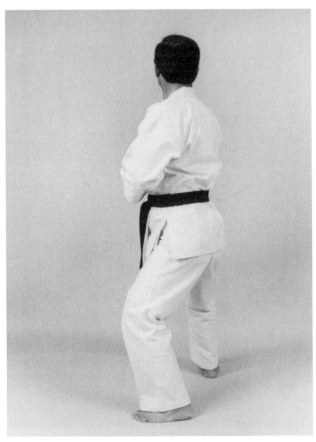

2. Knife-Hand Low Block

a. Hop half a step forward and at the same time hit your open left palm with your right wrist at stomach level.

b. Assume Right Back Stance.

c. Simultaneously execute a Right Knife-Hand Low Block, your open left hand placed in front of stomach, palm up.

Note: Twenty-First Position, 1 and 2, should be performed in a continuous motion.

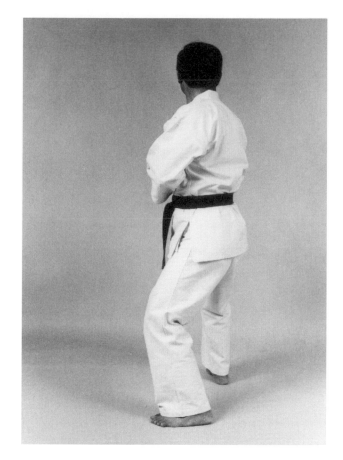

Twenty-Second Position: Diamond Side Punch (Keumgang-Yeop-Jiluki)

a. Slide your right foot slightly forward.

b. Assume Horseback Stance, body facing **R**, head continues to face **A**.

c. Simultaneously execute a Diamond Side Punch (High Block with your left hand and a Side Punch with your right hand).

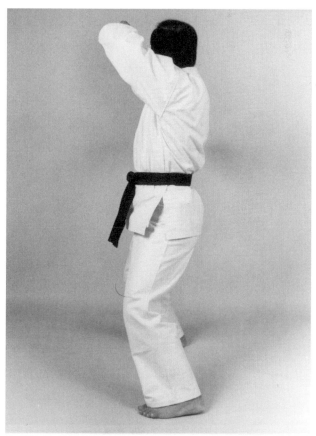

Twenty-Third Position:
Stamp and Jump, Target Kick, Diamond Side
Punch

1. Stamp and Jump
a. Stamping your right foot, jump and turn your body 360° to the left while in the air. Lift your leg high to help you jump.

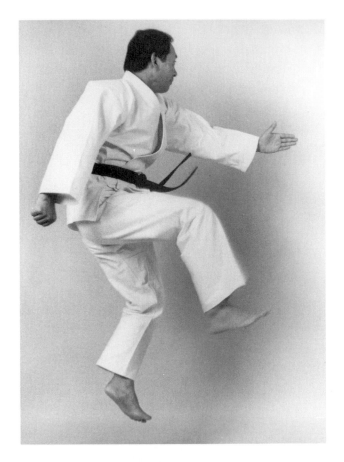

2. Target Strike
a. While in the air, execute a Target Kick with the arch of your right foot hitting your left palm.

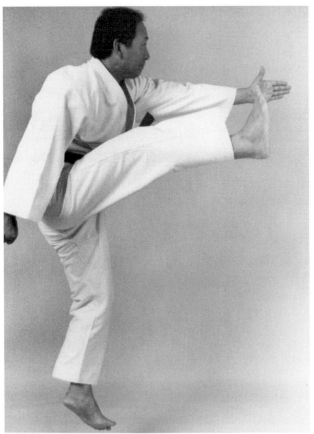

3. Diamond Side Punch

a. As your feet touch the floor, assume Horseback Stance, body facing **R**, and head facing **A**.

b. Simultaneously execute a Diamond Side Punch (High Block with your left hand and a Side Punch with your right hand).

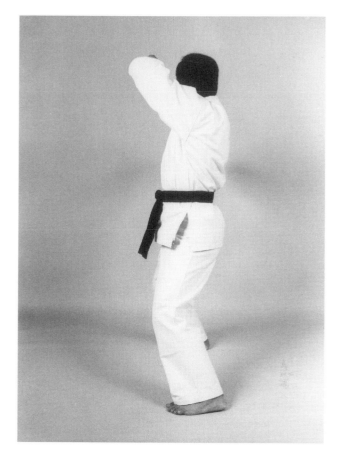

Twenty-Fourth Position: Knife-Hand Mountain Block (Sonnal-Oesanteul-Makki)

a. Maintaining your right foot in place, slide your left foot slightly backward and turn your face toward **B**.

b. Assume Left Back Stance (facing **B**).

c. Simultaneously cross your left arm, palm up, over your right arm, palm down, at chest level, and execute a Left Knife-Hand Low Block. At the same time execute a High Side Block with your right open hand, palm in. The block should be performed in slow motion with tension.

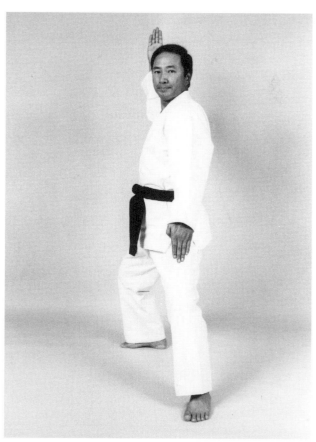

Twenty-Fifth Position:
Knife-Hand Mountain Block

a. Maintaining same stance, pivot to the right on the ball of your left foot and slide your right foot to the right and slightly out toward **A**.

b. Assume Right Back Stance. Head turns to face **A**, and body continues to face **R**.

c. Simultaneously cross your right arm, palm up, over your left arm, palm down, at chest level, and execute a Right Knife-Hand Low Block. At the same time execute a High Side Block with your left open hand, palm in. The block should be performed in slow motion with tension.

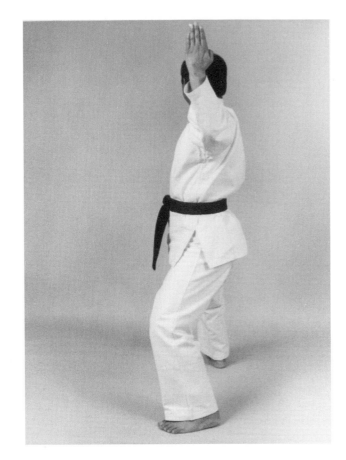

Twenty-Sixth Position:
Open-Hand Bull Block, Mountain Pushing (*Taesan-Milgi*)

Note: Twenty-Sixth Position, 1 and 2 should be performed in a continuous motion.

1. Open-Hand Bull Block

a. Pivoting to the left on the ball of your right foot, slide your left foot backward next to your right foot.

b. Assume Informal Stance (facing **B**).

c. Simultaneously cross both hands in front of abdomen, bring both hands up and circle outward, and execute an Open-Hand Bull Block.

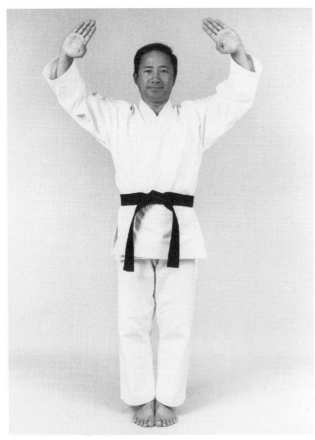

2. Mountain Pushing

a. Slide your right foot forward slightly.

b. Assume Right Cat Stance.

c. Simultaneously execute a Mountain Pushing motion. This motion is performed by bringing your left hand, palm out, next to your face and your right hand, palm out, next to your hip and then pushing both palms forward at the same time as if pushing an object like a mountain. This motion should be performed slowly with tension.

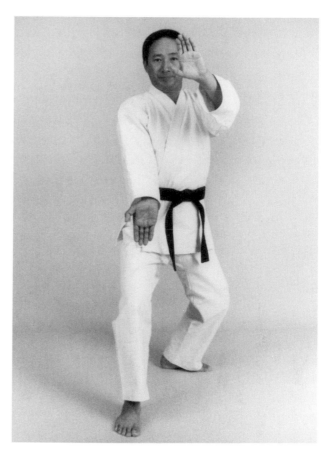

Twenty-Seventh Position: Open-Handed Bull Block, Mountain Pushing

Note: Twenty-Seventh Position, 1 and 2, should be performed in a continuous motion.

1. Open-Hand Bull Block

a. Slide your right foot backward next to your left foot.

b. Assume Informal Stance (facing **B**).

c. Simultaneously cross both hands in front of abdomen, bring both hands up and circle outward, and execute an Open-Hand Bull Block.

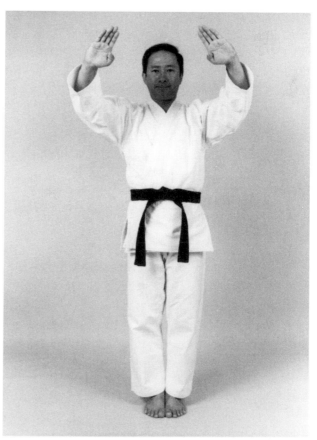

2. Mountain-Pushing

a. Slide your left foot forward slowly.

b. Assume Left Cat Stance.

c. Simultaneously execute a Mountain Pushing motion. (This motion is performed by bringing your right hand, palm out next to your face and your left hand, palm out, next to your hip and then pushing both palms forward at the same time as if pushing an object like a mountain.) This motion should be performed slowly with tension.

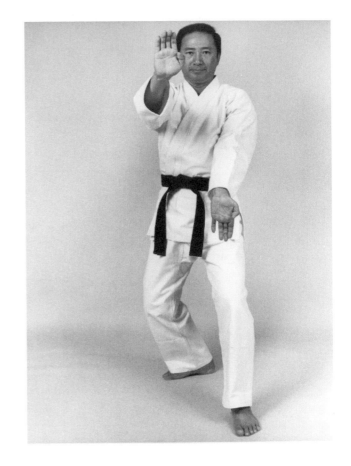

Stop

Sliding your left foot backward next to your right foot, maintain an Informal Stance, facing **B** at point **A**, with both open hands positioned in front of abdomen, palms in, right hand crossing over left hand.

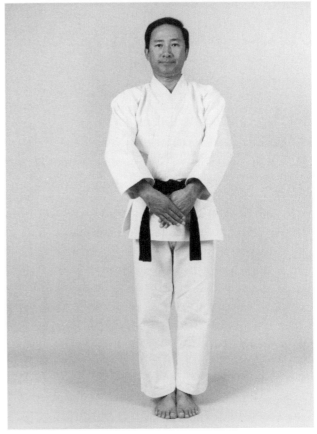

HANSOO (WATER)

Water is the source of life. It is also a substance of power. Water's power is not demonstrated by its ability to resist or to refuse to yield. Rather, because it adapts easily to flow around anything in its path, it cannot be stopped. And it overcomes obstacles not by destroying them with a sudden burst of force but with persistence, gradually wearing away the rocks in the bed of a river of the cliffs on the seacoast.

Like water, the strength of Taekwondo stems not from stubbornness and the refusal to yield but rather from fluidity and adaptability. The form Hansoo epitomizes these qualities; therefore, its forcefulness must come from its fluidity.

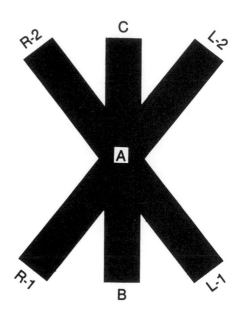

Hansoo

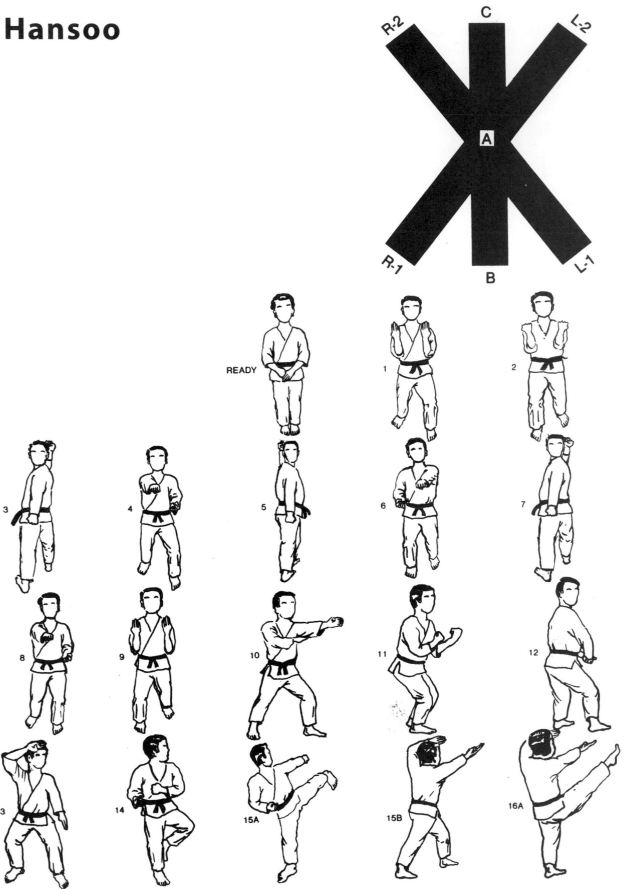

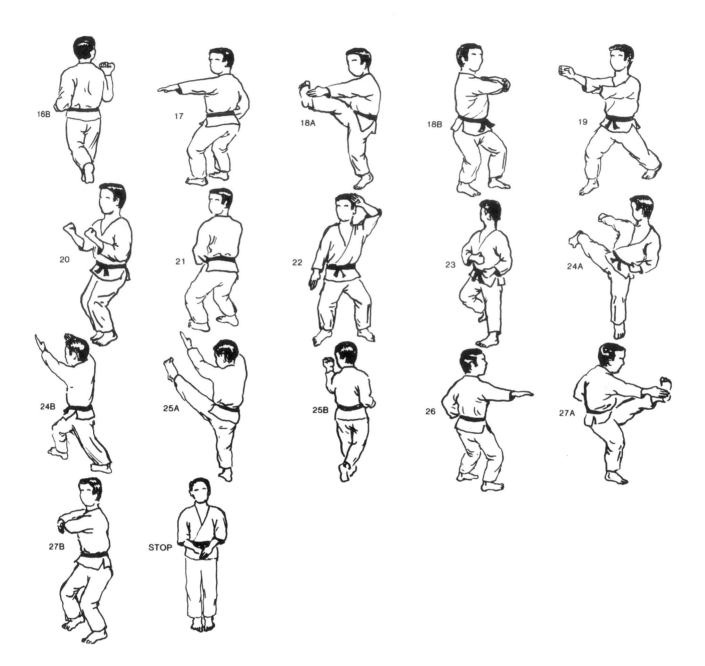

Ready (Cross-Hand Ready) *(Gyopsohn-Choonbi)*

Maintain an Informal Stance, facing **B** at point **A**, eyes focused straight ahead, with both open hands positioned in front of abdomen, palms in, left hand crossing over right hand.

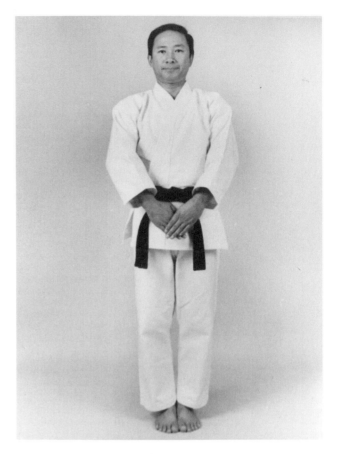

First Position:
Spread Knife-Hand Middle Block *(Sonnal-Deung-Momtong-Hechyo-Makki)*

a. Slide your left foot forward.

b. Assume Left Front Stance.

c. Simultaneously execute a Spread Knife-Hand Middle Block (palms in). The blocking surfaces are the inner forearms.

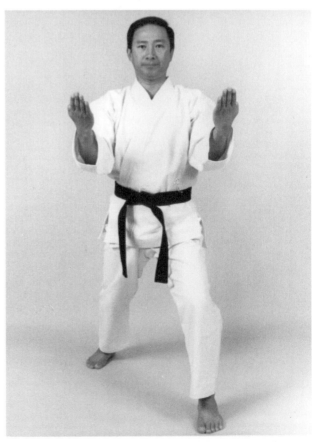

Second Position:
Double Hammer-Fist Strike

a. Slide your right foot forward

b. Assume Right Front Stance.

c. Simultaneously execute a Double Hammer-Fist Strike to the ribs.

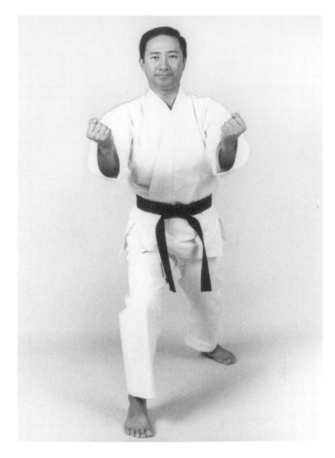

Third Position:
Single Mountain Block *(Oensanteul-Makki)*

a. Pivoting to the right on the ball of your left foot slide your right foot out and back in an arc toward **A**.

b. Assume Right Front Stance (toward **A**). Body faces **R**, and head continues facing **B**.

c. Simultaneously execute a Single Mountain Block (This is a Single Mountain Block with your right hand and Low Block to the side with your left hand.)

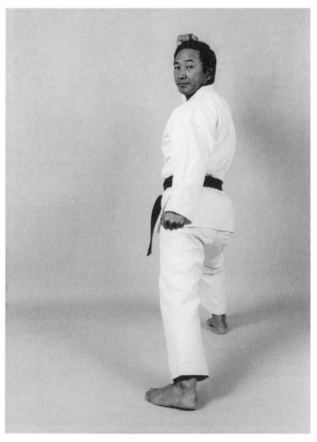

Fourth Position:
Reverse Middle Punch

a. Pivoting to the left on the ball of your right foot, slide your left foot one step to the left, facing **B**.

b. Assume Left Front Stance.

c. Simultaneously execute a Right-Hand Reverse Middle Punch (toward **B**)

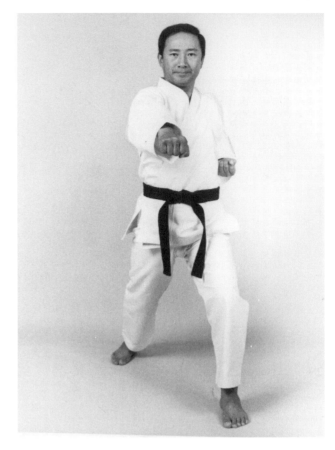

Fifth Position:
Single Mountain Block

a. Pivoting to the left on the ball of your right foot, slide your left foot out and back in an arch toward **A**.

b. Assume Left Front Stance (toward **A**). Body Faces **L**, and head continues facing **B**.

c. Simultaneously execute a Single Mountain Block

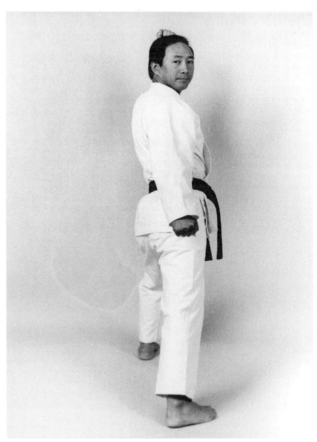

Sixth Position:
Reverse Middle Punch

a. Pivoting to the right on the ball of our left foot, slide your right foot one step to the right (facing **B**).

b. Assume Right Front Stance.

c. Simultaneously execute a Left-Hand Reverse Middle Punch.

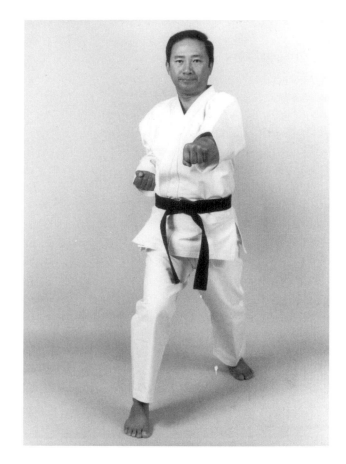

Seventh Position:
Single Mountain Block *(Oesanteul-Makki)*

a. Pivoting to the right on the ball of your left foot slide your right foot out and back in an arch toward **C**.

b. Assume Right Front Stance (toward **A**). Body faces **R**, and head continues facing **B**.

c. Simultaneously execute a Single Mountain Block.

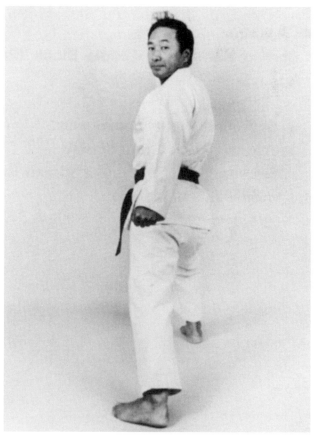

Eighth Position:
Reverse Middle Punch

a. Pivoting to the left on the ball of your right foot, slide your left foot one step to the left (facing **B**)

b. Assume Left Front Stance.

c. Simultaneously execute a Right-Hand Reverse Middle Punch (toward **B**).

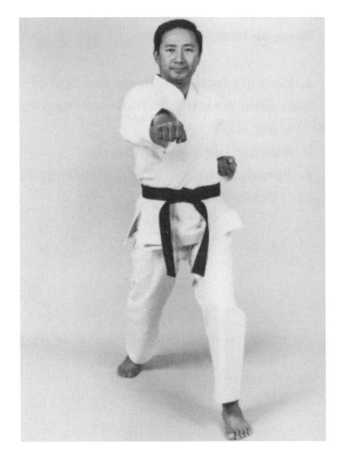

Ninth Position:
Spread Knife-Hand Middle Block

a. Slide your right foot forward.

b. Assume Right Front Stance.

c. Simultaneously execute a Spread Knife-Hand Middle Block (palms in).

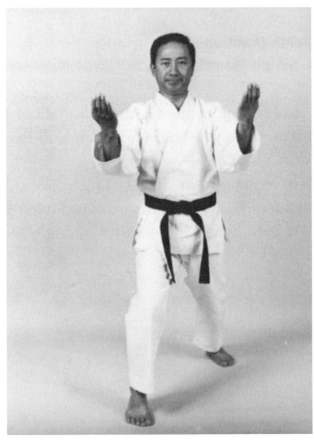

Tenth Position:

Tiger-Mouth Thrust *(Kaljaebi or Akum-sohn-Mokchiki)*

a. Pivoting slightly to the left on the ball of your right foot, slide your left foot forward at a 45° angle toward **L-1**.

b. Assume Left Front Stance.

c. Simultaneously execute a Tiger-Mouth Thrust with your left hand and place your right open hand under your left elbow, palm down.

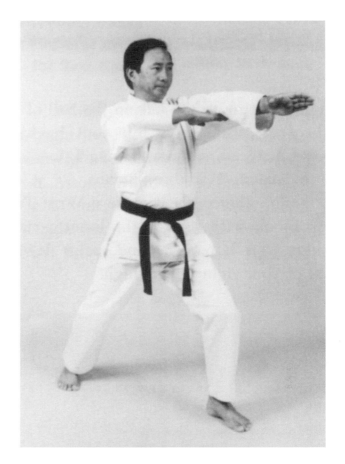

Eleventh Position:

Double Uppercut Punch *(Doojoomeok-Jeochyo-Jiruki)*

a. Leap one step forward with your right foot and immediately bring your left foot next to your right foot.

b. Assume Informal Stance with both knees bent (two-thirds of your weight is on your right foot).

c. Simultaneously execute a Double Uppercut Punch to the solar plexus.

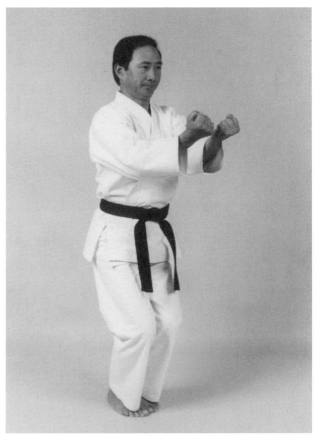

Twelfth Position:
Wrist-Target Low Block *(Palmok-Pyojeok-Arae-Makki)*

a. Pivoting to the left on the ball of your right foot, slide your left foot backward toward **A**. Head continues facing **L-1**.

b. Assume Horseback Stance.

c. Simultaneously execute a Wrist-Target Low Block with your right inner wrist by striking your left open hand, palm down, in front of your right upper thigh.

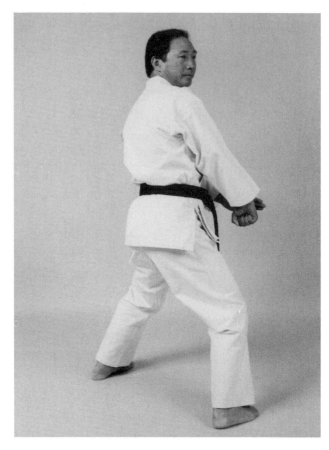

Thirteenth Position:
Knife-Hand Diamond Block *(Sohnal-Keumgang-Makki)*

a. Pivoting 90° to the right on the ball of your left foot, slide your right foot backward toward **A**. Head continues facing **L-1**.

b. Assume Left Back Stance.

c. Simultaneously execute a Knife-Hand Diamond Block. (This is a simultaneous Knife-Hand High Block with your right hand a Knife-Hand Low Block with your left hand.)

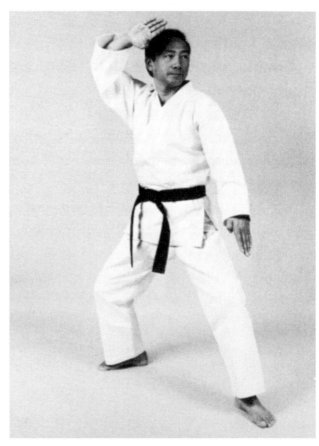

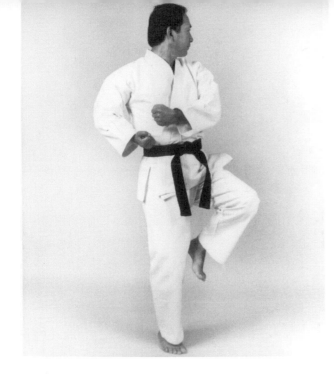

Fourteenth Position:
Right Crane Stance with Hand Position for Side Kick

a. Pivoting 90° to the left on the ball of your right foot, bring your left foot back next to your right knee, head turns toward **L-2**.

b. Assume Right Crane Stance.

c. Simultaneously bring both fists to your right side, right fist at waist level, palm up, and left fist, palm in, over your right fist.

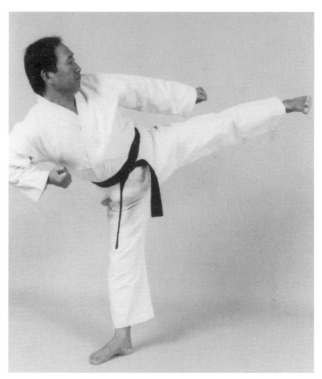

Fifteenth Position:
Side Kick, Left Knife-Hand High Block, and Right Knife-Hand Strike

1. Side Kick

a. Execute a Side Kick with your left foot and at the same time execute a Left Side Punch.

2. Left Knife-Hand High Block and Right Knife-Hand Strike

a. Step forward with your left foot toward **L-2**.

b. Assume Left Stance.

c. Simultaneously execute a Knife-Hand High Block with your left hand and a Knife-Hand Strike to the neck of your imaginary opponent with your right hand, palm up.

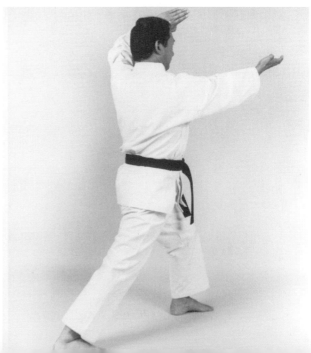

Sixteenth Position:
Front Kick, Back Fist Strike, and Yell

1. Front Kick

a. Execute a Front Kick with your right foot.

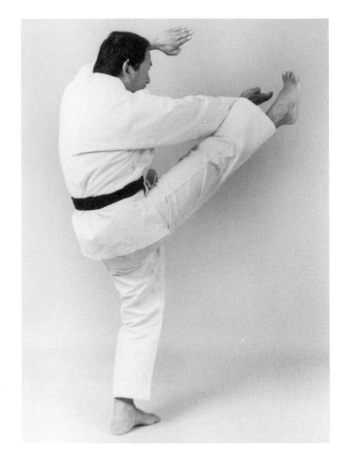

2. Back Fist Strike and Yell

a. Stamping your right foot one step forward, immediately bring your left foot behind your right foot.

b. Assume Right Cross Stance.

c. Simultaneously execute a Back Fist Strike to the face with your right hand and yell.

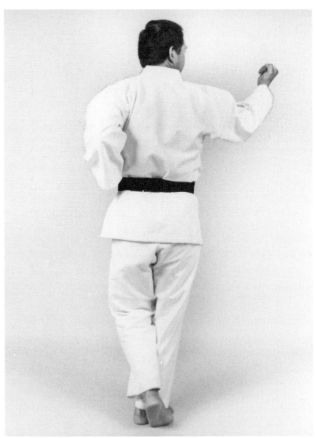

Seventeenth Position:
Knife-Hand Strike (Palm Down)

a. Pivoting to the left on the ball of your right foot, slide your left foot backward toward **A** (head turns toward **A**).

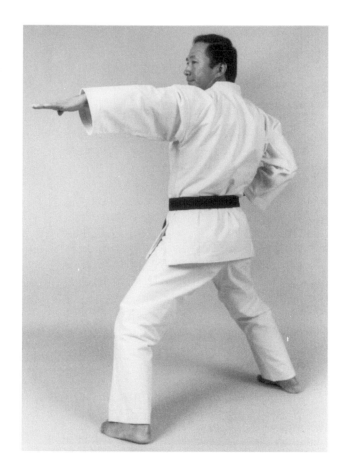

Eighteenth Position:
Target Kick, Elbow Target Strike

1. Target Strike

a. Execute a Target Kick with the arch of your right foot hitting your left palm.

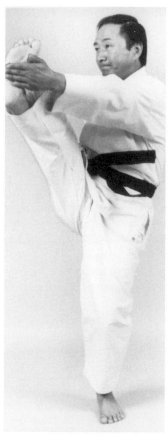

2. Elbow Target Strike

a. Step forward with your right foot toward **A**. Head turns toward **L-1**.

b. Assume Horseback Stance.

c. Simultaneously execute a Target Strike with your right elbow hitting your left palm.

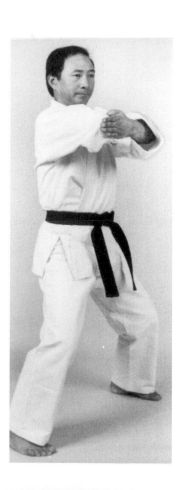

Nineteenth Position:
Tiger-Mouth Thrust

a. Keeping your right foot in place, slide your left foot to the right next to your right foot. Immediately pivot slightly to the right on the ball of your left foot and slide your right foot toward **R-1**. (Head turns toward **R-1**.)

b. Assume Right Front Stance.

c. Simultaneously execute a Tiger-Mouth Thrust with your right hand and place your left open hand under your right elbow, palm down.

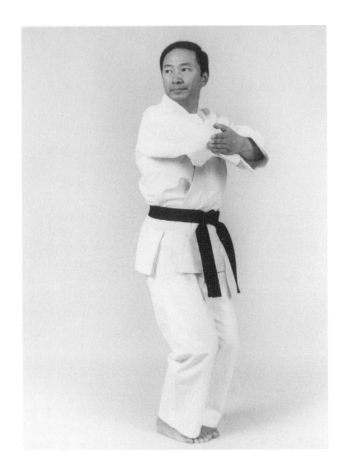

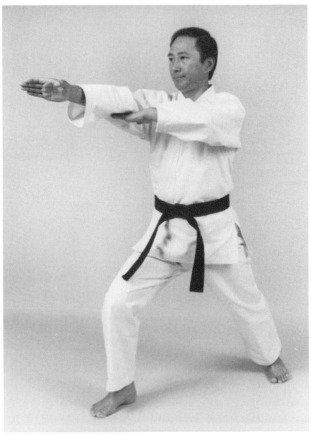

Twentieth Position:
Double Uppercut Punch *(Deung-Joomeok-Jechyo-Jiluki)*

a. Leap one step forward with your left foot and immediately bring your right foot next to your left foot.

b. Assume Informal Stance with both knees bent (two-thirds of your weight is on your left foot).

c. Simultaneously execute a Double Uppercut Punch to the solar plexus.

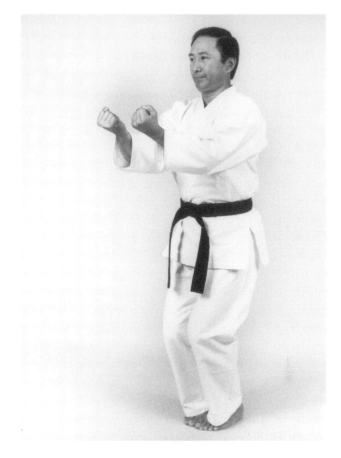

Twenty-First Position:
Wrist-Target Low Block

a. Pivoting to the right on the ball of your left foot, slide your right foot backward toward **A**. Head continues to face **R-1**.

b. Assume Horseback Stance.

c. Simultaneously execute a Wrist-Target Low Block with your left inner wrist by striking your right open hand, palm down, in front of your left upper thigh.

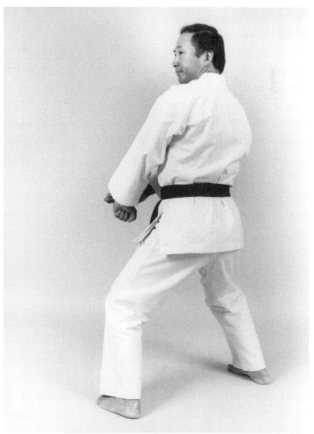

Twenty-Second Position:
Knife-Hand Diamond Block

a. Pivoting 90° to the right on the ball of your right foot, slide your left foot backward toward **A**. Head continues to face **R-1**.

b. Assume Right Back Stance.

c. Simultaneously execute a Knife-Hand Diamond Block

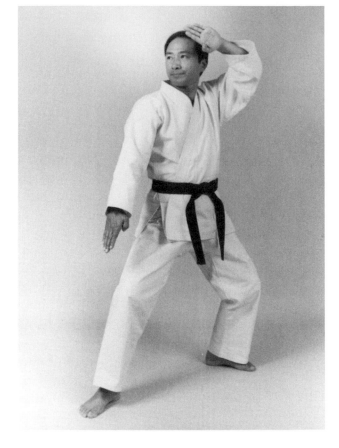

Twenty-Third Position:
Left Crane Stance

a. Pivoting 90° to the right on the ball of your left foot, bring your right foot back next to your left knee (head turns toward **R-2**).

b. Assume Right Crane Stance toward **R-2**.

c. Simultaneously bring both fists to your left side, left fist at waist level, palm up, and right fist, palm in, over your left fist.

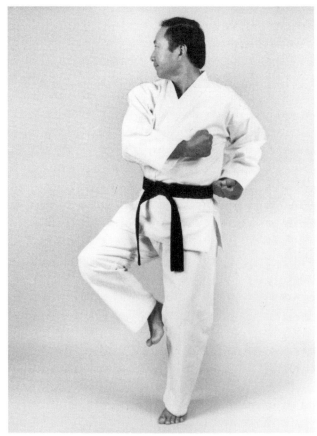

Twenty-Fourth Position:
Side Kick, Right Knife-Hand High Block, and Left Knife-Hand Strike *(Jebipoom-Mok-Chiki)*

1. Side Kick

a. Execute a Side Kick with your right foot and at the same time execute a Right Side Punch.

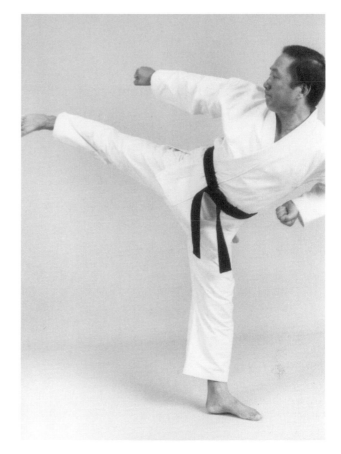

2. Right Knife-Hand High Block and Left Knife-Hand Strike

a. Step forward with your right foot toward **R-2**.

b. Assume Right Front Stance.

c. Simultaneously execute a Knife-Hand High Block with your right hand and a Knife-Hand Strike to the neck of your imaginary opponent with your left hand palm-up.

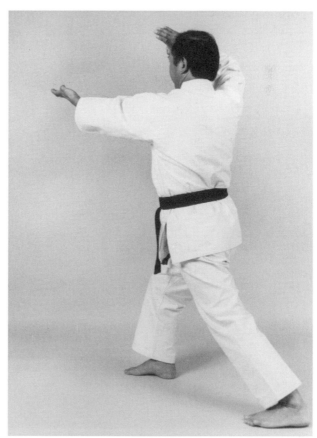

Twenty-Fifth Position:
Front Kick, Back Fist Strike, and Yell

1. Front Kick

a. Execute a Front Kick with your left foot.

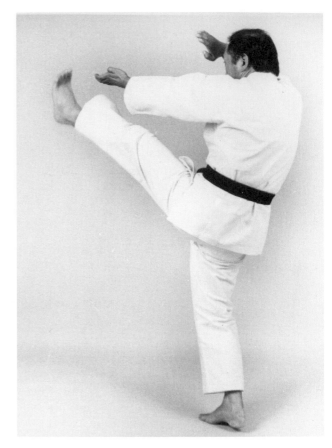

2. Back Fist Strike and Yell

a. Stamping your left foot one step forward, immediately bring your right foot behind your left foot.

b. Assume Left Cross Stance.

c. Simultaneously execute a Back Fist Strike to the face with your left hand and yell.

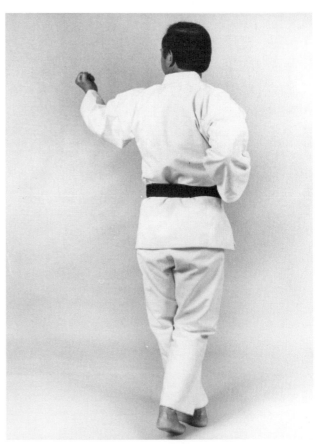

Twenty-Sixth Position:
Knife-Hand Strike (Palm Down)

a. Pivoting to the right on the ball of your left foot slide your right foot backward toward **A** (head turns toward **A**.)

b. Assume Horseback Stance.

c. Simultaneously execute a Knife-Hand Strike, palm down, with your right hand.

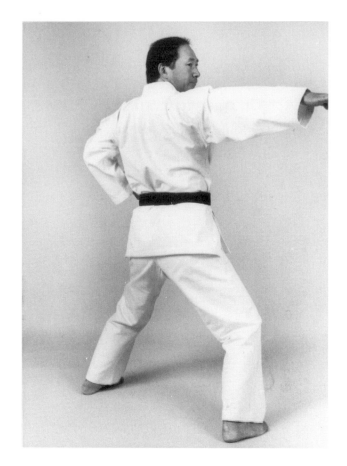

Twenty-Seventh Position:
Target Kick, Elbow Target Strike

1. Target Kick

a. Execute a Target Kick with the arch of your left foot hitting your right palm.

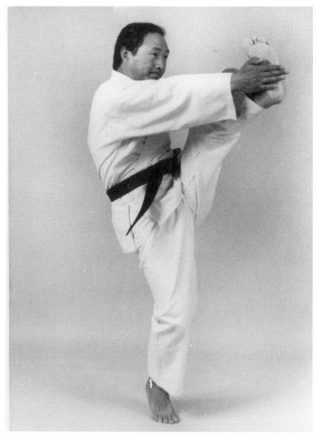

2. Elbow Target Strike

a. Step forward with your left foot toward **A** (head turns toward **R-1**).

b. Assume Horseback Stance.

c. Simultaneously execute a Target Strike with your left elbow hitting your right palm.

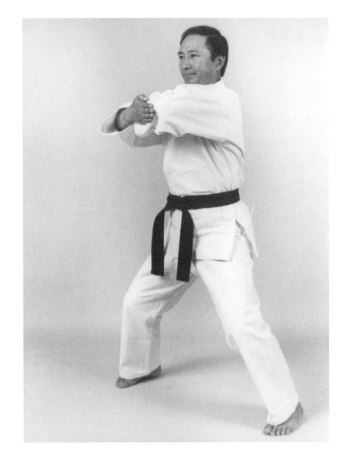

Stop

Pivoting slightly to the left on the ball of your right foot, slide your left foot to the right next to your right foot and assume an Informal Stance, facing **B** at point **A**, eyes focused straight ahead, with both open hands positioned in front of abdomen, palms in, left hand crossing over right hand.

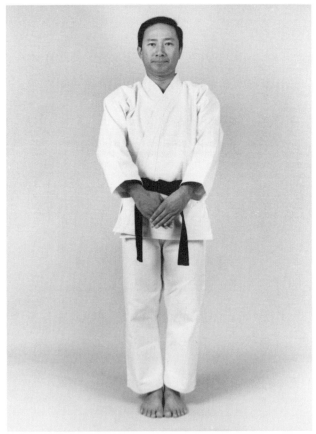

ILYO (ONENESS)

In Buddhism, the goal of the spiritual life is said to be *Ilyo*—oneness, or nirvana. To arrive at this state of purity one must discard all worldly desires, leaving oneself with a profound faith and a complete unity of body and mind. Only in this state is the ego overcome. Buddha taught that the entire perceptible universe has no permanent being and because everything is impermanent, including the individual self, it is all in a state of becoming, moving from birth to death and subject to pain and sorrow. The ego, or self, suffers because of its desires, its attempt to cling to objects and people and to life itself. This clinging, given the inevitable ongoing cycle of birth and death, can only bring pain. So the first step to freedom is to realize that the self has no reality; then it is easy to shed the desires that the self clings to.

The ideal of Taekwondo is this state of Ilyo. It is a discipline in which you concentrate your attention on every movement and in so doing shed all worldly thoughts and preoccupations. The Ilyo form begins and ends at a center, moving outward but eventually returning to its center to achieve oneness. The spirit must be kept within the confines of the form, allowing no distraction.

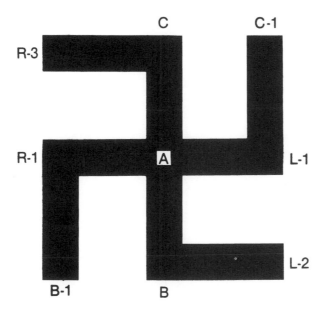

Ilyo

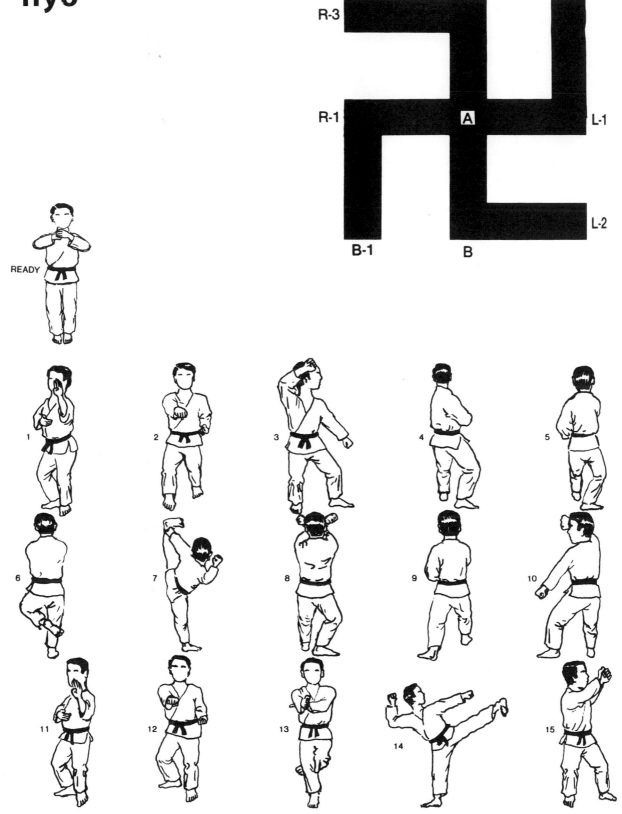

READY

C   C-1
R-3

R-1   A   L-1

L-2
B-1   B

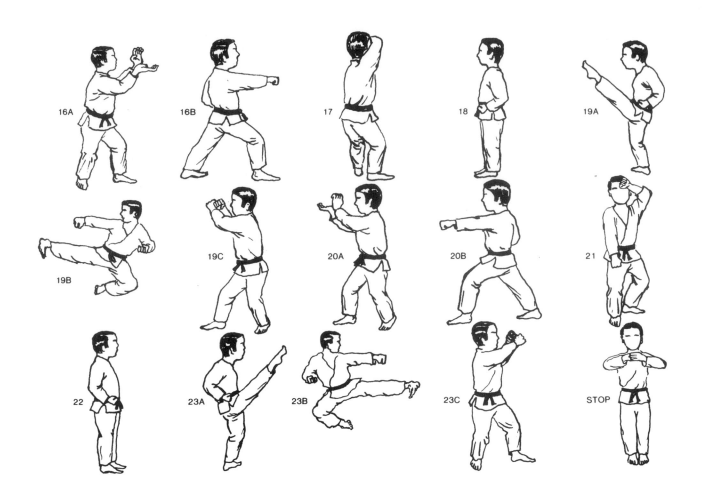

Ready (Covered-Fist Ready) *(Bojoomeok)*

Maintain an Informal Stance, facing **B** at point **A**, eyes focused straight ahead, with both hands positioned in front of upper chest, palms in, and left hand wrapped around right fist.

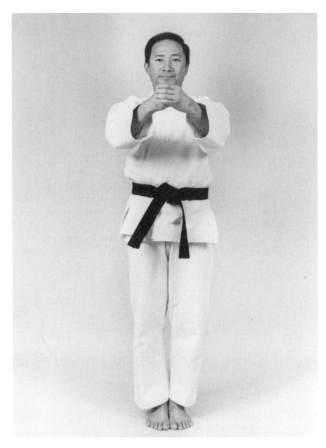

First Position:
 Knife-Hand High Block

 a. Slide your left foot forward

 b. Assume Left Back Stance.

 c. Simultaneously execute a Left Knife-Hand High Block.

Note: This motion should be performed rapidly.

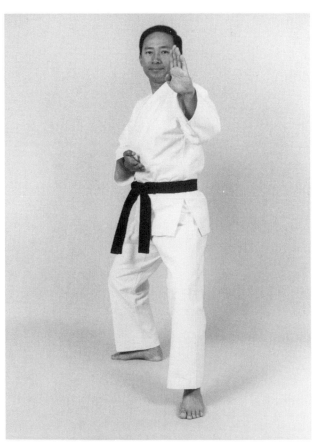

Second Position:
Middle Punch

a. Slide your right foot forward

b. Assume Right Front Stance.

c. Simultaneously execute a Right-Hand Middle Punch.

Note: This motion should be performed rapidly.

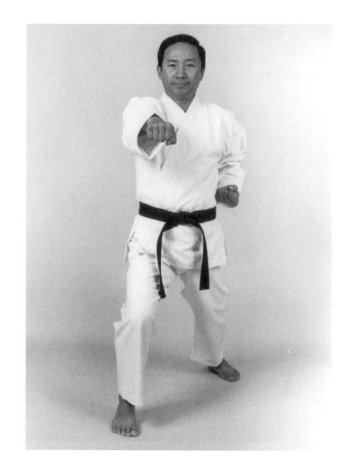

Third Position:
Diamond Block *(Keumgang-Makki)*

a. Keeping your right foot in place, slide your left foot forward and to the left, pointing toward **L-2**.

b. Assume Left Back Stance (toward **L-2**).

c. Simultaneously execute a Diamond Block. (This is a simultaneous Right-Hand High Block and a Left-Hand Low Block.)

Note: This motion should be performed in slow motion and with full body tension.

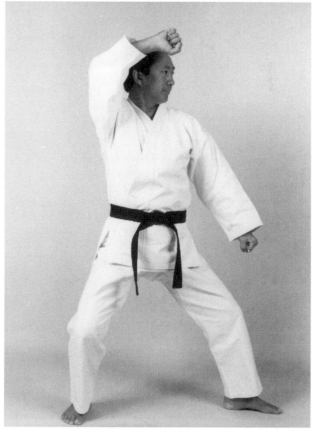

Fourth Position:
Knife-Hand Middle Block

a. Pivoting to the left on the ball of your right foot, slide your left foot out, turning 90° to the left (toward **A**).

b. Assume Left Back Stance.

c. Simultaneously execute a Left Knife-Hand Middle Block.

Note: This motion should be performed rapidly.

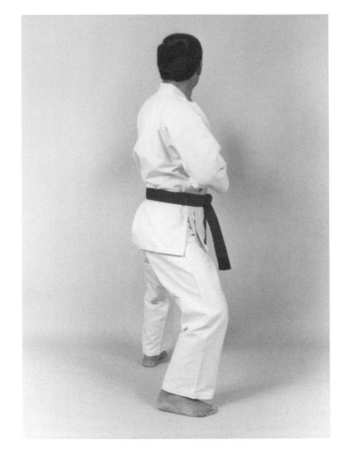

Fifth Position:
Reverse Middle Punch

a. Maintain the same stance.

b. Execute a Reverse Middle Punch with your right hand.

Note: This motion should be performed rapidly.

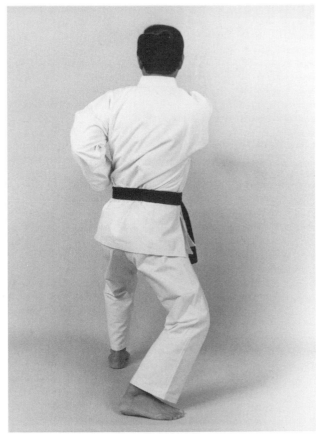

Sixth Position:
Vertical Spear-Hand Thrust and Yell

a. Leaping one step forward with your right foot, bring your left instep to the back your right knee.

b. Assume Right Crane Stance, left foot behind.

c. Simultaneously execute a Left Vertical Spear-Hand Thrust and yell.

Note: This motion should be performed rapidly.

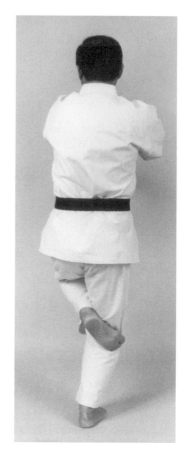
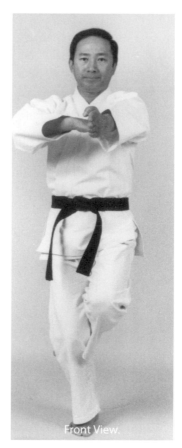

Front View.

Seventh Position:
Single Mountain Side Kick (Oesanteul-Yeopchaki)

a. Maintaining the same stance, pivot 90° to the right on the ball of your right foot. Body turns toward **L**, in slow motion with tension.

b. Assume Right Crane Stance, left foot behind. Body faces **L**, and head continues facing **A**.

c. Simultaneously execute a Single Mountain Block with your right hand and at the same time execute a Left Side Kick and Left Side Punch, palm down, over your kicking leg.

Note: This motion should be performed with full body tension.

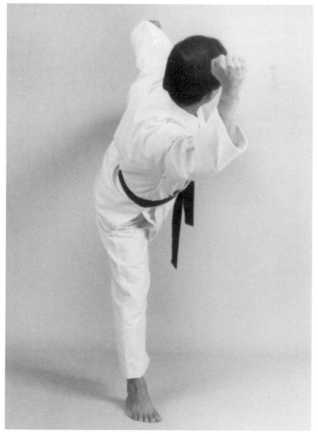

Eighth Position:
Double-Fist X High Block *(Eotgeoreo-Eolgool-Makki)*

a. Step forward with your left foot.

b. Assume Left Back Stance.

c. Simultaneously execute a Double-Fist X High Block, right wrist over left.

Note: This motion should be performed rapidly.

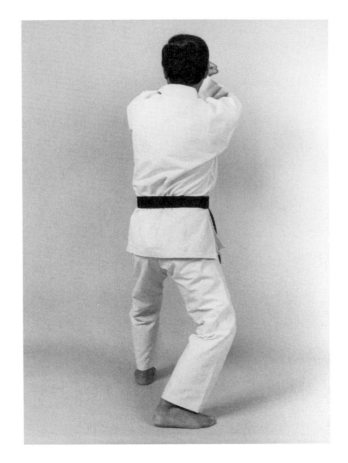

Ninth Position:
Middle Punch

a. Twisting your wrists clockwise, open your hands as if grabbing your opponent's arm. Then slide your right foot forward toward **C** and bring your left fist to the waist.

b. Assume Right Front Stance.

c. Simultaneously execute a Right-Hand Middle Punch.

Note: This motion should be performed in slow motion with full body tension.

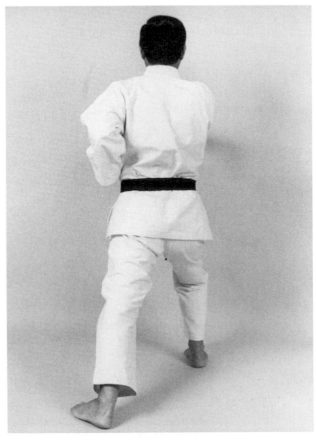

Tenth Position:
Diamond Block

a. Keeping your right foot in place, slide your left foot forward and to the left, pointing toward **R-3**.

b. Assume Left Back Stance.

c. Simultaneously execute a Diamond Block. (This is a simultaneous Right-Hand Block and a Left-Hand Low Block.)

Note: This motion should be performed in slow motion with full body tension.

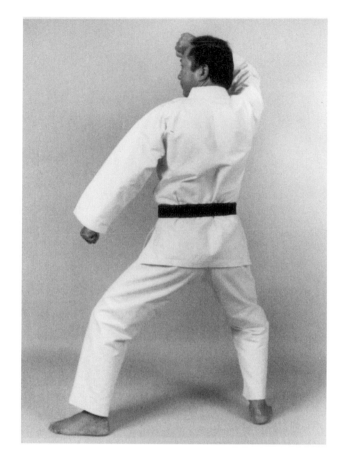

Eleventh Position:
Knife-Hand Middle Block

a. Keeping your right foot in place, slide your left foot 90° to the left toward **A**. (Face turns toward **A**.)

b. Assume Left Back Stance.

c. Simultaneously execute a Left Knife-Hand Middle Block.

Note: This motion should be performed rapidly.

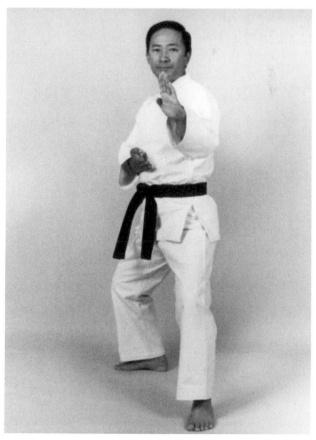

Twelfth Position:
Reverse Middle Punch

    a. Maintain the same stance.

    b. Execute a Reverse Middle Punch with your right hand.

Note: This motion should be performed rapidly.

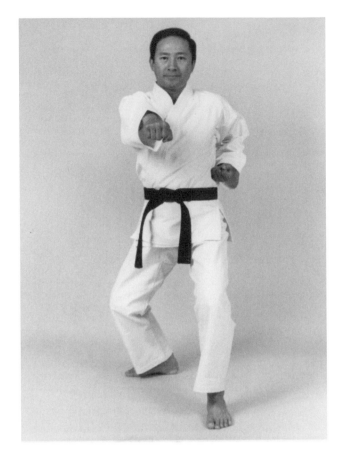

Thirteenth Position:
Vertical Spear-Hand Thrust and Yell

    a. Leaping one step forward with your right foot, bring your left instep to the back of your right knee.

    b. Assume Right Crane Stance, left foot behind.

    c. Simultaneously execute a Left Vertical Spear-Hand Thrust and yell.

Note: This motion should be performed rapidly.

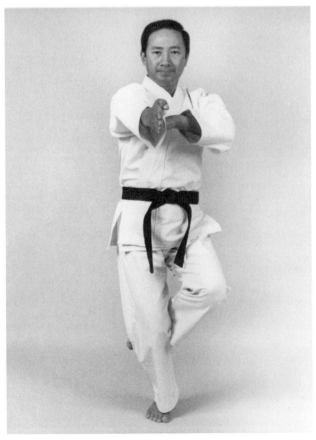

Fourteenth Position:
Single Mountain Side Kick

a. Turning your head toward **L-1**, execute a Single Mountain Block with your right hand and at the same time execute a Left Side Kick and a Left Side Punch, palm down, over your kicking leg.

Note: This motion should be performed with full body tension.

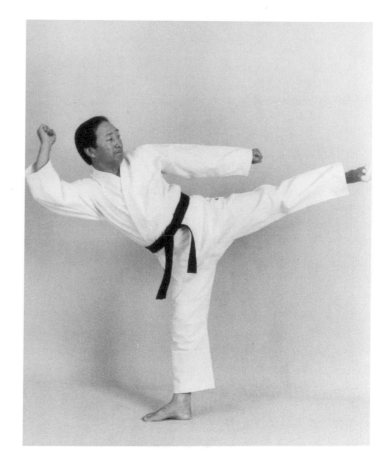

Fifteenth Position:
Double-Fist X High Block

a. Step forward with your left foot toward **C-1**.

b. Assume Left Back Stance.

c. Simultaneously execute a Double-Fist X High Block.

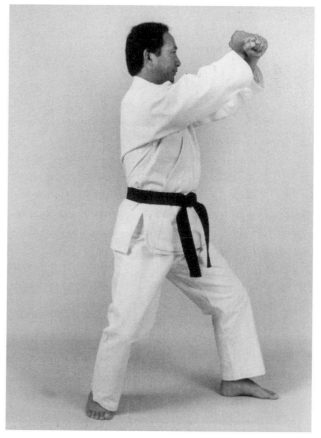

Sixteenth Position:
Wrist-Twist Middle Punch

1. Wrist Twist
a. Twisting your wrists clockwise, open hands to grab your opponent's arm

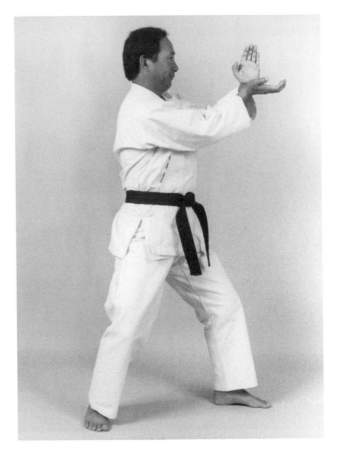

2. Middle Punch
a. Sliding your right foot forward, grab with your left hand in place and bring your right fist to your waist.

b. Assume Right Front Stance.

c. Simultaneously execute a Right-Hand Middle Punch and at the same time pull your left fist back to your waist.

Note: This motion should be performed in slow motion with full body tension.

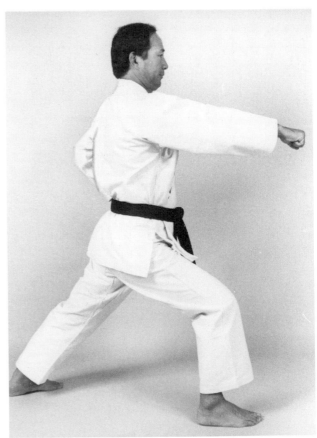

Seventeenth Position:
Diamond Block

a. Keeping your right foot in place, slide your left foot forward and to the left, pointing toward **C-1**.

b. Assume Left Back Stance.

c. Simultaneously execute a Diamond Block (Right-Hand High Block and Left-Hand Low Block).

Note: This motion should be performed in slow motion with full body tension.

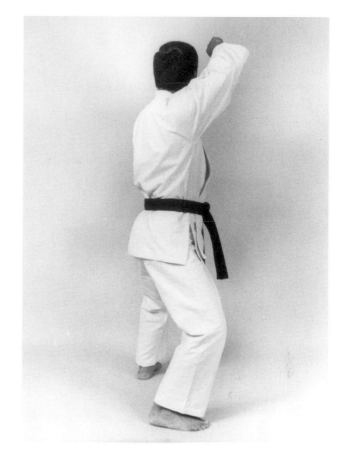

Eighteenth Position:
Fists at Waist (*Doo-Joomeok-Heori*)

a. Pivoting 180° to the left on the ball of your right foot, slide your left foot backward, next to your right foot, in slow motion, facing **R-1**.

b. Assume Informal Stance (body facing **R-1**).

c. Simultaneously bring both your fists to waist level, palms up.

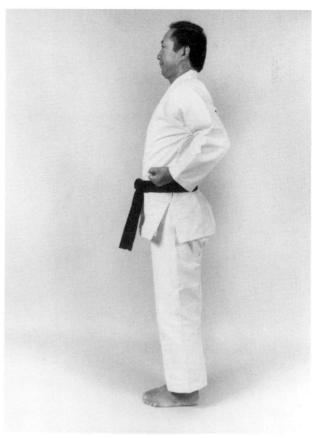

Nineteenth Position:
Front Kick, One-Step Jumping Side Kick
(*Tdwiyo-Doobal-Yeopchaki*)

1. Front Kick
a. Execute a Front Kick with your left foot.

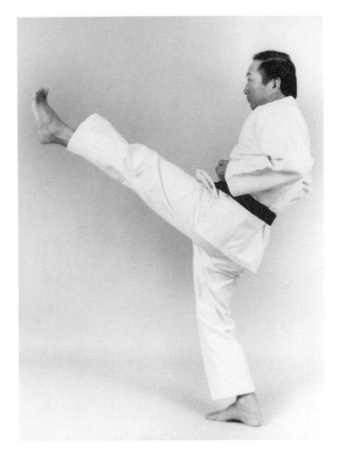

2. One-Step Jumping Side Kick
a. Stamping your left foot one step forward, jump to prepare for Jumping Side Kick.

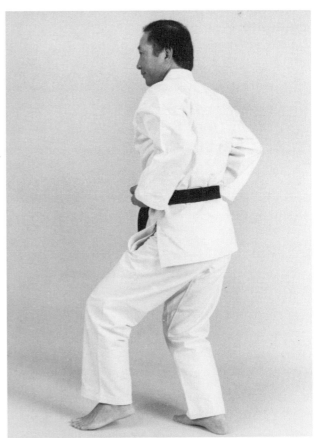

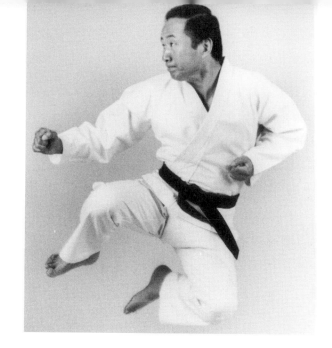

b. Execute a One-Step Jumping Side Kick with your right foot. (Kick should be performed while both feet are in the air.)

Note: The above motions, 1 and 2, should be performed rapidly.

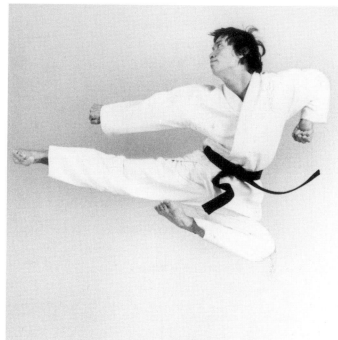

3. Double-Fist X High Block

a. As your feet touch the floor, assume Right Back Stance.

b. Simultaneously execute a Double-Fist X High Block

Note: Motion 3 should be performed with full body tension.

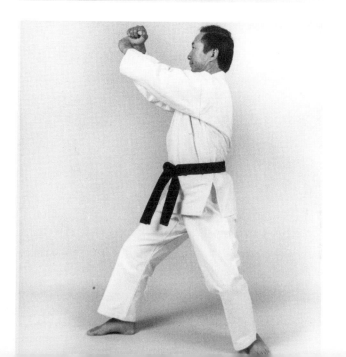

Twentieth Position:
Wrist-Twist Middle Punch

1. Wrist Twist

a. Twisting your wrists clockwise, open your hands to grab your opponent's arm.

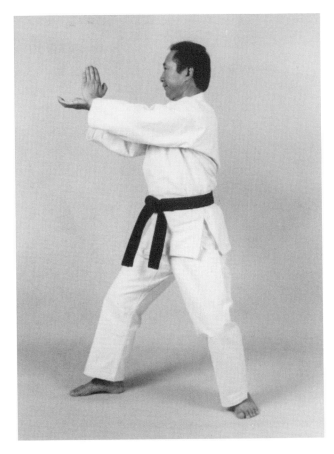

2. Middle Punch

a. Sliding your left foot forward, grab with your left hand in place and bring your right fist to the waist.

b. Assume Left Front Stance.

c. Simultaneously execute a Left-Hand Middle Punch and pull your right hand back to your waist.

Note: This motion should be performed in slow motion with full body tension

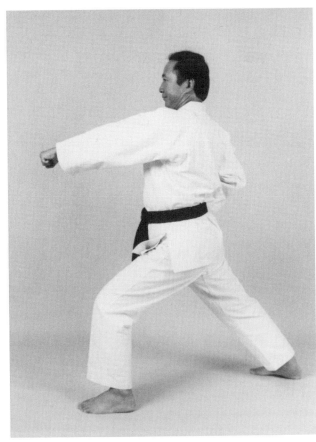

Twenty-First Position:
Diamond Block

a. Pivoting 180° to the right on the ball of your left foot, slide your right foot backward to the right and out in a arc (toward **B-1**).

b. Assume Right Back Stance.

c. Simultaneously execute a Diamond Block (Left-Hand High Block and Right-Hand Low Block).

Note: This motion should be performed in slow motion with full body tension.

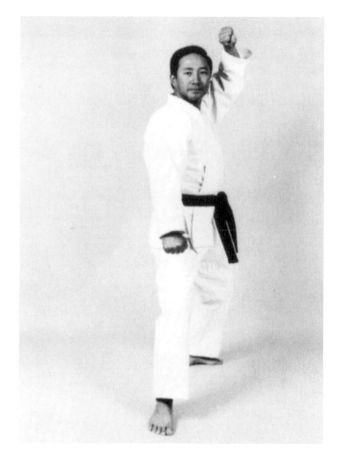

Twenty-Second Position:
Fists at Waist

a. Keeping your left foot in place, slide your right foot backward next to your left foot, facing **A**.

b. Assume Informal Stance.

c. Simultaneously bring both your fists to waist level, palms up.

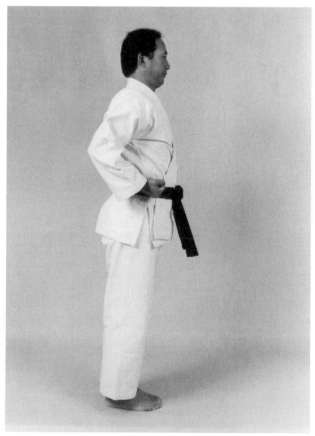

Twenty-Third Position:
Front Kick, One-Step Jumping Side Kick,
Double-Fist X High Block

1. Front Kick

a. Execute a Front Kick with your right foot.

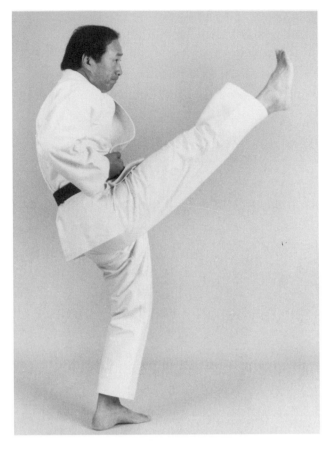

2. One-Step Jumping Side Kick

a. Stamping your right foot one step forward, jump to prepare for Jumping Side Kick.

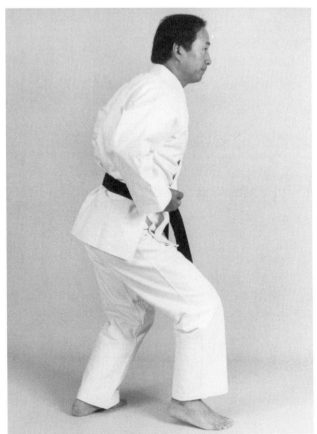

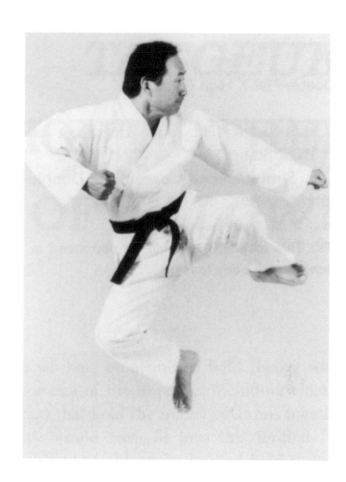

b. Execute a One-Step Jumping Side Kick with your left foot. (Kick should be performed while both feet are in the air.)

Note: The above motions, 1 and 2, should be performed rapidly.

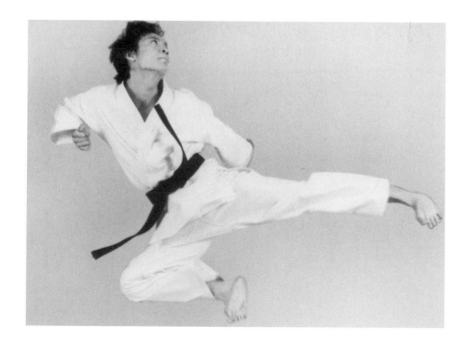

3. Double-Fist X High Block

a. As your feet touch the floor, assume Left Back Stance.

b. Simultaneously execute a Double-Fist X High Block.

Note: This motion, 3, should be performed in slow motion with full body tension.

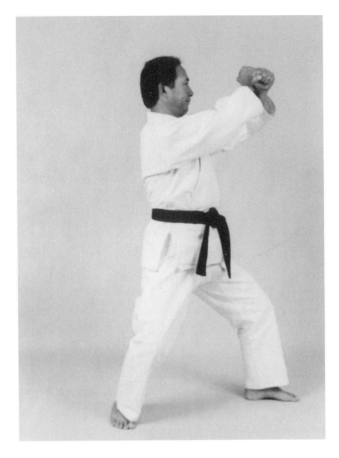

Stop

Keeping your right foot in place, slide your left foot next to your right foot. Assume an informal Stance, facing **B** at point **A**, eyes focused straight ahead, with both hands positioned in front of upper chest, palms in, and left hand wrapped around right fist.

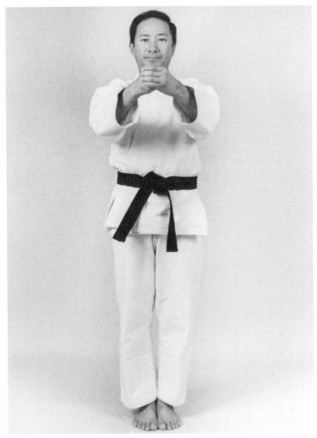

Taeguek:
The Eight Other Branches of Palgwe

When Albert Einstein died, he was working on a unified theory, which would explain all of the basic phenomena of the universe, including electricity, magnetism, gravity, and the forces that hold the nuclei of atoms together. His magnificent theory of relativity would have fit into this unified field theory. However, Einstein was not able to complete the unified field theory.

For the practitioner of Taekwondo, the phenomena of the Universe are explained by the ancient philosophy of Um (Yin) and Yang, as described in the *Joo-Yeok,* the *Book of Changes.* In this ancient Oriental work, the Palgwe symbolizes the phenomena of man and the Universe.

Palgwe means "law" or "command." It symbolizes the eternal duality of all that exists—the interdependence of good and evil, of plus and minus, of North and South, of Heaven and Earth. These are opposite, yet they are part of the same whole. They are in constant dynamic struggle with each other, yet they can never break apart.

Consider the nucleus of an atom, the basic building block of the Universe. This nucleus is composed of positively and negatively charged particles in extreme proximity. The forces with which like particles repel one another are measured in billions of electron volts, yet they do not fly apart, for they are bound together by an even greater yet unexplained force. This nuclear force binds them together no matter how they struggle to break apart. It is truly cosmic force cohesion—like the force that joins the opposing Um and Yang forces into a single duality.

In Taekwondo, the infinite and unknowable constancy of Truth and the truth of constant change are expressed in the Palgwe forms. These forms have a deep philosophical root. They express the mutually contradictory concepts which are forever developing and growing by combining and changing. Within this struggle, there is Truth, which is the integral strength, and cosmic Order, which brings harmony out of chaos.

The principle of Palgwe is that he who knows himself and his environment will find the path of harmony between the changeable forces of the world in which he lives. As the Taekwondo practitioner executes the Palgwe forms, he must bear in mind the reciprocal commands they represent.

These commands may be translated as:

1. Know yourself and be in harmony with the Universe.

2. Be responsible for yourself and loyal to your commitments.

3. Be respectful of our relationships; know the limits beyond which your freedom encroaches on the freedom of another.

4. Be pure in motive and direct in action.

Palgwe, in its most profound philosophical sense, symbolically expresses all of the phenomena of man and the Universe. It is the most basic philosophic principle contained in the ancient *Book of Changes*.

Within Palgwe, there are sixty-four *gwes,* or commands, which naturally flow from its basic, all encompassing law. These *gwes* are grouped into eight trigrams, or branches, which are called *Taegeuk.*

Taegeuk is written 太極.

Tae (太) means "bigness," *geuk* (極) means "eternity." Thus, Taegeuk has no form, no beginning, and no end. It is the eternal infinity whose vastness contains the essence of everything, and from which everything in the Universe originates.

TAEGEUK 1 JANG

In Taekwondo, there are eight Taegeuk forms corresponding to the eight aspects of eternity.

The first of these is Taegeuk 1 Jang, which applies the actions of Keon (乾) to Palgwe. Keon is the principle *gwe* in the *Book of Changes.* It represents Heaven and Light. It is the powerful and manly *gwe*, the source of creation and the symbol of the father. As Heaven, it is the symbol of pure creativity. Keon originally meant "dry," and since the dry is light, it floats up to heaven. Thus Keon came to be identified with Heaven.

From the time that *Homo sapiens* became aware of their ability to think, mankind has followed divergent paths in its search for the true meaning of existence and of the origin and meaning of the Universe. Sometimes however, those paths converge. Compare, for instance, the concept of Keon with the Biblical account found in *Genesis* 1:2-3: "And the earth was without form, and void.... And God said, 'Let there be light.' And there was light."

Keon signifies the infinite concentration of Yang energy.

This form represents the source of creation by presenting the most basic techniques—the Low Block, Inside Middle Block, Middle Punch, and Reverse Kick. These techniques can be easily learned by the beginning student but are practical throughout the study of Taekwondo. Taegeuk 1 Jang, therefore is the foundation from which the other forms build. Most of this form is performed in High Front Stance, which is easy for a beginner to maintain. However, the Front Stance is introduced, and the student learns to shift from one stance to another.

All eight forms, Taegeuk 1 Jang through Taegeuk 8 Jang, follow the same I-shaped floor pattern, which can be used as a reference for all eight forms

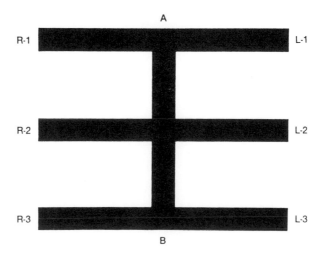

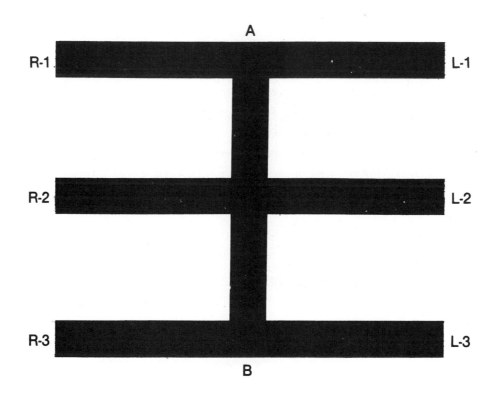

Center
(Starting Point)

A

R-1   L-1

R-2   L-2

R-3   L-3

B

Taeguek 1 Jang

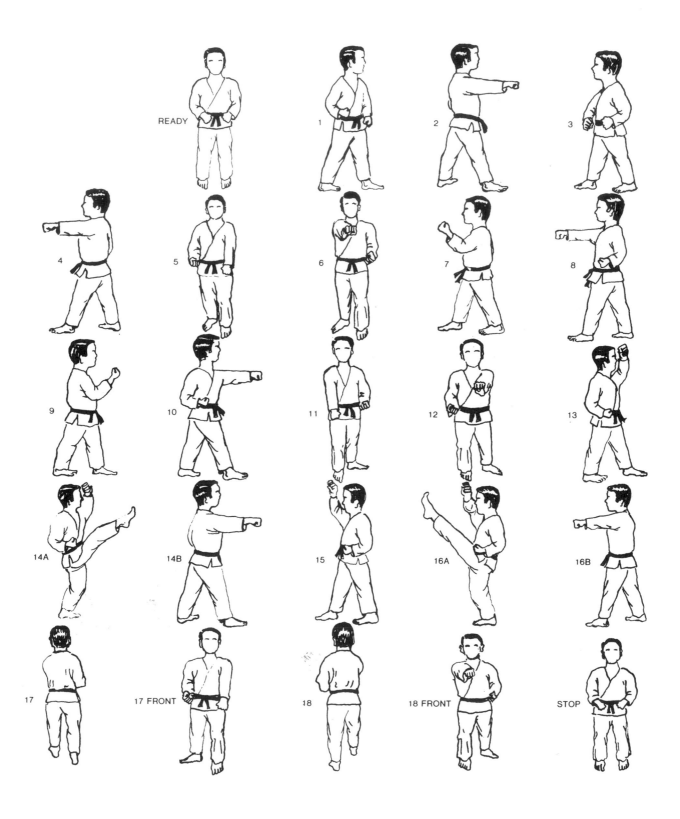

READY 1 2 3
4 5 6 7 8
9 10 11 12 13
14A 14B 15 16A 16B
17 17 FRONT 18 18 FRONT STOP

Assume Ready Stance (at center, A)

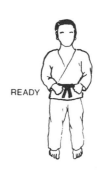

READY

1. Turn your body 90° to the left toward L-1 while sliding out with your left foot forward into a Left High Front Stance, simultaneously executing a Left-Hand Low Block.

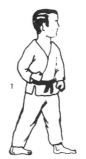

2. Slide your right foot forward toward L-1 into a Right High Front stance, simultaneously executing a Right-Hand Middle Punch.

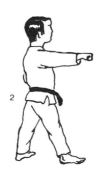

3. Turn your body 180° to the right toward **R-1** while pivoting on the ball of your left foot and stepping forward toward **R-1** into a Right High Front Stance, simultaneously executing a Right-Hand Low Block.

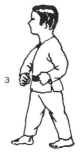

4. Slide your left foot towards **R-1** into a Left High Front Stance, simultaneously executing a Left-Hand Middle Punch.

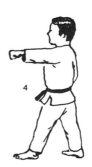

5. Turn your body 90° to the left toward **B** while sliding out with your left foot forward into a Left Front Stance, simultaneously executing a Left-Hand Low Block.

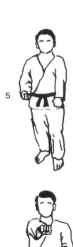

Note: Fifth and Sixth positions should be performed in a rapid, continuous motion.

6. Maintain the Left Front stance and execute a Reverse Right-Hand Middle Punch.

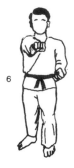

7. While turning your face and body 90° to the right, pivot to the right on the ball of your left foot and slide your right foot forward toward **R-2** into a Right High Front Stance, simultaneously executing a Left-Hand Middle Block (outside to inside).

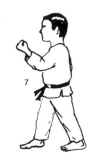

8. Slide your left foot forward toward **R-2** into a Left High Front Stance, simultaneously executing a Reverse Right-Hand Middle Punch.

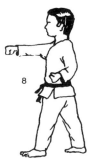

9. Turn your body 180° to the left toward **L-2** while pivoting on the ball of your right foot and sliding out with your left foot forward toward L-2 into a Left High Front Stance, simultaneously executing a Right-Hand Middle Block (outside to inside).

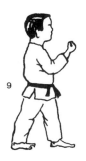

10. Slide your right foot forward toward **L-2** into a Right High Front Stance, simultaneously executing a Reverse Left-Hand Middle Punch.

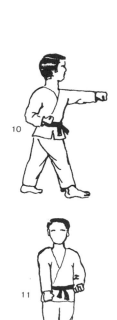

11. Turn your body 90° to the right toward **B** while sliding out with your right foot forward toward **B** into a Right Front stance, simultaneously executing a Right-Hand Low Block.

Note: Eleventh and Twelfth Positions should be performed in a rapid, continuous motion.

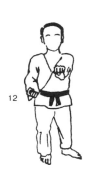

12. Maintain the Right Front Stance and execute a Left-Hand Reverse Middle Punch.

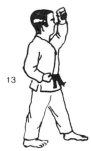

13. While turning your face and body 90° to the left, pivot to the left on the ball of your right foot and slide your left foot forward toward **L-3** into a Left High Front Stance, simultaneously executing a Left-Hand High Block.

14. a. Execute a Right Front Kick toward **L-3**.

b. Step forward with your right foot toward **L-3** into a Right High Front Stance, simultaneously executing a Right-Hand Middle Punch.

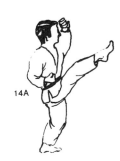
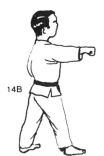

15. Turn your body 180° to the right toward **R-3** while pivoting on the ball of your left foot and sliding out with your right foot forward toward **R-3** into a Right High Front Stance, simultaneously executing a Right-Hand High Block.

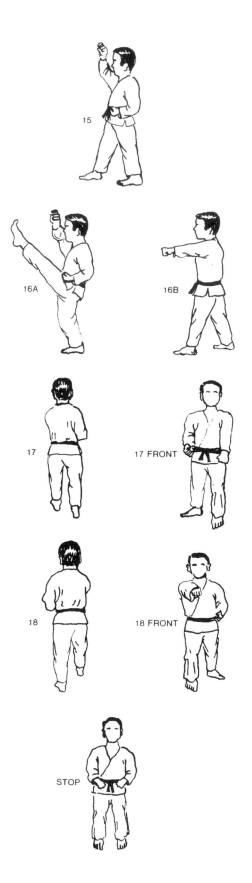

16. a. Execute a Left Front Kick toward **R-3**.

    b. Step forward with your left foot toward R-3 into a High Front stance, simultaneously executing a Left-Hand Middle Punch.

17. While turning your face and body to the right toward **A**, pivot to the right on the ball of your right foot and slide your left foot in an arc forward, toward **A**, into a Left Front stance, simultaneously executing a Left-Hand Low Block.

Note: Positions Seventeen and Eighteen should be performed in a rapid, continuous motion.

18. Slide your right foot forward toward **A** into a Right Front Stance, simultaneously executing a Right-Hand Middle Punch and yell.

Stop

While turning your face and body 180° to the left toward **B**, pivot to the left on the ball of your right foot and slide your left foot around behind the right foot toward center **A** into a Ready Stance, facing **B**.

TAEGEUK 2 JANG

The second aspect of Taegeuk is the principle *Tae* (兌)of Palgwe. (This Tae, as seen by its Chinese character, is different from the Tae (太)in Taeguek). Tae (兌)means joyfulness. Its form represents the state of mind, which is serene and gentle, yet firm within, the state from which true virtue smiles.

Tae is feminine, it is symbolized by lake. Tae is not silent but bubbling with joy.

The second form, representing joyfulness, consists of movements that are made softly yet firmly with control. The student shifts from a High Front Stance to a Front Stance more frequently than in Taegeuk 1 and emphasizes the Front Kick, learning to move more freely. This emphasis on movements of the lower parts of the body allows the student to learn balance and the proper stances, and strengthens the muscles in the proper stances, and strengthens the muscles in the legs.

Taegeuk 2 Jang introduces the High Block as a new technique.

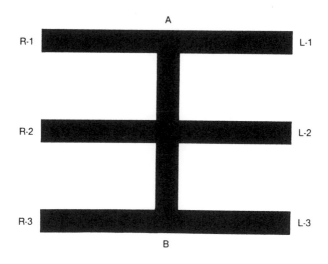

Taeguek 2 Jang

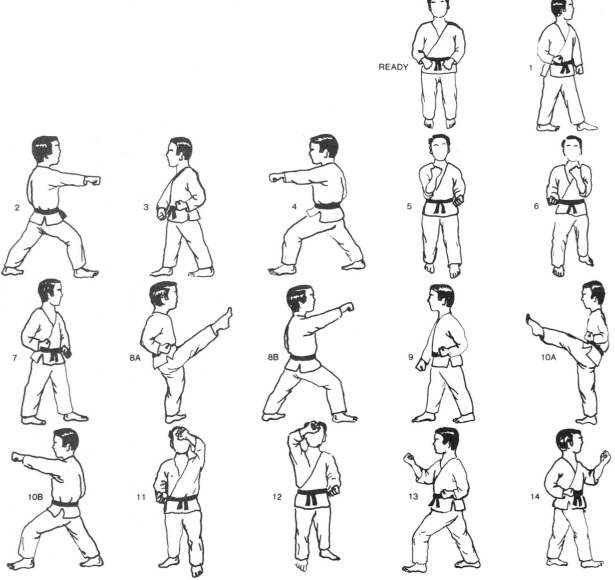

READY 1 2 3 4 5 6 7 8A 8B 9 10A 10B 11 12 13 14

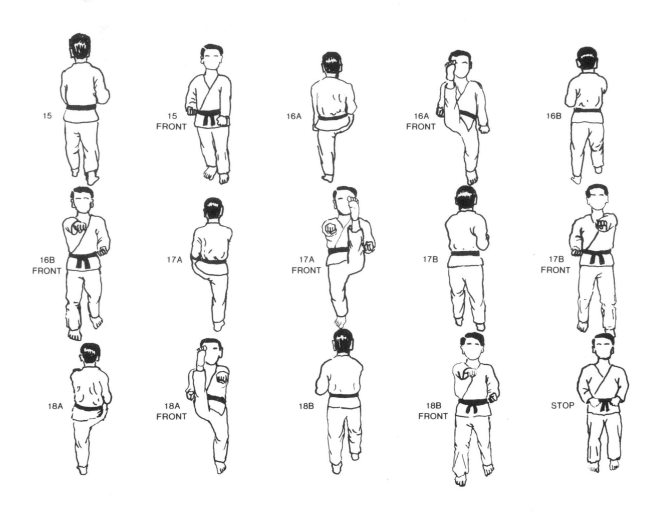

15

15
FRONT

16A

16A
FRONT

16B

16B
FRONT

17A

17A
FRONT

17B

17B
FRONT

18A

18A
FRONT

18B

18B
FRONT

STOP

Assume Ready Stance (at center, A).

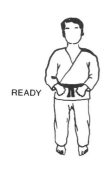

READY

1. Turn your body 90° to the left toward **L-1** while sliding out with your left foot forward toward **L-1** into a Left High Front Stance, simultaneously executing a Left-Hand Low Block.

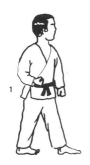

1

2. Slide your right foot forward toward **L-1** into a Right Front Stance, simultaneously executing a Right-Hand Middle Punch.

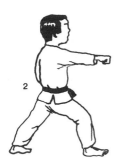

2

3. Turn your body 180° to the right toward **R-1** while pivoting on the ball of your left foot and sliding out with your right foot forward toward **R-1** into a Right High Front Stance, simultaneously executing a Right-Hand Low Block.

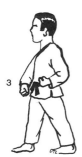

3

4. Slide your left foot forward towards **R-1** into a Left Front Stance, simultaneously executing a Left-Hand Middle Punch.

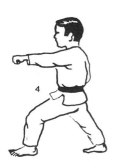

4

5. Turn your body 90° to the left toward **B** while sliding out with your left foot forward toward **B** into a Left High Front Stance, simultaneously executing a Right-Hand Middle Block, outside to inside.

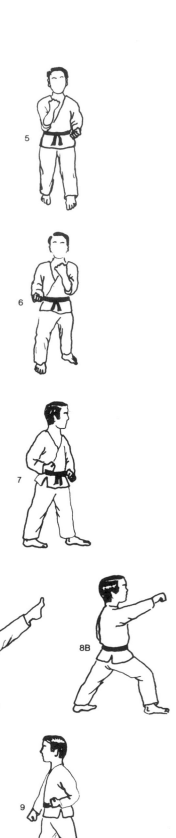

6. Slide your right foot forward toward **B** into a Right-Hand Front Stance, simultaneously executing Left-Hand Middle Block (outside to inside).

7. While turning your face and body 90° to the left, pivot to the left on the ball of your right foot and slide your left foot forward toward **L-2** into a Left High Front Stance, simultaneously executing a Left-Hand Low Block.

8. a. Execute a Right Front Kick toward **L-2**.

   b. Step forward with your right foot toward L-2 into a Right Front Stance, simultaneously executing a Right-Hand High Punch.

9. Turn your body 180° to the right toward **R-2** while pivoting on the ball of your left foot and sliding out with your right foot forward toward **R-2** into a Right High Front Stance, simultaneously executing a Right-Hand Low Block.

10. a. Execute a Left Front Kick toward **R-2**.

b. Step forward with your left foot toward R-2 into a Left Front Stance, simultaneously executing a Left-Hand High Punch.

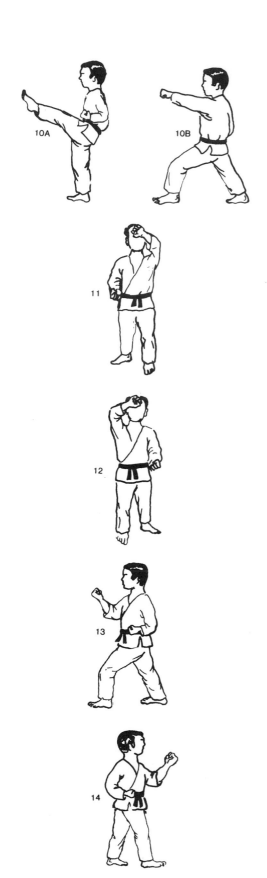

11. Turn your body 90° to the left toward **B** while sliding out with your left foot forward toward **B** into a Left High Front Stance, simultaneously executing a Left-Hand High Block.

12. Slide your right foot toward **B** into a Right High Front stance, simultaneously stance executing a Right-Hand High Block.

13. Turn your body 270° to the left toward **R-3** while pivoting to the left on the ball of your right foot and sliding out with your left foot, crossing in an arc behind the right foot toward **R-3** into a Left High Front Stance, simultaneously executing a Right-Hand Middle Block (outside to inside).

14. Turn your body 180° to the right toward **L-3** while pivoting to the right on the ball of your left foot and sliding out to the right with your right foot toward **L-3** into a Right High Front Stance, simultaneously executing a Left-Hand Middle Block (outside to inside).

15. Turn your face and body 90° to the left toward A while pivoting to the left on the ball of your right foot and sliding your left foot near the right foot forward toward A into a Left-High Front Stance, simultaneously executing a Left-Hand Low Block.

16. a. Execute a Right Front Kick toward A.

    b. Step forward with your right foot toward A into a Right High Front Stance, simultaneously executing a Right-Hand Middle Punch. (The punch should be delivered as quickly as possible and follow the Front Kick as a continuous motion.)

Note: Sixteenth position, a and b, should be performed in a rapid, continuous motion.

17. a. Execute a Left Front Kick toward **A**.

    b. Step forward with your left foot toward **A** into a Left High Front Stance, simultaneously executing a Left-Hand Middle Punch. (The punch should be delivered as quickly as possible and follow the Front Kick as a continuous motion.)

Note: Seventeenth position, a and b, should be performed in a rapid, continuous motion.

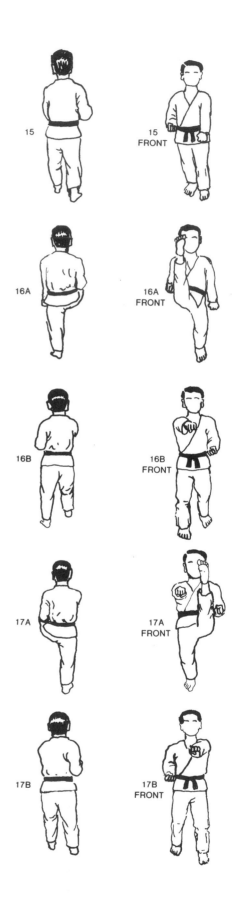

18. a. Execute a Right Front Kick toward **A**.

b. Step forward with your right foot toward **A** into a Right High Front Stance, simultaneously executing a Right-Hand Middle Punch. (The punch should be delivered as quickly as possible and follow the front kick as a continuous motion) and yell.

Note: Eighteenth position, a and b, should be performed in a rapid, continuous motion.

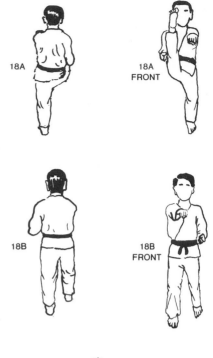

Stop

While turning your face and body 180° to the left toward **B**, pivot to the left on the ball of your right foot and slide your left foot around behind the right foot toward center **A** into a Ready Stance, facing **B**.

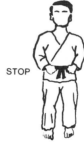

TAEGEUK 3 JANG

Taegeuk 3 Jang applies the principle of *Ri* (肉) of Palgwe. It symbolizes fire and sun, and their characteristics of warmth, enthusiasm, and hope.

Ri is feminine; it represents South. The actions of Ri should be performed with variety and passion, like the flickering of a fire.

Like the fire, which it represents Taegeuk 3 Jang is filled with changing bursts of power connected with a continuous flow of motion. It teaches combinations, specifically those hand combinations that are used in free fighting, such as Front Kick followed by a Double Punch, a Front Kick followed by a Low Block and a Reverse Middle Punch, and a Single Knife-Hand Block followed by a Reverse Middle Punch. After practicing these combinations in this form, they can be applied in free sparring.

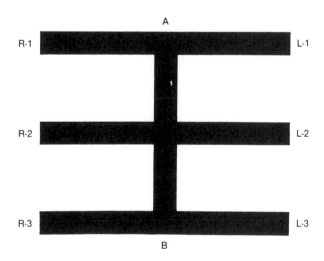

Taeguek 3 Jang

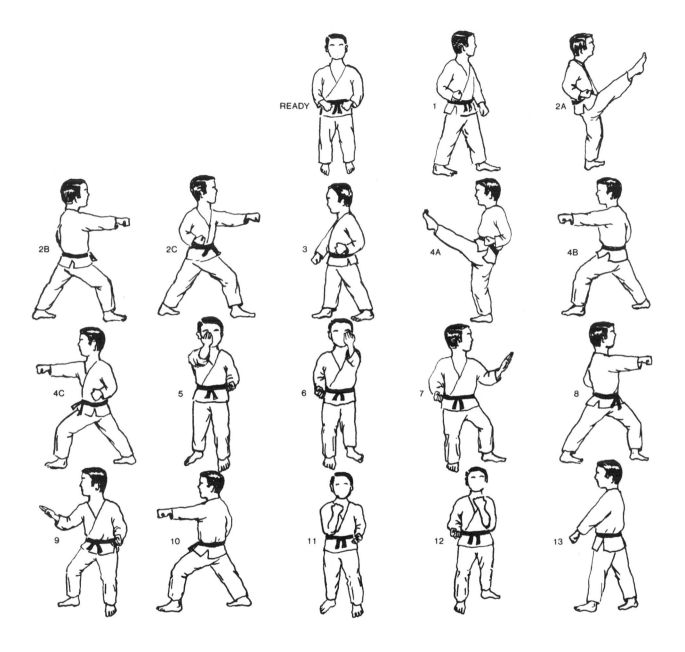

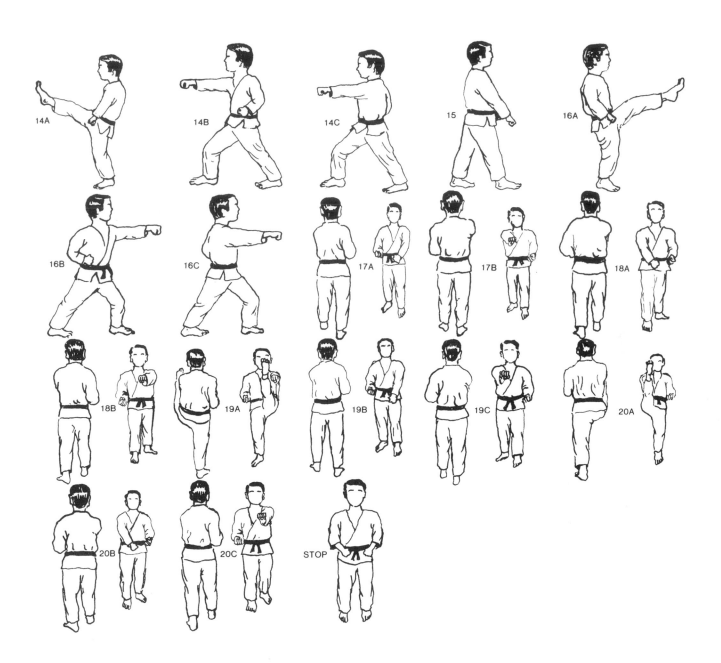

Assume Ready Stance (at center, A).

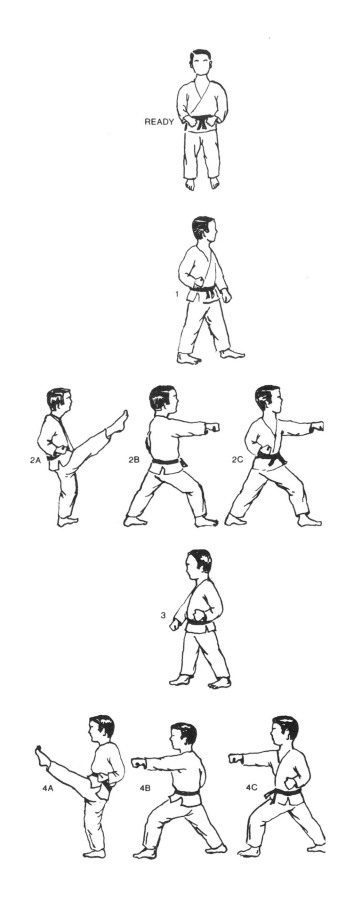

1. Turn your body 90° to the left toward **L-1** while sliding out with your left foot forward toward **L-1** into a Left High Front Stance, simultaneously executing a Left-Hand Low Block.

2. a. Execute a Right Front Kick toward **L-1**.

   b. Step forward with your right foot toward **L-1** into a Right Front Stance, simultaneously executing a Right-Hand Middle Punch.

   c. Maintain the Right Front Stance and execute a Reverse Left-Hand Middle Punch.

Note: Second position a, b, and c, should be performed in a rapid, continuous motion.

3. Turn your body 180° to the right toward **R-1** while pivoting on the ball of your left foot and sliding out with your right foot forward toward **R-1** into a Right High Front Stance simultaneously executing a Right-Hand Low Block.

4. a. Execute a Left Front Kick toward **R-1**.

   b. Step forward with your left foot toward **R-1** into a Left Front Stance simultaneously executing a Left-Hand Middle Punch.

   c. Maintain the Left Front Stance and execute a Reverse Hand Middle Punch.

Note: Fourth Position a, b, and c should be performed in a rapid, continuous motion.

5. Turn your body 90° to the left toward **B** while sliding out with your left foot forward toward **B** into a Left High Front stance, simultaneously executing a Right Knife-Hand Strike (palm up) to the temple.

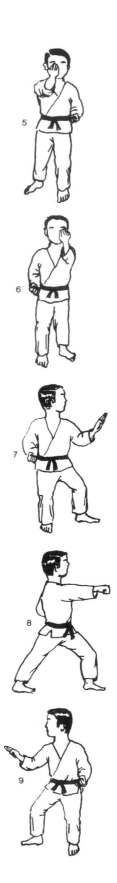

6. Slide your right foot forward toward **B** into a Right High Front Stance, simultaneously executing a Left Knife-Hand Strike (palm-up) to the temple.

7. While turning your face 90° to the left, slide your left foot forward toward **L-2** into a Left Back Stance, simultaneously executing a Single Left Knife-Hand Middle Block (inside to outside).

Note: Seventh and Eighth Positions should be performed in a rapid, continuous motion.

8. While pivoting to the left on the ball of your right foot, slide your left foot forward toward **L-2** into a Left Front Stance, simultaneously executing a Reverse Right-Hand Middle Punch.

9. Turn your body 180° to the right toward **R-2** while pivoting to the right on the ball of your left foot and sliding out with your right foot toward **R-2** into a Right Back Stance, simultaneously executing a Single Right Knife-Hand Middle Block (inside to outside).

Note: Ninth and Tenth Positions should be performed in a rapid, continuous motion.

10. While pivoting to the right on the ball of your left foot, slide your right foot forward toward **R-2** into a Right Front Stance, simultaneously executing a Reverse Left-Hand Middle Punch.

11. Turn your face and body 90° to the left toward **B** while pivoting to the left on the ball of your right foot and sliding your left foot near the right foot forward toward **B** into a Left High Front Stance, simultaneously executing a Right-Hand Middle Block (outside to inside).

12. Slide your right foot forward toward **B** into a Right High Front Stance, simultaneously executing a Left-Hand Middle Block (outside and inside).

13. Turn your body 270° to the left toward **R-3** while pivoting to the left on the ball of your right foot and sliding out with your left foot, crossing in an arc behind the right foot toward **R-3**, into a Left High Front Stance, simultaneously executing a Left-Hand Low Block.

14. Execute a Right Front Kick toward **R-3**.

   b. Step forward with your right foot toward **R-3** into a Right Front Stance simultaneously execute a Right-Hand Middle Punch.

   c. Maintain the Right Front Stance and execute a Reverse Left-Hand Middle Punch.

Note: Fourteenth Position, a, b, and c, should be performed in a rapid, continuous motion.

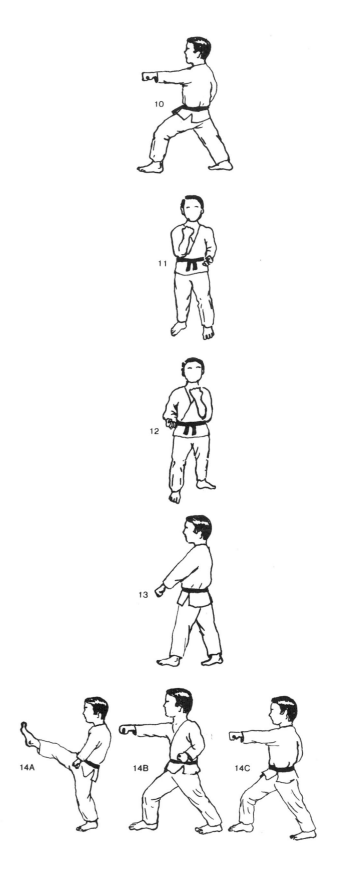

15. Turn your body 180° to the right toward **L-3** while pivoting to the right on the ball of your left foot and sliding out with your right foot forward toward **L-3** into a Right High Front Stance, simultaneously executing a Right-Hand Low Block.

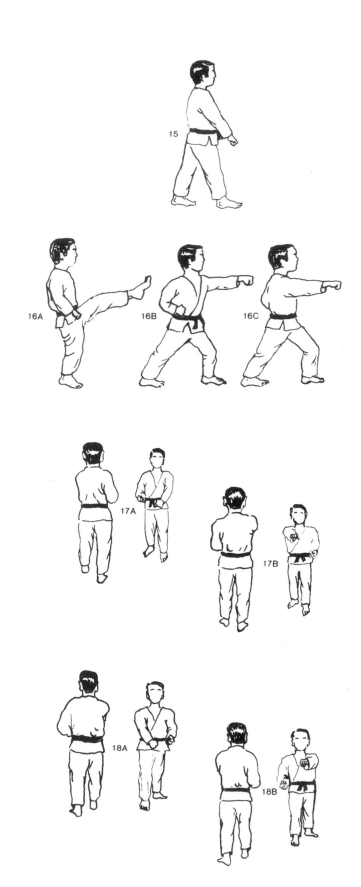

16. a. Execute a Left Front Kick toward R-3.

    b. Step forward with your left foot toward R-3 into a Left Front Stance, simultaneously executing a Left-Hand Middle Punch.

    c. Maintain the Left Foot Front Stance and execute a Reverse Right-Hand Middle Punch.

Note: Sixteenth Position a, b, and c should be performed in a rapid, continuous motion.

17. a. Turn your body 90° to the left toward **A** while sliding out with your left foot toward **A** into a Left High Front Stance, simultaneously executing a Left-Hand Low Block.

    b. Maintain the Left High Front Stance and execute a Reverse Right-Hand Middle Punch.

Note: Seventeenth Position a and b should be performed in a rapid, continuous motion.

18. a. Slide your right foot forward toward **A** into a Right High Front Stance, simultaneously executing a Right-Hand Low Block.

    b. Maintain the Right High Front Stance and execute a Reverse Left-Hand Middle Punch.

Note: Eighteenth Position a and b should be performed in a rapid, continuous motion.

19. a. Execute a Left Front Kick toward **A**.

b. Step forward with your left foot toward **A** into a Left High Front Stance, simultaneously executing a Left-Hand Low Block.

c. Maintain the Left High Front Stance and execute a Reverse Right-Hand Middle Punch.

Note: Nineteenth Position a, b, and c should be performed in a rapid, continuous motion.

20. a. Execute a Right Front Kick toward **A**.

b. Step forward with your right foot toward **A** into a Right High Front Stance, simultaneously executing a Right-Hand Low Block.

c. Maintain the Right High Front Stance and execute a Reverse Left-Hand Middle Punch and yell.

Note: Twentieth Position a, b, and c should be performed in a rapid, continuous motion.

Stop

While turning your face and body 180° to the left toward **B**, pivot to the left on the ball of your right foot and slide your left foot around behind the right foot toward center **A** into a Ready Stance, facing **B**.

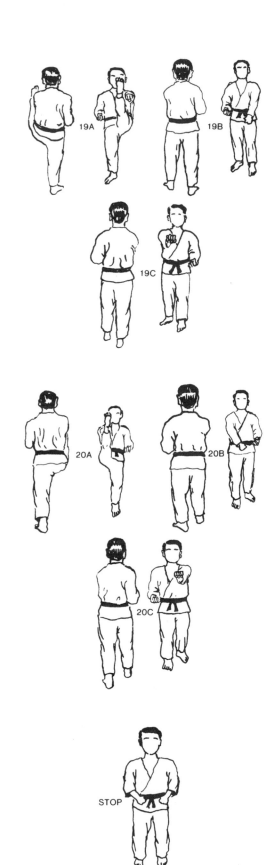

TAEGEUK 4 JANG

Taegeuk 4 Jang applies the principle of *Jin* (震) of Palgwe. Jin is male. It represents thunder, which with lightening, evokes fear and trembling but reminds us that danger—like a thunderstorm—passes as suddenly as it comes, leaving a blue sky, sunshine, and rain-freshened air in its wake.

The practice of this form should help one act calmly and bravely in the face of loud and terrifying dangers—real or imagined—knowing that they, too, shall pass.

In Taegeuk 4 Jang, one is responding calmly to threats of danger. In performing all forms, you should think not of executing techniques in a vacuum but rather of responding to attacks from a number of opponents surrounding you. You should always turn your head first, look at your imaginary opponent, then perform the required block or attack. For example, this form begins with a Knife-Hand Block. Imagine you are blocking a punch and thrust a Spear-Hand into your opponent's midsection. Then you block an imaginary attack to your head with a High Knife-Hand Block, palm out, and simultaneously execute a Knife-Hand Strike to your imaginary opponent's neck. (This double move is called *Jebi Poom Mokchiki*).

This form introduces the Outside Middle Block, palm out, many Knife Hand techniques, and the student's first kicking combinations—two Side Kicks, first right, then left. This kicking combination requires the student to practice balance and coordination without sacrificing power.

This form also trains the coordination of the entire body with the arms and legs, particularly in steps 10a and 10b, and 12a and 12b. Here the student must execute a Front Kick and step back with the kicking leg into a Back Stance, and hop back. Then, when this combination is mastered, the student will be able to slide back smoothly and quickly as one motion rather than step back and hop. This combination is followed by a Reverse Inside Middle Block, in which the body is twisted 45° toward the imaginary opponent.

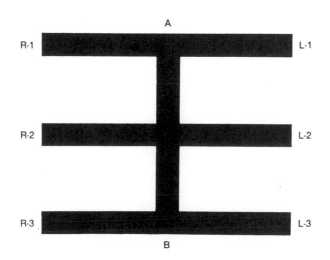

Taeguek 4 Jang

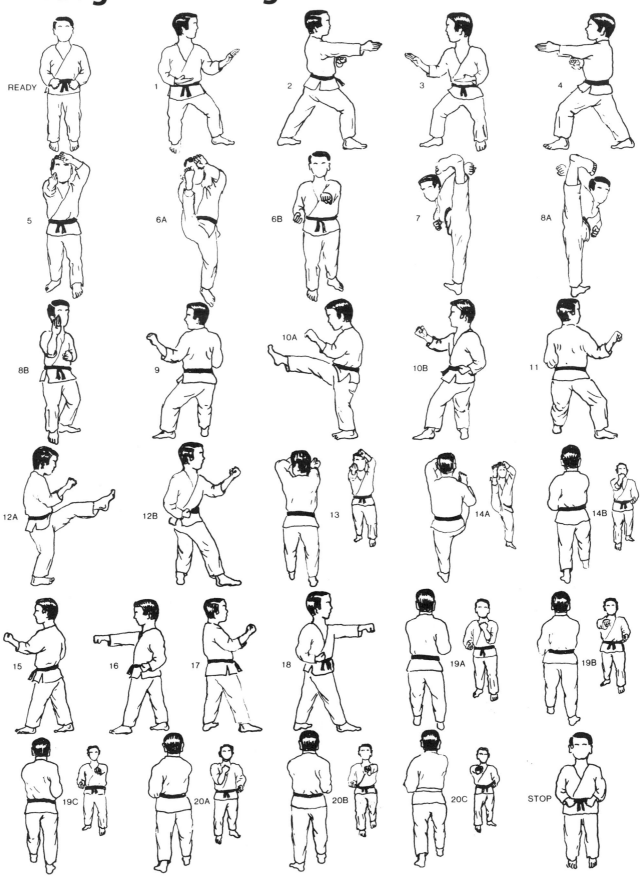

READY   1   2   3   4
5   6A   6B   7   8A
8B   9   10A   10B   11
12A   12B   13   14A   14B
15   16   17   18   19A   19B
19C   20A   20B   20C   STOP

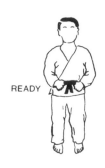

1. Turn your body 90° to the left toward **L-1** while sliding out with your left foot forward into a Left Back Stance, simultaneously executing a Left Knife-Hand Middle Block.

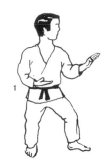

2. Slide your right foot forward toward **L-1** into a Right Front Stance, simultaneously executing a Right Spear-Hand Middle Thrust (with open left hand under your right elbow. Palm down).

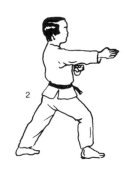

3. Turn your body 180° to the right toward **R-1** while pivoting on the ball of your left foot and sliding out with your right foot forward toward **R-1** into a Right Back Stance, simultaneously executing a Right Knife-Hand Middle Block.

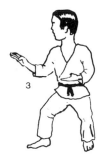

4. Slide your left foot forward toward **R-1** into a Left Front Stance, simultaneously executing a Left Spear-Hand Middle Thrust (with open right hand under your left elbow, palm down).

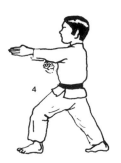

5. Turn your body 90° to the left toward **B** while sliding out with your left foot forward into a Left Front Stance, simultaneously executing a Left Knife-Hand High Block with a Right Knife-Hand Strike (outside to inside, palm up) at the neck level.

6. a. Execute a Right Front Kick toward **B**.

   b. Step forward with your right foot forward toward **B** into a Right High Front Stance simultaneously executing a Reverse Left-Hand Middle Punch.

7. Execute a Left Side Kick toward **B** and a Left-Hand Side Punch toward **B**, parallel to your kicking leg.

Note: Seventh and Eighth Positions should be performed in a rapid, continuous motion.

8. a. Step down with your left foot and turn your body 180° to the left and execute a Right Side Kick toward **B** and a Right-Hand Side Punch.

   b. Step forward with your right foot toward **B** into a Right Back Stance simultaneously executing a Right-Hand Middle Block.

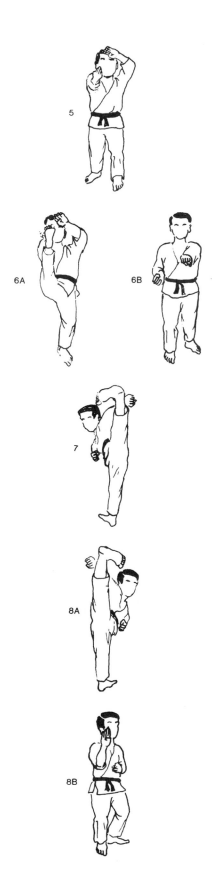

9. Turn your body 270° to the left Toward **R-3** while pivoting on the ball of your right foot and sliding out with your left foot, crossing in an arc behind your right leg, into a Left Back Stance simultaneously executing a Left-Hand Middle Block (inside to outside, palm out). Blocking surface is the outer edge of the forearm.

10. a. Execute a Right Front Kick toward **R-3**.

    b. Bring your kicking left (right foot) one step back and slide backward on both feet into a Left Back Stance simultaneously executing a Right-Hand Middle Block (outside to inside). Turn your upper body 45° to the left.

Note: Tenth position, a and b, should be performed in a rapid, continuous motion.

11. While remaining in place, turn your body 180° to the right toward **L-3** into a Right Back Stance, simultaneously executing a Right-Hand Middle Block (inside to outside, palm out). Blocking surface is the outer edge of the forearm.

12. a. Execute a Left Front Kick toward **L-3**.

    b. Bring your kicking leg (left foot) one step back and slide backward on both feet into a Right Back Stance, simultaneously executing a Left-Hand Middle Block (outside to inside). Turn your upper body 45° to the right.

Note: Twelfth Position a and b, should be performed in a rapid continuous motion.

13. While keeping your right foot in place, turn your body 90° to the left toward **A** and slide forward with your left foot into Left Front Stance simultaneously executing a Left-Knife-Hand High Block and a Right Knife-Hand Strike (outside to inside, palm up) at neck level.

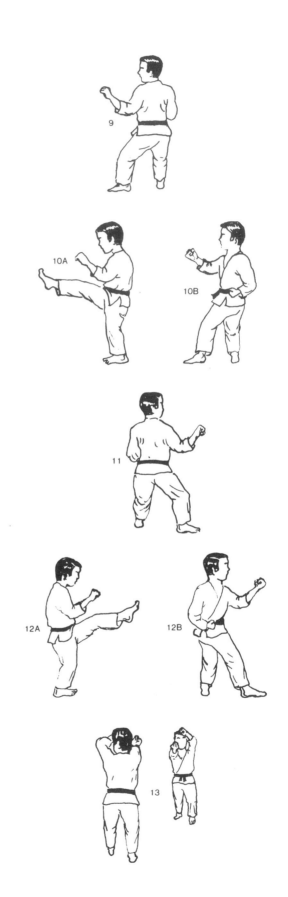

14. a. Execute a Right Front Kick toward **B**.

 b. Step forward with your right foot toward **A** into a Right Front Stance, simultaneously executing a Right Back Fist Strike to the face.

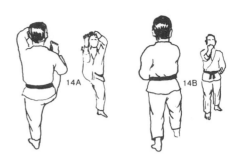

15. While keeping your right foot in place, turn your body 90° to the left toward **R-2** and step forward with your left foot into a Left High Front Stance, simultaneously executing a Left-Hand Middle Block (outside to inside).

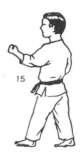

Note: Fifteenth and Sixteenth Positions should be performed in a rapid, continuous motion.

16. Maintain the Left High Front Stance and execute a Reverse Right-Hand Middle Punch.

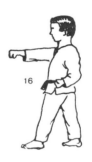

17. While remaining in place, turn your body 180° to the right toward **L-2** into a Right High Front Stance, simultaneously executing a Right-Hand Middle Block (outside to inside).

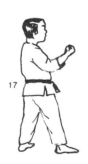

Note: Seventeenth and Eighteenth Positions should be performed in a rapid, continuous motion.

18. Maintain the Right High Front Stance and execute a Reverse Left-Hand Middle Punch.

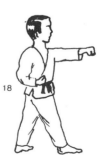

19. a. While keeping your right foot in place, turn your body 90° to the left toward **A** and step forward with your left foot into a Left Front Stance, simultaneously executing a Left-Hand Middle Block (outside to inside).

b. Maintain Left Front Stance and execute a Reverse Right-Hand Middle Punch.

c. Execute a Left-Hand Middle Punch immediately following the Reverse Right-Hand Middle Punch (punch should be delivered as one continuous motion).

Note: Nineteenth Position a, b, and c, should be performed in a rapid, continuous motion.

20. a. Slide your right foot forward toward **A** into a Right Front Stance, simultaneously executing a Right-Hand Middle Block (outside to inside).

b. Maintain the Right Front Stance and execute a Reverse Left-Hand Middle Punch.

c. Execute a Right-Hand Middle Punch immediately following the Reverse Left-Hand Middle Punch (punch should be delivered as one continuous motion) and yell.

Note: Twentieth Position, a, b, and c, should be performed in a rapid, continuous motion.

Stop

While turning your face and body 180° to the left toward **B**, pivot to the left on the ball of your right foot and draw your left foot around behind the right leg toward center **A** into a Ready Stance, facing **B**.

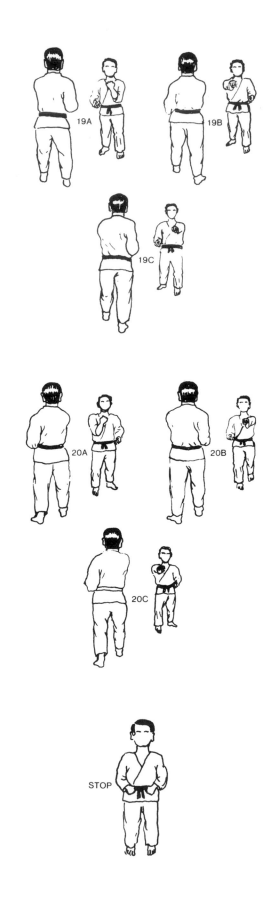

TAEGEUK 5 JANG

Taegeuk 5 Jang is a series of actions applying to the *Seon* (巽) of Palgwe.

Seon is female. It symbolizes the wind. Although there are horrible and destructive winds—such as the typhoon, hurricane, and tornado—the wind's true nature is gentle but penetrating. Spring breezes softly caress the willow, but the willow does not stop the wind, rather it bends willingly in its path.

Thus, wind symbolizes humility and good—natures actions. Seon can be alternately gentle and flexible as a breeze, or powerful and unyielding as a cyclone. Again, this form expresses the duality implicit in all the Palgwe forms.

Like a gentle breeze, Taegeuk 5 Jang is simple. Yet like a storm, it is strong and powerful. Its techniques sweep through the air, pushing away resistance, and then penetrating like the wind. These penetrating techniques include a Hammer Strike to the face, and Elbow Strike, and the execution of a Back Fist while leaping into a Crossed Stance. Taegeuk 5's powerful combinations include a Front Kick, Inside Middle Block, Back Fist Strike and High Block, Side Kick, Elbow Strike.

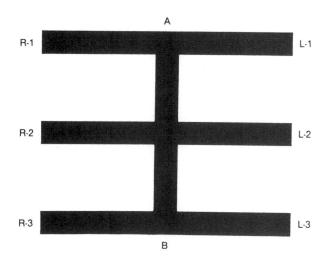

Taeguek 5 Jang

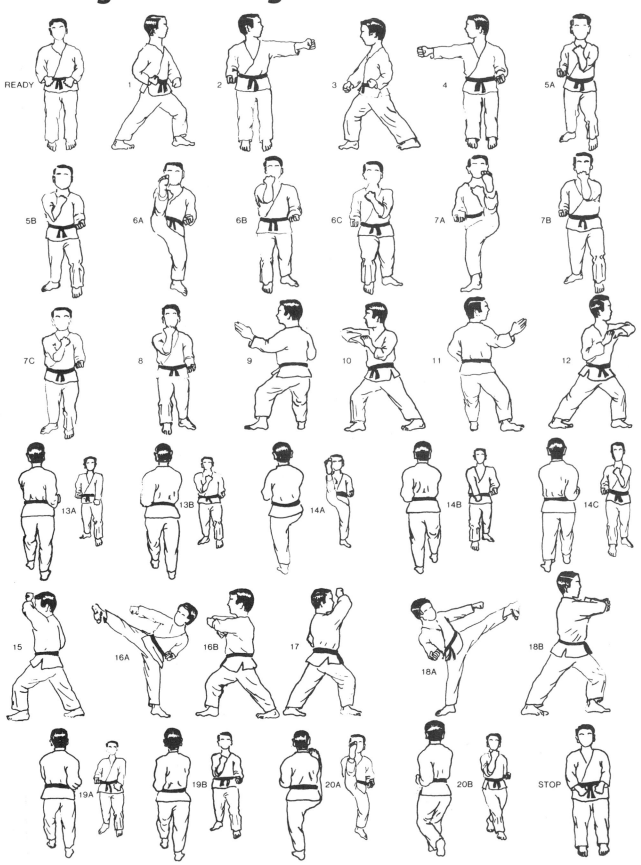

READY   1   2   3   4   5A

5B   6A   6B   6C   7A   7B

7C   8   9   10   11   12

13A   13B   14A   14B   14C

15   16A   16B   17   18A   18B

19A   19B   20A   20B   STOP

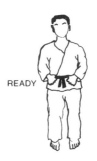

Assume Ready Stance (at center, A)

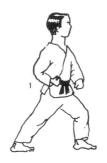

1. Turn your body 90° to the left while sliding out with your left foot forward into a Left Front Stance, simultaneously execute a Left-Hand Low Block.

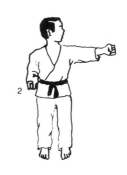

2. Draw your left foot back to center **A** into a Ready Stance, with body facing **B** and face still turned toward **L-1**, simultaneously drawing your left fist across your stomach and swinging it upward in an arc toward **L-1**, executing a downward Hammer Fist Strike. (Strike should be delivered as rapidly as possible.)

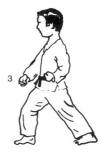

3. Turn your face and body toward **R-1** while stepping out with your right foot forward toward **R-1** into a Right Front Stance, simultaneously execute a Right-Hand Low Block.

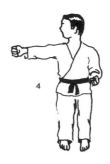

4. Draw your right foot back to center **A** into a Ready Stance, with your body facing **B** and face still turned toward **R-1**, simultaneously drawing your right fist across your stomach, and swinging it upward in an arc, toward **R-1**, execute a downward Hammer Fist Strike (strike should be delivered as rapidly as possible).

5. a. Slide your left foot forward toward **B**, into a Left Front Stance, simultaneously execute a Left-Hand Middle Block (outside to inside).

b. Maintain the Left Front Stance and execute a Right-Hand Middle Block (outside to inside).

Note: Fifth Position, a and b, should be performed in a rapid, continuous motion.

6. a. Execute a Right Front Kick toward **B**.

b. Step forward with your right foot toward **B** into a Right Front Stance, simultaneously execute a Right Back Fist Strike to the face.

c. Maintain the Right Front stance and execute a Left-Hand Middle Block (outside to inside).

Note: Sixth Position, a, b, and c, should be performed in a rapid, continuous, motion.

7. a. Execute a Left Front Kick toward **B**.

b. Step forward with left foot toward **B** into a Left Front Stance, simultaneously execute a Left Back Fist Strike to the face.

c. Maintain the Left Front Stance and execute a Right-Hand Middle Block (outside to inside).

Note: Seventh Position a, b and c, should be performed in a rapid, continuous motion.

8. Slide your right foot forward toward **B** into a Right Front Stance, simultaneously execute a Right Back Fist Strike to the face.

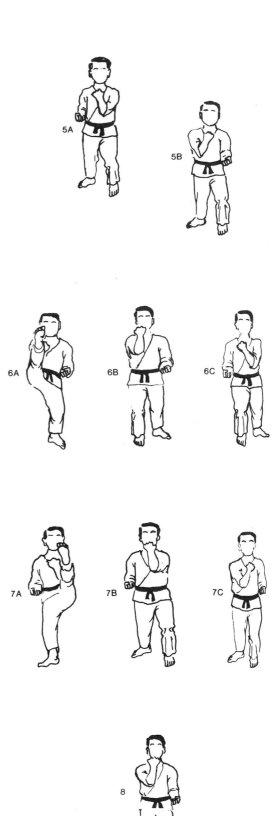

9. Turn your body 270° to the left toward **R-3** while pivoting on the ball of the right foot and sliding out with your left foot, crossing in an arc behind your right foot into a Left Back Stance, simultaneously execute a Left Single Knife-Hand Middle Block (right fist at waist level, palm up).

10. Slide your right foot forward toward **R-3** into a Right Front Stance, simultaneously execute a Right Elbow Strike to the mid-area (with left hand holding right back fist).

11. Turn your body 180° to the right toward **L-3**, while pivoting on the ball of your left foot and sliding out with your right foot forward into a Right Back Stance, simultaneously, execute a Right Single Knife-Hand Middle Block (left fist at waist level, palm up).

12. Slide your left foot forward toward **L-3** into a Left Front Stance, simultaneously execute a Left Elbow Strike to the mid-area (with right hand holding your left back fist).

13. a. Turn your body 90° to the left toward **A** while sliding out with your left foot forward into a Left Front Stance, simultaneously execute a Left-Hand Low Block.

   b. Maintain the Left Front Stance and execute a Right-Hand Middle Block (outside to inside).

Note: Thirteenth Position a and b, should be performed in a rapid, continuous motion.

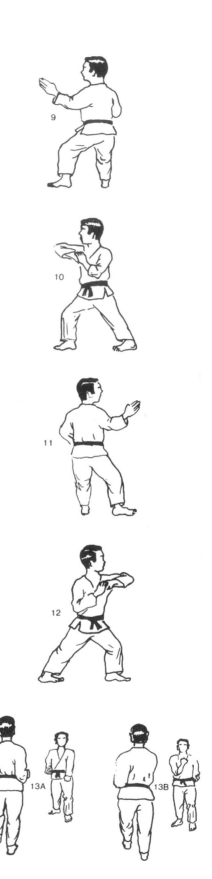

14. a. Execute a Right Front Kick toward **A**.

   b. Step forward with your right foot toward **A** into a Right Front Stance, simultaneously execute a Right-Hand Low Block.

   c. Maintain the Right Front Stance and execute a Left-Hand Middle Block (outside to inside).

Note: Fourteenth Position, a, b and c, should be performed in a rapid, continuous motion.

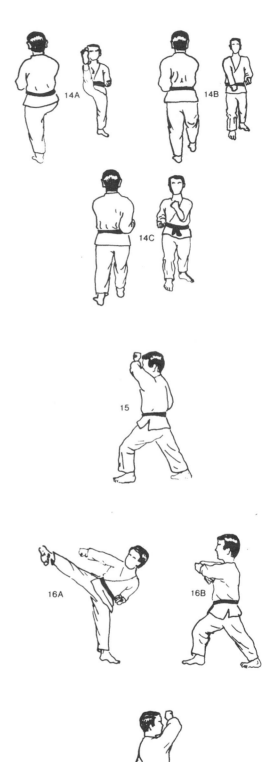

15. While keeping your right foot in place, turn your body 90° to the left toward **R-2** and slide forward with your left foot into a Left Front Stance, simultaneously execute a Left-Hand High Block.

16. a. Execute a Right Side Kick toward **R-2**.

   b. Step down with your right foot toward **R-2** into Right Front Stance, simultaneously execute a Left Elbow Strike to the mid-area (striking your right palm with your left elbow).

17. Turn your body 180° to the right toward **L-2** while pivoting on the ball of your left foot and sliding out with your right foot forward into a Right Front Stance, simultaneously execute a Right-Hand High Block.

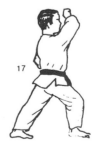

18. a. Execute a Left Side Kick toward **L-2**.

b. Step down with your left foot toward **L-2** into a Left Front Stance, simultaneously execute a Right Elbow Strike to the mid-area (striking your left palm with your right elbow).

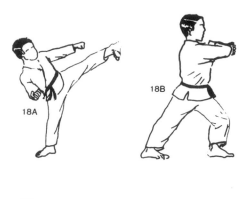

19. a. Turn your body 90° to the left toward **L-2** while sliding out with your left foot forward into a Left Front Stance, simultaneously execute a Left-Hand Low Block.

b. Maintain the Left Front Stance and execute a Right-Hand Middle Block (outside to inside) as rapidly as possible.

Note: Nineteenth Position, a and b, should be performed in a rapid, continuous motion.

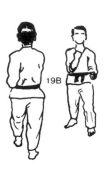

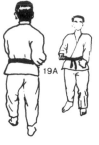

20. a. Execute a Right Front Kick toward **A**.

b. Leap forward with your right foot toward **A** and draw your left foot forward, behind your right leg, into a Right Cross Stance, simultaneously execute a Right Back Fist strike to the face as rapidly as possible and yell.

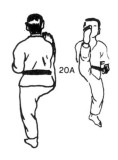

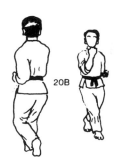

Stop

While turning your face and body 180° to the left toward **B**, pivot to the left on the balls of both of your feet and step to the left with your left foot toward center **A** into a Ready Stance facing **B**.

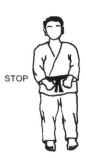

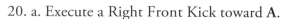

TAEGEUK 6 JANG

Taegeuk 6 Jang applies to the principle of *Gam* (坎) of Palgwe.

Gam is water, which is liquid and formless yet never loses its nature, though it may conform to the vessel in which it finds itself. Water always flows downward and, in time, can wear away the hardest granite.

Gam is male. It symbolizes North. Through Gam, we learn that we can overcome every difficulty if we go forward with self-confidence and persistence, easy to bend but not break.

Like water, Taegeuk 6 Jang is flowing and gentle yet destructive. It teaches that man, when faced with a challenge, can overcome it by persistence and unwavering belief. To give this form the appearance of continuity, its separate sequences of motion are connected by the Front Kick.

This form uses the Outside High Block, palm out, and Middle and High Reverse Single Knife-Hand Blocks, which demand fluidity, as the hip and body must twist 45° toward the target. It introduces a Round Kick, followed by an immediate change of direction, which requires great balance and coordination to remain fluid, like water.

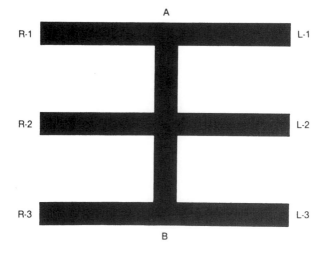

Taeguek 6 Jang

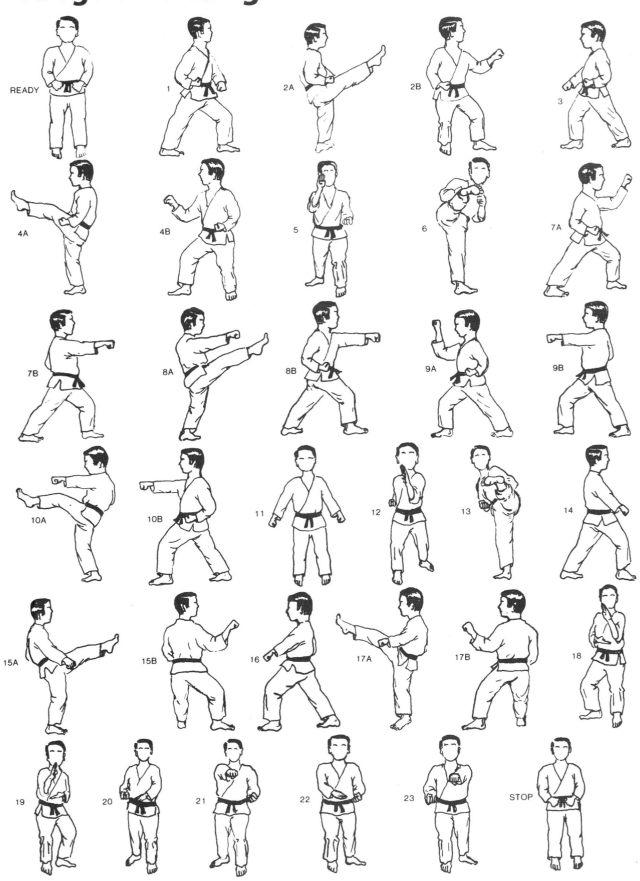

READY   1   2A   2B   3

4A   4B   5   6   7A

7B   8A   8B   9A   9B

10A   10B   11   12   13   14

15A   15B   16   17A   17B   18

19   20   21   22   23   STOP

Assume Ready Stance (at center, A).

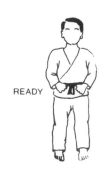

READY

1. Turn your body 90° to the left toward **L-1** while sliding out with your left foot forward into a Left Front Stance, simultaneously execute a Left-Hand Low Block.

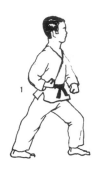

2. a. Execute a Right Front Kick toward **L-1**.

   b. Bring your right foot back to center **A** and slide your left foot backward into a Left Back Stance, simultaneously execute a Left-Hand Middle Block (inside to outside, palm out). Blocking surface is the outer edge of the Forearm.

Note: Second Position, a and b, should be performed in rapid, continuous motion.

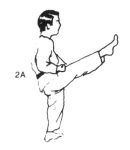

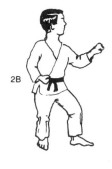

3. Turn your body 180° to the right toward **R-1** while pivoting to the right on the ball of your left foot and sliding out with your right foot forward toward **R-1** into a Right Front Stance, simultaneously execute a Right-Hand Low Block.

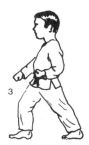

4. a. Execute a Left Front Kick toward **R-1**.

   b. Bring your left foot back to center **A** and slide your right foot backward into a Right Back Stance, simultaneously execute a Right-Hand Middle Block (inside to outside, palm out). Blocking surface is the outer edge of the forearm.

Note: Fourth Position, a and b, should be performed in a rapid, continuous motion.

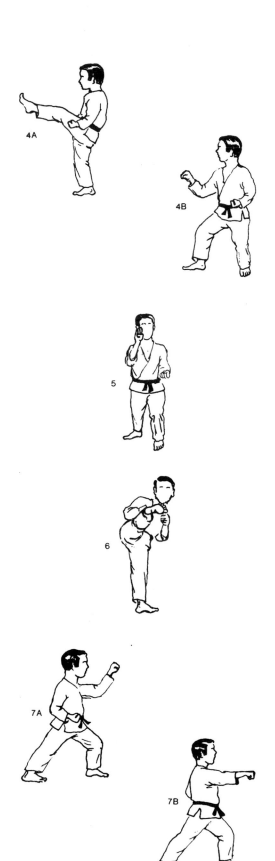

5. Turn your face 90° to the left toward **B** and slide forward toward **B** with your left foot into a Left Front Stance, simultaneously execute a Right Single Knife-Hand Hand Block (with your hip twisting sharply to the left as the block is executed), and withdraw left fist at waist level.

6. Execute a Right Round Kick.

7. a. Step down toward **B** with your right foot and step forward toward **L-2** with your left foot into a Left Front Stance, simultaneously execute a Left-Hand Outside High Block, palm out.

   b. Maintain the Left Front Stance and execute a Reverse Right-Hand Middle Punch as rapidly as possible, simultaneously withdraw left fist in at waist level.

Note: Seventh Position, a and b, should be performed in a rapid, continuous motion.

8. a. Execute a Right Front Kick toward **L-2**.

  b. Step forward with your right foot toward **L-2** into a Right Front Stance, simultaneously execute a Reverse Left-Hand Middle Punch as rapidly a possible.

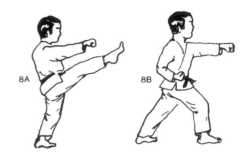

9. a. Turn your body 180° to the right toward **R-2** while pivoting on the ball of your left foot and sliding out with your right foot forward into a Right Front Stance, simultaneously execute a Right-Hand Outside High Block, palm out.

  b. Maintain the Right Front Stance and execute a Reverse Left-Hand Middle Punch as rapidly as possible, simultaneously withdraw right fist in at waist level.

Note: Ninth Position, a and b, should be performed in a rapid continuous motion.

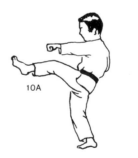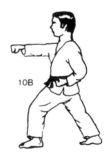

10. a. Execute a Left Front Kick toward **R-2**

  b. Step forward toward **R-2** with your left foot into a Left Front Stance, simultaneously execute a Reverse Right-Hand Middle Punch as rapidly as possible.

11. Turn your body 90° to the left toward **B** while pivoting to the left on the ball of your right foot and sliding your left foot back next to your right foot into a Ready Stance, simultaneously execute a Spread Low Block to the sides in slow motion.

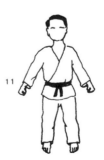

12. Slide your right foot forward toward **B** into a Right Front Stance simultaneously execute a Left Single Knife-Hand High Block (with your hip twisting sharply to the right as the block is executed), and withdraw right fist in at waist level.

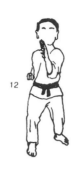

13. Execute a Left Round Kick and yell.

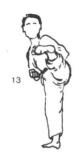

14. Step down toward **B** with your left and turn your body 270° to the right toward **L-3** while pivoting on the ball of your left foot and sliding out with your right foot, crossing in an arc behind your left leg into a Right Front Stance toward **L-3**, simultaneously execute a Right-Hand Low Block as rapidly as possible.

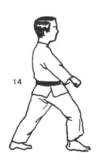

15. a. Execute a Left Front Kick, toward **L-3**.

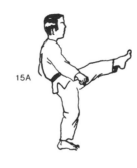

b. Bring your left foot back behind the right foot (as if into a Right Front Stance), and slide your right foot backward into a Right Back Stance, simultaneously execute a Right-Hand Middle Block (inside to outside, palm out). Blocking surface is the outer edge of the forearm.

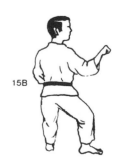

Note: Fifteenth position, a and b, should be performed in a rapid, continuous motion.

16. Turn your body 180° to the left toward **R-3** while pivoting to the left on the ball of your right foot and sliding out with your left foot forward toward **R-3** into a Left Front Stance, simultaneously execute a Left-Hand Low block as rapidly as possible.

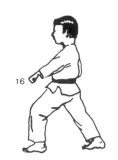

17. a. Execute a Right Front Kick toward **R-3**.

   b. Bring your right foot back behind the left foot (as if into a Left Front Stance) and slide your left foot backward into a Left Back Stance, simultaneously execute a Left-Hand Middle block (inside to outside, palm out). Blocking surface is the outer edge of the forearm.

Note: Seventeenth Position, a and b, should be performed in a rapid, continuous motion.

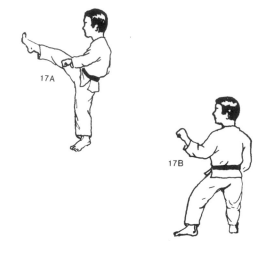

18. Turn your face and body 90° to the left toward **B** and slide in toward **A** with your right foot crossing behind your left foot into a Left Back Stance facing **B**, simultaneously execute a Left-Knife-Hand Middle Block.

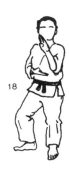

19. Slide your left foot backward toward **A** behind the right foot into a Right Back Stance facing **B**, simultaneously execute a Right Knife-Hand Middle Block.

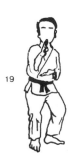

20. Slide your right foot backward behind the left foot into a Left Front Stance facing **B**, simultaneously execute a Left Palm-Heel Middle Block.

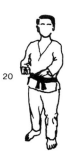

21. Maintain the Left Front Stance and execute a Reverse Tight-Hand Middle Punch.

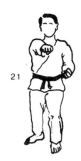

22. Slide backward with your left foot toward **A** into a Right Front Stance facing **B**, simultaneously execute a Right Palm-Heel Middle Block.

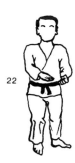

23. Maintain the Right Front Stance and execute a Reverse Left-Hand Middle Punch.

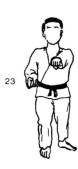

Stop
Slide your right foot backward toward center **A** into a Ready Stance, facing **B**.

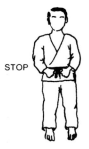

TAEGEUK 7 JANG

Taegeuk 7 Jang applies to the *Gan* (艮)principle of Palgwe.

Gan means "top stop" and symbolizes a mountain. It is male, taciturn, and steady. Like a mountain it is totally stable and cannot be moved.

One should not act hastily—the principle expressed by Gan. We must know when to forge ahead but also when to stop and rest in order to achieve our goals.

Representing the mountain, this form teaches the student to move only when it is necessary to move (and then to move rapidly) and to stop suddenly and solidly, standing like a rock. It teaches commitment to motion and to immobility, for one must not waver. This concept can be applied in sparring, to eliminate superfluous motions that waste energy.

This form is the first of the Taegeuks to be performed in a cat stance, which can easily be held still but out of which one can also move quickly.

It introduces the Knee Kick and the Crescent Kick as well as a number of blocks designed to stop an opponent's motion without being rocked—like the unwavering power of a mountain. These blocks include the Palm-Heel Center Block, Scissor Blocks, C-Blocks, and Spread Blocks, both palm out and palm in.

Its spurts of rapid motion include alternating Scissor Blocks, followed by a dead stop, and repeat, and Spread Middle Block, followed by a Knee Kick and Double Uppercut and stop.

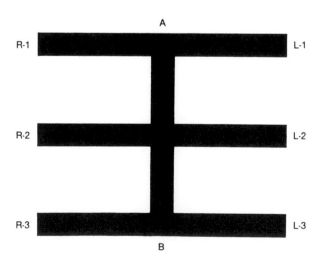

Taeguek 7 Jang

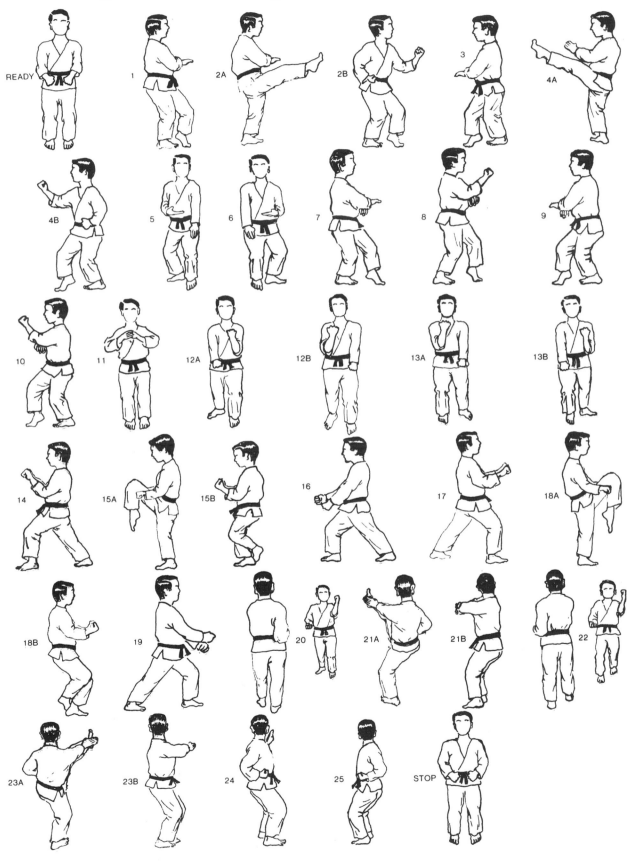

READY 1 2A 2B 3 4A
4B 5 6 7 8 9
10 11 12A 12B 13A 13B
14 15A 15B 16 17 18A
18B 19 20 21A 21B 22
23A 23B 24 25 STOP

Assume Ready Stance (at center, A).

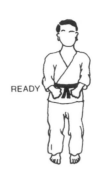

READY

1. Turn your body 90° to the left toward **L-1** while sliding out with your left foot forward into a Left Cat Stance, simultaneously execute a Right Palm-Heel Middle Block.

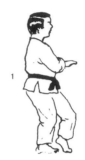

1

2. a. Execute a Right Front Kick, toward **L-1**.

   b. Bring your right foot back behind the left foot into a Left Cat Stance facing **L-1**, simultaneously execute a Left-Hand Middle Block, outside to inside.

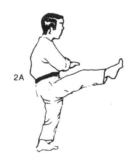

2A

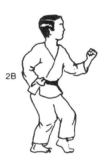

2B

3. Turn your body 180° to the right toward **R-1** while pivoting to the right on the ball of your left foot and sliding to the right with your right foot toward **R-1** into a Right Cat Stance, simultaneously execute a Left Palm-Heel Middle Block.

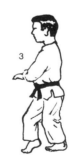

3

4. a. Execute a Left Front Kick toward **R-1**.

   b. Bring your left foot back behind the right foot into a Right Cat Stance (facing **R-1**), simultaneously execute a Right-Hand Middle Block (outside to inside).

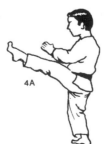

4A

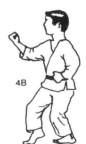

4B

5. Turn your face 90° to the left toward **B** while sliding forward with your left foot toward **B** into a Left Back Stance, simultaneously execute a Lefty Knife-Hand Low Block.

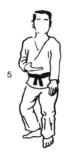

6. Slide your right foot forward toward **B** into a Right Back Stance, simultaneously execute a Right Knife-Hand Low Block.

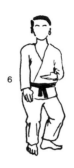

7. Turn your face and body 90° to the left toward **L-2** while sliding to the left with your left foot toward **L-2** into a Left Cat Stance, simultaneously execute a Right Palm-Heel Middle Block (with left fist placed under the right elbow, palm down).

Note: Seventh and Eighth Positions should be performed in a rapid, continuous motion.

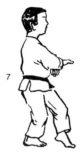

8. Maintain the Left Cat Stance and execute a Right Back-Fist Snap Punch to the face as rapidly as possible (with the left fist placed under the right elbow, palm down).

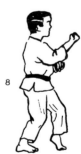

9. Turn your body 180° to the right toward **R-2** while pivoting to the right on the ball of your left foot and sliding to the right toward **R-2** with your right foot into a Right Cat Stance, simultaneously execute a Left Palm-Heel Middle Block (with right fist placed under left elbow, palm down).

Note: Ninth and Tenth Positions should be performed in a rapid, continuous motion.

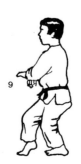

10. Maintain the Right Cat Stance and execute a Left Back Fist Snap Punch to the face as rapidly as possible (with right fist placed under left elbow, palm down).

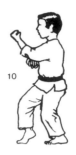

11. Turn your face and body 90° to the left toward **B** and slide your left foot next to your right foot into an Informal Ready Stance (feet together) facing **B**, simultaneously cover your left fist with your right hand, palms in, in front of your body at chin level.

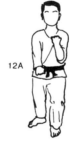

12. a. Slide your left foot forward toward **B** into Left Front Stance, simultaneously execute a Scissor Block (Right-Hand Low Block and Left-Hand Middle Block).

   b. Maintain the Left Front Stance and execute a Scissor Block (Left-Hand Low Block and Right-Hand Middle Block) as rapidly as possible.

Note: Twelfth Position, a and b, should be performed in a rapid, continuous motion.

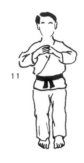

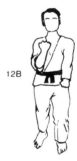

13. a. Slide your right foot forward toward **B** into a Right Front Stance, simultaneously execute a Scissor Block (Left-Hand Low Block and Right-Hand Middle Block).

   b. Maintain the Right Front Stance and execute a Scissor Block (Right-Hand Low Block and Left-Hand Middle Block) as rapidly as possible.

Note: Thirteenth Position, a and b, should be performed in a rapid, continuous motion.

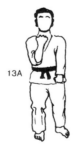

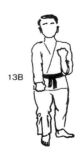

14. Turn your body 270° to the left toward **R-3** while pivoting to the left on the ball of your right foot and sliding out with your left foot, crossing into a Left Front Stance, simultaneously execute a Spread Middle Block, palms out.

15. a. Execute a Right Knee Kick toward **R-3**.

    b. Leap one step forward with your right foot toward **R-3** into a Right Cross Stance, simultaneously execute a Double Fist Middle punch, palms up. The motion resembles Uppercut, but aimed at midsection.

16. Slide your left foot backward into a Right Front Stance facing **R-3**, simultaneously execute a Low X Block, right fist over left toward **R-3**, as rapidly as possible.

17. Turn your body 180° to the right toward **L-3** while pivoting to the right on the ball of your left foot and sliding out with your right foot forward into a Right Front Stance, simultaneously execute a Double Hand Spread Middle Block, palms out.

18. a. Execute a Left Knee Kick toward **L-3**.

    b. Leap one step forward with your left foot toward **L-3** into a Left Cross Stance, simultaneously execute a Double Fist Middle Punch, palm up. The motion resembles Uppercut, but aimed at midsection.

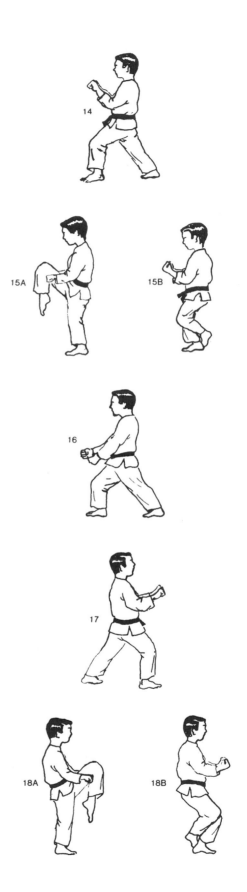

19. Slide your right foot backward into a Left Front Stance (facing **L-3**), simultaneously execute a Low X Block, right fist over left, as rapidly as possible.

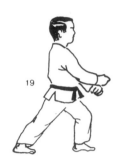

20. Turn your body 90° to the left toward **A** while sliding out with your left foot forward into a Left High Front Stance, simultaneously execute a Left Back Fist Strike (to the side of the face).

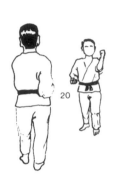

21. a. Execute a Right Crescent Kick toward **A** (striking the palm of your open left hand with the arch of your right foot).

   b. Step forward with your right foot toward **A** into a Horseback Stance (body facing **R** and face turned toward **A**), simultaneously execute a Right Elbow Strike to the palm of your left hand (with face still turned toward **A**).

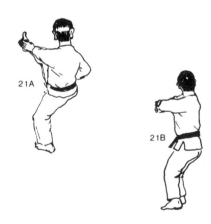

22. Turn your body 90° toward **A** and pivot to the right on the ball of your right foot while sliding your left foot forward toward **A** into a Right High Front Stance (facing **A**), simultaneously execute a Right Back Fist Strike (to the side of the face).

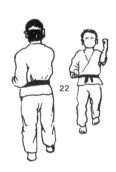

23. a. Execute a Left Crescent Kick toward **A** (striking the palm of your open right hand with the arch of your left foot at shoulder-high level).

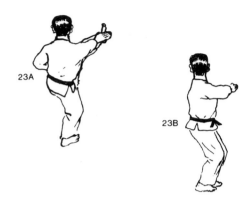

   b. Step forward with your left foot toward **A** into a Horseback Stance (body facing **L** and face turned toward **A**), simultaneously execute a Left Elbow Strike to the palm of your hand (with face still turned toward **A**).

24. Maintain the Horseback Stance and execute a Left Single Knife-Hand Middle Block toward **A**.

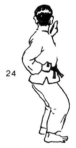

25. Slide your right foot forward toward **A** into a Horseback Stance (body facing **R** and face still turned toward **A**), simultaneously execute a Right Side Punch while clenching your left fist (as if grabbing your opponent) and pull your left fist back to waist level, palm up, and yell.

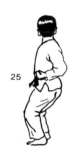

Stop

While turning your body 90° to the left toward **B** pivot to the left on the ball of your right foot and slide your left foot back in an arc to center **A** into a Ready Stance, facing **B**.

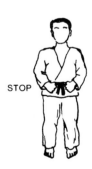

TAEGEUK 8 JANG

Taegeuk 8 Jang applies the *Gon* (坤) principle of Palgwe.

Gon symbolizes the earth, the source of life. As Keon is father, Gon is mother. The earth is where the creative force of heaven is realized.

Gon represents the receptivity of the earth. It is moist and heavy, sinking into the ground. Gon is also gentle and nurturing.

Gon signifies the infinite concentration of Um energy. The earth hugs and grows everything. It nurtures in silence and in strength. Gon teaches us the importance of the life force within ourselves and to respect life in all forms.

As the last of the Palgwe forms, Gon acts as a mother, testing our knowledge, reassuring us, passing on her energy as we prepare to move on to higher forms.

Representing the mother earth, from which all life comes, Taegeuk 8 Jang contains *all* the basic elements of Taekwondo, serving both as a review of the beginning forms and as foundation for the first black belt form. Besides reviewing techniques already introduced, it adds a Lifting Outside Middle Block, a simultaneous Grab and Uppercut, and a Single Mountain Block.

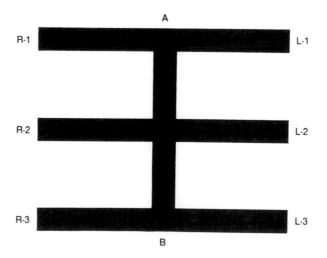

Taeguek 8 Jang

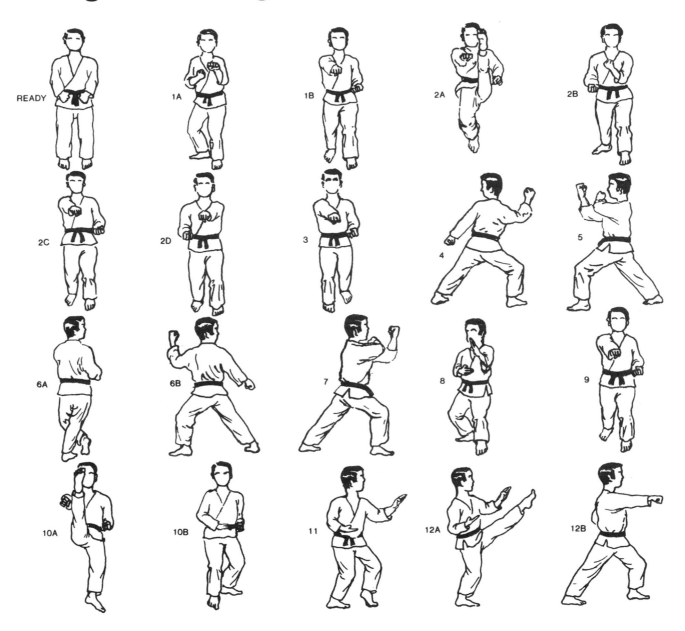

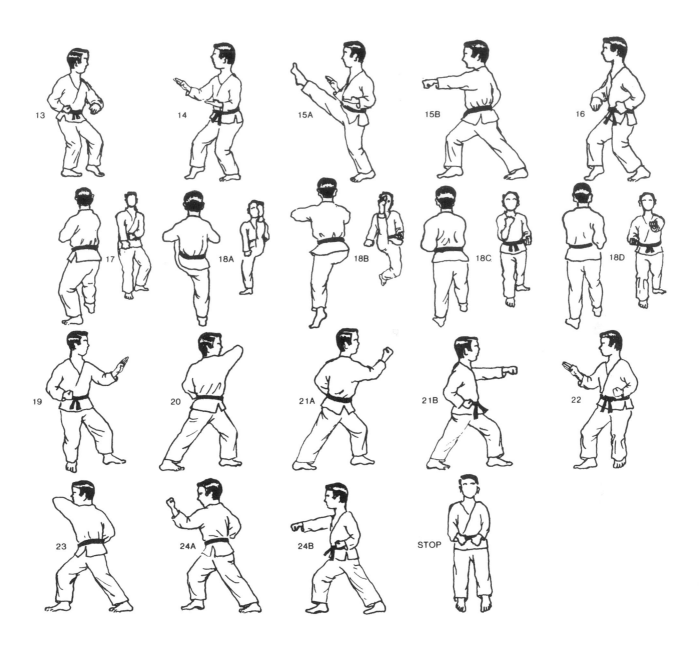

13 14 15A 15B 16

17 18A 18B 18C 18D

19 20 21A 21B 22

23 24A 24B STOP

Assume Ready Stance (at center, A).

1. a. Slide your left foot forward toward **B** into a Left Back Stance, simultaneously execute a Left-Hand Lifting Middle Block, palm out (right hand assisting, palm up).

   b. Slide your left foot slightly forward toward **B** into a Left Front Stance, simultaneously execute a Reverse Right-Hand Middle Punch.

Note: First Position, a and b, should be performed in a rapid, continuous motion.

2. a. First, execute a Double Jumping Front Kick toward **B** (a Right Jumping High Front Kick and consecutively a Left Jumping High Front Kick) and yell.

   b. Step down with your left foot forward toward **B** into a Left Front Stance, simultaneously execute a Left-Hand Middle Block (outside to inside).

   c. Maintain the Left Front Stance and execute a Reverse Right-Hand Middle Punch.

   d. Maintain the Left Front Stance and execute a Left-Hand Middle Punch.

Note: Second Position, a, b, c and d, should be performed in a rapid, continuous motion.

3. Slide your right foot forward toward **B** into a Right Front Stance, simultaneously execute a Right-Hand Middle Punch.

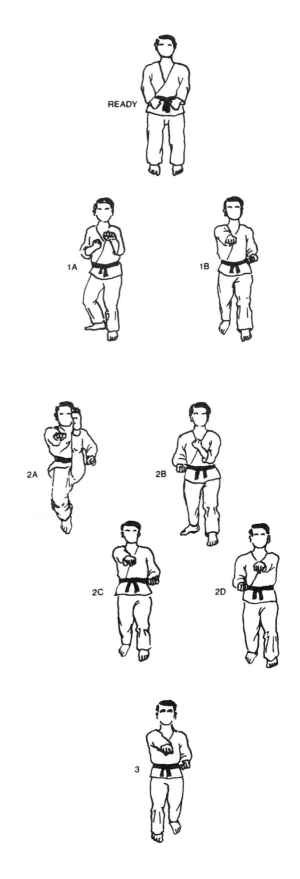

4. Turn your body 180° to the left toward **A** and turn your face 270° toward **R-3** while pivoting to the left on the ball of your right foot and sliding your left foot back toward **R-3** into a Right Front Stance (with toes pointed toward **L-3**, body facing **A**, toward **R-3**) and face turned to the left), simultaneously execute a Single Mountain Block (simultaneous High Side Block with your right hand and Low Side Block with your left hand).

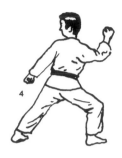

5. Turn your body 90° to the left toward **R-3** while pivoting to the left on the ball of your right foot and sliding to the left with your left foot into a Left Front Stance, simultaneously pull your left fist in toward your right shoulder, palm up, while pulling your right fist downward and execute an Uppercut Thrust to the chin with your right fist in slow motion.

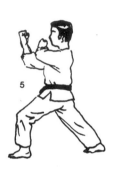

6. a. Turn your body 90° to the right facing **A** and turn your face 180° to the right toward **L-3** while pivoting to the right on the ball of your right foot and moving your left foot to the right into a Left Cross Stance, simultaneously bring your right fist back at the right chest level, palm in, and your left forearm across your body with your left fist, palm in, placed in front of your stomach, palm in.

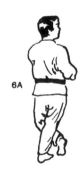

b. Maintaining face and body in same position, move your right foot sideways toward **L-3** and pivot 90° to the left toward **R-3** on the ball of your left foot into a Left Front Stance (face still turned toward **L-3** and body facing **A**), simultaneously execute a Single Mountain Block (simultaneous High Side Block with your left hand and Low Side Block with your right hand).

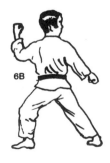

Note: Sixth Position, a and b, should be performed in a rapid, continuous motion.

7. Turn your body 90° to the right toward **L-3** while pivoting to the right on the ball of your left foot and sliding to the right with your right foot into a Right Front Stance, simultaneously pull your right fist in toward your left shoulder, palm up, while pulling your left fist downward and execute an Uppercut Thrust to the chin with your left fist in slow motion.

8. Turn your body 270° to the left toward **B** while pivoting to the left on the ball of your left foot and sliding your right foot to the left in an arc toward **A**, body facing **B** into a Left Back Stance, simultaneously execute a Left Knife-Hand Middle Block.

Note: Eighth and Ninth Positions should be performed in a rapid, continuous motion.

9. Slide slightly forward with your left foot toward **B** into a Left Front Stance, simultaneously execute a Reverse Right-Hand Middle Punch.

10. a. Execute a Right Front Kick toward **B**.

 b. Bring your right foot (kicking leg) back to the original position and immediately slide one step backward toward **A** with your left foot. At the same time slide backward slightly with your right foot and assume a Right Cat Stance, simultaneously execute a Right Palm-Heel Middle Block.

11. Turn your face 90° to the left toward **L-2** while sliding your left foot forward toward **L-2** into a Left Cat Stance, simultaneously execute a Left Knife-Hand Middle Block.

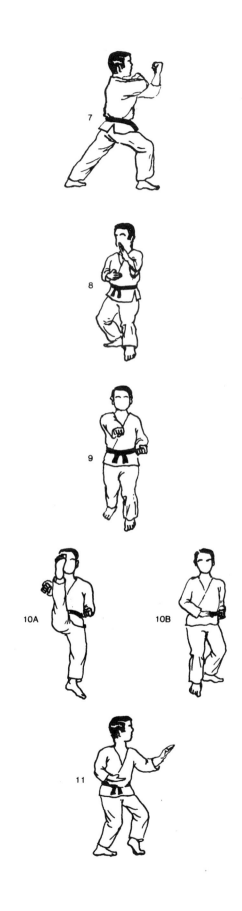

12. a. Execute a Left Front Kick (with your front foot) toward **L-2**.

 b. Step forward with your left foot toward **L-2** into a Left Front Stance, simultaneously execute a Reverse Right-Hand Middle Punch.

13. While keeping your right foot in place, slide your left foot backward into a Left Cat Stance, simultaneously execute a Left Palm-Heel Middle Block.

14. Turn your body 180° to the right toward **R-2** while pivoting to the right on the ball of your left foot and slide to the right with you right foot into a Right Cat Stance facing **R-2**, simultaneously execute a Right Knife-Hand Middle Block.

15. a. Execute a Right Front Kick (with your front foot) toward **R-2**.

 b. Step forward with your right foot toward **R-2** into a Right Front Stance, simultaneously execute a Reverse Left-Hand Middle Punch.

16. While keeping your left foot in place, slide your right foot backward into a Right Cat Stance facing **R-2**, simultaneously execute a Right Palm-Heel Middle Block.

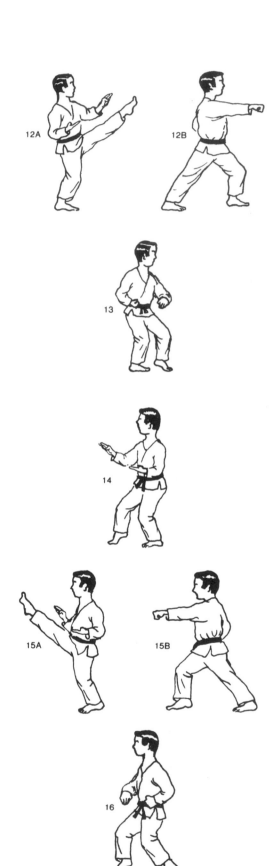

17. Turn your body 90° to the right toward **A** while pivoting to the right on the ball of your left foot and sliding to the right in an arc, with your right foot forward toward **A**, into a Right Back Stance, simultaneously execute a Right Double-Hand Low Block, palm down (left hand assisting, palm up).

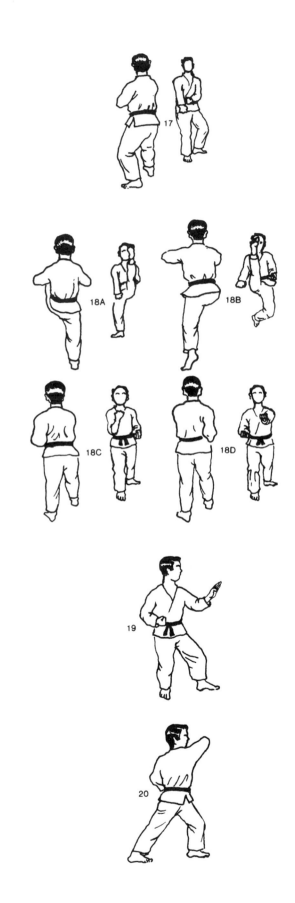

18. a. Execute a Left Front Kick toward **A**.

   b. Execute a Right Jumping Kick toward **A** while left foot is still in the air.

   c. Step down with your right foot toward **A** into a Right Front Stance (with your left foot placed where your right had been before, executing the Right Jumping Front Kick), simultaneously execute a Right-Hand Middle Block (outside to inside).

   d. Maintain the Right Front Stance and execute a Reverse Left-Hand Middle Punch and yell.

Note: Eighteenth Positions, a, b, c, and d ,should be performed in a rapid, continuous motion.

19. Turn your body 270° to the left toward **L-1** while pivoting to the left on the ball of your right foot and sliding out with your left foot, crossing in an arc behind your right foot, into a Left Back Stance, simultaneously execute a Left Single Knife-Hand Middle Block.

20. Slide forward with your left foot toward **L-1** into a Left Front Stance, simultaneously execute a Right Elbow Strike inward to the face toward **L-1** with your body twisting to the left.

Note: Twentieth and Twenty-First Positions a and b should be performed in a rapid, continuous motion.

21. a. Maintain the left front Stance and execute a Right Back-Fist Strike to the face toward **L-1** while twisting your body to the right.

b. Maintain the Left Front Stance and execute a Left-Hand Middle Punch.

22. Turn your body 180° to the right while pivoting to the right toward **R-1** on the ball of your left foot and sliding out to the right with your right foot toward **R-1** into a Right Back Stance, simultaneously execute a Right Single Knife-Hand Middle Block.

23. Slide forward with your right foot toward **R-1** into a Right Front Stance, simultaneously execute a Left Elbow Strike inward to the face toward **R-1** with your body twisting to the right.

Note: Twenty-Third and Twenty-Fourth Positions, a and b, should be performed in a rapid, continuous motion.

24. a. Maintain the Right Front Stance and execute a Left Back Fist Strike to the face toward **R-1** while twisting your body to the left.

b. Maintain the Right Front Stance and execute a Right-Hand Middle Punch.

Stop

While turning your face and body 90° to the left toward **B**, slide your left foot to center **A** into a Ready Stance facing **B**.

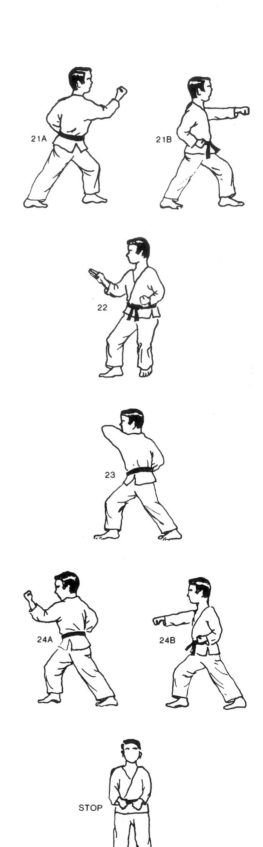

Index

About the Author

Richard Chun began studying Taekwondo at the age of 11 under two highly respected teachers in Seoul, Korea: Chong Soo Hong and Ki Whang Kim. He progressed to 9th Dan by Kukkiwon (World Taekwondo Federation) and Moo Duk Kwan after more than fifty years of study, establishing him as one of the highest ranking master instructors in the United States. (9th Dan by Kukkiwon in 1989 and by Moo Duk Kwan in 1981)

A graduate of Yon Sei University in Seoul in 1957, he organized and served as team captain of the Taekwondo Club. Immigrating to the United States in 1962, he earned an M.B.A. in marketing from the School of Business Administration at Long Island University and a Ph.D. in Education. He has been a Professor of Health and Physical Education at Hunter College City University of New York. Dr. Chun has been teaching Taekwondo at his center in New York City for four decades.

He was instrumental in organizing the Annual Universal Taekwondo Championships in the 1960's. He was appointed head coach of the U.S.A. Taekwondo team in 1973 for the first World Taekwondo Championships in Seoul. He has traveled and lectured extensively at local Taekwondo schools around the country as well as made appearances on TV talk shows. He went on to establish the United States Taekwondo Association in 1980 and has served as its President as well as assisted in the organization of Taekwondo as an event in the 1988 Olympics. Dr. Chun has since served as Senior International Referee for championships and the Olympics. In the fall of 1999, Dr. Chun was appointed as a Special Assistant to the President of the World Taekwondo Federation, Dr. Un Yong Kim. He continues to train senior black belts around the world and was inducted into the Black Belt Hall of Fame by *Black Belt Magazine* in 1979.

Advancing in Tae Kwon Do is his second book, originally published in 1983 by Harper-Collins. His other books are *Tae Kwon Do*, published by Harper-Collins; *Tae Kwon Do Moo Duk Kwan, Volumes I and II,* published by Ohara Publications; and *Taekwondo Spirit and Practice,* published by YMAA Publication Center. He has also produced a number of instructional videos on self-defense.

Dr. Chun has served various New York communities to help make them a better place to live in. Dr. Chun was elected District Governor of New York, Lions Clubs International Association in 1988 and has served the Association as an International Committee member for the Campaign Sight First Program to help prevent the curable blindness worldwide. For his outstanding community services he has received the "Lion of the Year" Award, several International President Awards from the Lions Clubs International, and the Presidential Award from the resident and the Government of Korea. Richard Chun is married with two children.

BOOKS FROM YMAA

VIDEOS FROM YMAA

more products available from...
YMAA Publication Center, Inc. 楊氏東方文化出版中心
4354 Washington Street Roslindale, MA 02131
1-800-669-8892 • ymaa@aol.com • www.ymaa.com

VIDEOS FROM YMAA (CONTINUED)

DEFEND YOURSELF 1 — UNARMED	T010/343
DEFEND YOURSELF 2 — KNIFE	T011/351
EMEI BAGUAZHANG 1	T017/280
EMEI BAGUAZHANG 2	T018/299
EMEI BAGUAZHANG 3	T019/302
EIGHT SIMPLE QIGONG EXERCISES FOR HEALTH 2ND ED.	T005/54X
ESSENCE OF TAIJI QIGONG	T006/238
MUGAI RYU	T050/467
NORTHERN SHAOLIN SWORD — SAN CAI JIAN & ITS APPLICATIONS	T035/051
NORTHERN SHAOLIN SWORD — KUN WU JIAN & ITS APPLICATIONS	T036/06X
NORTHERN SHAOLIN SWORD — QI MEN JIAN & ITS APPLICATIONS	T037/078
QIGONG: 15 MINUTES TO HEALTH	T042/140
SCIENTIFIC FOUNDATION OF CHINESE QIGONG — LECTURE	T029/590
SHAOLIN KUNG FU BASIC TRAINING — 1	T057/0045
SHAOLIN KUNG FU BASIC TRAINING — 2	T058/0053
SHAOLIN LONG FIST KUNG FU — TWELVE TAN TUI	T043/159
SHAOLIN LONG FIST KUNG FU — LIEN BU CHUAN	T002/19X
SHAOLIN LONG FIST KUNG FU — GUNG LI CHUAN	T003/203
SHAOLIN LONG FIST KUNG FU — YI LU MEI FU & ER LU MAI FU	T014/256
SHAOLIN LONG FIST KUNG FU — SHI ZI TANG	T015/264
SHAOLIN LONG FIST KUNG FU — XIAO HU YAN	T025/604
SHAOLIN WHITE CRANE GONG FU — BASIC TRAINING 1	T046/440
SHAOLIN WHITE CRANE GONG FU — BASIC TRAINING 2	T049/459
SHAOLIN WHITE CRANE GONG FU — BASIC TRAINING 3	T074/0185
SIMPLIFIED TAI CHI CHUAN — 24 & 48	T021/329
SUN STYLE TAIJIQUAN	T022/469
TAI CHI CHUAN & APPLICATIONS — 24 & 48	T024/485
TAI CHI FIGHTING SET	T078/0363
TAIJI BALL QIGONG — 1	T054/475
TAIJI BALL QIGONG — 2	T057/483
TAIJI BALL QIGONG — 3	T062/0096
TAIJI BALL QIGONG — 4	T063/010X
TAIJI CHIN NA	T016/408
TAIJI CHIN NA IN DEPTH — 1	T070/0282
TAIJI CHIN NA IN DEPTH — 2	T071/0290
TAIJI CHIN NA IN DEPTH — 3	T072/0304
TAIJI CHIN NA IN DEPTH — 4	T073/0312
TAIJI PUSHING HANDS — 1	T055/505
TAIJI PUSHING HANDS — 2	T058/513
TAIJI PUSHING HANDS — 3	T064/0134
TAIJI PUSHING HANDS — 4	T065/0142
TAIJI SABER	T053/491
TAIJI & SHAOLIN STAFF — FUNDAMENTAL TRAINING — 1	T061/0088
TAIJI & SHAOLIN STAFF — FUNDAMENTAL TRAINING — 2	T076/0347
TAIJI SWORD, CLASSICAL YANG STYLE	T031/817
TAIJI WRESTLING — 1	T079/0371
TAIJI WRESTLING — 2	T080/038X
TAIJI YIN & YANG SYMBOL STICKING HANDS–YANG TAIJI TRAINING	T056/580
TAIJI YIN & YANG SYMBOL STICKING HANDS–YIN TAIJI TRAINING	T067/0177
TAIJIQUAN, CLASSICAL YANG STYLE	T030/752
WHITE CRANE HARD QIGONG	T026/612
WHITE CRANE SOFT QIGONG	T027/620
WILD GOOSE QIGONG	T032/949
WU STYLE TAIJIQUAN	T023/477
XINGYIQUAN — 12 ANIMAL FORM	T020/310
YANG STYLE TAI CHI CHUAN AND ITS APPLICATIONS	T001/181

DVDS FROM YMAA

ANALYSIS OF SHAOLIN CHIN NA	D0231
BAGUAZHANG 1,2, & 3 —EMEI BAGUAZHANG	D0649
CHIN NA IN DEPTH COURSES 1 — 4	D602
CHIN NA IN DEPTH COURSES 5 — 8	D610
CHIN NA IN DEPTH COURSES 9 — 12	D629
EIGHT SIMPLE QIGONG EXERCISES FOR HEALTH	D0037
THE ESSENCE OF TAIJI QIGONG	D0215
QIGONG MASSAGE—FUNDAMENTAL TECHNIQUES FOR HEALTH AND RELAXATION	D0592
SHAOLIN KUNG FU FUNDAMENTAL TRAINING 1&2	D0436
SHAOLIN LONG FIST KUNG FU — BASIC SEQUENCES	D661
SHAOLIN WHITE CRANE GONG FU BASIC TRAINING 1&2	D599
SIMPLIFIED TAI CHI CHUAN	D0630
SUNRISE TAI CHI	D0274
TAI CHI FIGHTING SET—TWO PERSON MATCHING SET	D0657
TAIJI BALL QIGONG COURSES 1&2—16 CIRCLING AND 16 ROTATING PATTERNS	D0517
TAIJI PUSHING HANDS 1&2—YANG STYLE SINGLE AND DOUBLE PUSHING HANDS	D0495
TAIJIQUAN CLASSICAL YANG STYLE	D645
TAIJI SWORD, CLASSICAL YANG STYLE	D0452
WHITE CRANE HARD & SOFT QIGONG	D637

more products available from...

YMAA Publication Center, Inc. 楊氏東方文化出版中心

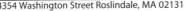

4354 Washington Street Roslindale, MA 02131
1-800-669-8892 • ymaa@aol.com • www.ymaa.com